ISSUES AND RESOURCES FOR THE CANCER NURSE

A NOTE FROM THE PUBLISHER

Cancer Nursing: Principles and Practice, Second Edition by Groenwald, Frogge, Goodman, and Yarbro is the best-selling text ever published for oncology nurses. Nurses around the world commonly refer to this landmark text as the "encyclopedia" of cancer nursing.

Over the years, oncology nurses have expressed a desire to have *Cancer Nursing* available in smaller, more specialized parts. Today, with the growing specialization within the oncology nursing field, this demand has increased.

In light of the tremendous demand, we are pleased to publish the individual parts from *Cancer Nursing*. All eight Parts are available in paperback format. (Parts VIII and IX have been combined).

In order to maximize the utility of the individual parts we have structured them as follows:

1. All parts have complete front matter (preface, foreword, and table of contents) from the main text. This helps the user understand how and where the individual part fits into the scope of the main text. In addition, the foreword by Vincent T. DeVita Jr., MD provides an interesting insight into the oncology field and should be read by all oncology nurses.
2. All parts have the complete index from the main text. This allows the user to identify additional topics available in *Cancer Nursing* and in the individual parts.
3. All parts maintain their page numbers from the main text. Therefore, the pages of the individual part will start on a page number consistent with the main text and not necessarily from page one.

Thank you for supporting our oncology nursing series.

ISSUES AND RESOURCES FOR THE CANCER NURSE

Parts VIII and IX from
CANCER NURSING
Principles and Practice
Second Edition

EDITED BY

Susan L. Groenwald, RN, MS

Assistant Professor of Nursing—Complemental
Department of Medical Nursing
Rush University College of Nursing

Rush-Presbyterian-St. Luke's Medical Center
Chicago, Illinois

Michelle Goodman, RN, MS

Assistant Professor of Nursing
Rush University College of Nursing
Teacher / Practitioner
Department of Surgical Nursing
Section of Medical Oncology

Rush-Presbyterian-St. Luke's Medical Center
Chicago, Illinois

Margaret Hansen Frogge, RN, MS

Senior Vice President, Clinical Services
Coordinator, Community Cancer Program

Riverside Medical Center
Kankakee, Illinois

Connie Henke Yarbro, RN, BSN

Editor, *Seminars in Oncology Nursing*
Clinical Associate Professor
Department of Medicine
Division of Hematology / Oncology

University of Missouri—Columbia
Columbia, Missouri

JONES AND BARTLETT PUBLISHERS
BOSTON

Editorial, Sales, and Customer Service Offices
Jones and Bartlett Publishers
20 Park Plaza
Boston, MA 02116

ISBN 0-86720-307-2

The selection and dosage of drugs presented in this book are in accord with standards accepted at the time of publication. The authors and publisher have made every effort to provide accurate information. However, research, clinical practice, and government regulations often change the accepted standard in this field. Before administering any drug, the reader is advised to check the manufacturer's product information sheet for the most up-to-date recommendations on dosage, precautions, and contraindications. This is especially important in the case of drugs that are new or seldom used.

Printed in the United States of America
95 94 93 92 91   10 9 8 7 6 5 4 3 2 1

Katherine T. Alkire, RN, MN
Oncology Clinical Nurse Specialist
St. Luke's Regional Medical
 Center
Boise, ID

Barbara D. Blumberg, ScM
Director of Education
Komen Alliance Clinical Breast
 Center
Charles A. Sammons Cancer
 Center
Baylor University Medical Center
Dallas, TX

Joy H. Boarini, RN, MSN, CETN
Professional Education Manager
Hollister Incorporated
Libertyville, IL

Ann Rohman Booth, RN, BSN
Clinical Research Nurse
Hematology and Oncology
University of Arizona Cancer
 Center
Tucson, AZ

Jean K. Brown, RN, MS,
 PhD Cand.
University of Rochester
School of Nursing
Rochester, NY

Patricia Corcoran Buchsel, RN,
 BSN
Director, Outpatient Nursing
Fred Hutchinson Cancer
 Research Center
Seattle, WA

Candace Carter-Childs, RN, MS
AIDS Project Case Manager
Hospice of Marin
Marin County, CA
Assistant Clinical Professor
University of California
San Francisco, CA

Jane C. Clark, RN, MN, OCN
Oncology Clinical Nurse Specialist
Assistant Professor
Emory University
Atlanta, GA

Rebecca F. Cohen, RN, EdD,
 CPQA
Instructor, Community Health
School of Allied Health Profes-
 sions
Northern Illinois University
DeKalb, IL

Mary Barton Cook, RN, BSN,
 OCN
Director of Nursing
Oncology Program Coordinator
CPS Pharmaceutical Services
IV and Nutritional Services Divi-
 sion
Mountain View, CA

Vincent T. DeVita, Jr, MD
Physician-in-Chief
Memorial Sloan-Kettering Cancer
 Center
New York, NY

Kathy A. Dietz, RN, MA, MS
Nurse Clinician—Hematology
Memorial Sloan-Kettering Cancer
 Center
Associate
Columbia University School of
 Nursing
New York, NY

Joanne M. Disch, RN, PhD
Clinical Director
Department of Medical Nursing,
 Emergency Services and Dialy-
 sis
Hospital of the University of
 Pennsylvania
Assistant Professor of Nursing
University of Pennsylvania School
 of Nursing
Philadelphia, PA

Michele Girard Donehower, RN,
 MSN
Student, Nurse Practitioner Pro-
 gram
University of Maryland School of
 Nursing
Baltimore, MD

Constance T. Donovan, RN,
 MSN, FAAN
Oncology Clinical Nurse Specialist
Yale New Haven Hospital
Associate Clinical Professor
Yale University School of Nursing
New Haven, CT

Diane Scott Dorsett, RN, PhD,
 FAAN
Director
Comprehensive Support Services
 for Persons with Cancer
Associate Clinical Professor
University of California
San Francisco, CA

Susan Dudas, RN, MSN
Associate Professor
College of Nursing
University of Illinois at Chicago
Chicago, IL

Ellen Heid Elpern, RN, MSN
Clinical Nurse Specialist
Section of Pulmonary Medicine
Assistant Professor of Nursing
Rush University
Rush-Presbyterian-St. Luke's
 Medical Center
Chicago, IL

Dolores Esparza, RN, MS
President
Esparza Oncology Consultants,
 Inc.
San Antonio, TX

Betty Rolling Ferrell, RN, PhD, FAAN
Research Scientist, Nursing Research
City of Hope National Medical Center
Duarte, CA

Anne Marie Flaherty, RN, MS
Administrative Nurse Clinician
Adult Day Hospital
Memorial Sloan-Kettering Cancer Center
New York, NY

Arlene E. Fleck, RN, MNEd
Clinical Cancer Research Coordinator
Cancer Prevention Center
Kelsey-Seybold Foundation
Houston, TX

Marilyn Frank-Stromborg, RN, EdD, Nurse Practitioner, FAAN
Coordinator
Oncology Clinical Specialist Program
Professor
School of Nursing
Northern Illinois University
DeKalb, IL

Margaret Hansen Frogge, RN, MS
Senior Vice President, Clinical Services
Coordinator, Community Cancer Program
Riverside Medical Center
Kankakee, IL

Gayling Gee, RN, MS
Director, Outpatient Nursing
San Francisco General Hospital
Assistant Clinical Professor
School of Nursing
University of California
San Francisco, CA

Barbara Holmes Gobel, RN, MS
Oncology Clinical Nurse Specialist
Lake Forest Hospital
Faculty, Complemental
Rush University College of Nursing
Chicago, IL

Michelle Goodman, RN, MS
Oncology Clinical Nurse Specialist
Section of Medical Oncology
Assistant Professor of Nursing
Rush University
Rush-Presbyterian-St. Luke's Medical Center
Chicago, IL

Marcia M. Grant, RN, DNSc, OCN
Director of Nursing Research and Education
City of Hope National Medical Center
Duarte, CA

Susan L. Groenwald, RN, MS
Oncology Nurse Consultant
Assistant Professor of Nursing—Complemental
Rush University College of Nursing
Chicago, IL

Shirley M. Gullo, RN, MSN, OCN
Oncology Nurse
The Cleveland Clinic Foundation
Cleveland, OH

Patricia Hakius, RN, MSN
Cancer Care Consultant
Doctoral Student
University of San Diego
San Diego, CA

Nancy E. Harte, RN, MS
Oncology Clinical Nurse Specialist
Section of Medical Oncology
Rush-Presbyterian-St. Luke's Medical Center
Instructor
Rush University College of Nursing
Chicago, IL

Laura J. Hilderley, RN, MS
Oncology Clinical Nurse Specialist
Private Practice of Philip G. Maddock, MD
Radiation Oncology
Warwick, RI

Barbara Hoffman, JD
Private Consultant
Cancer Survivorship and Discrimination
Princeton, NJ

Catherine M. Hogan, RN, MN, OCN
Oncology Clinical Nurse Specialist
Department of Hematology/ Oncology
University of Michigan
Ann Arbor, MI

Susan Molloy Hubbard, RN, BA
Director
International Cancer Information Center
National Cancer Institute
Bethesda, MD

Patricia F. Jassak, RN, MS, CS
Oncology Clinical Nurse Specialist
Foster G. McGaw Hospital
Loyola University of Chicago
Chicago, IL

Judith (Judi) L. Bond Johnson, RN, PhD
Nursing Director
North Memorial Medical Center
Minneapolis, MN

Paula R. Klemm, RN, DNSc Cand.
Nursing Instructor II
The Johns Hopkins Oncology Center
Baltimore, MD

Linda U. Krebs, RN, MS, OCN
Oncology Nursing Program Leader
University of Colorado Cancer Center
Denver, CO

Charles E. Kupchella, PhD
Dean
Ogden College of Science, Technology and Health
Western Kentucky University
Bowling Green, KY

Jennifer M. Lang-Kummer, RN, MS
Oncology Clinical Nurse Specialist
Beaumont County Hospital
Washington, NC

Susan Leigh, RN, BSN
Cancer Survivorship Consultant
Tucson, AZ

Julena M. Lind, RN, MN
Executive Director
Center for Health Information,
    Education and Research
California Medical Center
Adjunct Assistant Professor of
    Nursing
University of Southern California
Los Angeles, CA

Ada M. Lindsey, RN, PhD
Dean and Professor
School of Nursing
University of California
Los Angeles, CA

Lois J. Loescher, RN, MS
Research Specialist
Program Coordinator
Cancer Prevention and Control
University of Arizona Cancer
    Center
Tucson, AZ

Alice J. Longman, RN, EdD
Associate Professor
College of Nursing
University of Arizona
Tucson, AZ

Jean McNicholas Lydon, RN, MS
Oncology Clinical Nurse Specialist
Department of Therapeutic
    Radiology
Rush-Presbyterian-St. Luke's
    Medical Center
Chicago, IL

Mary B. Maxwell, RN, C, PhD
Oncology Clinical Nurse Specialist
Nurse Practitioner
Veterans' Administration Medical
    Center
Portland, OR

Mary Dee McEvoy, RN, PhD
Robert Wood Johnson Clinical
    Nurse Scholar
Hematology/Oncology Section
Division of Nursing
Hospital of the University of
    Pennsylvania
Philadelphia, PA

Rose F. McGee, RN, PhD
Professor
American Cancer Society
    Professor of Oncology Nursing
Emory University
Atlanta, GA

Deborah B. McGuire, RN, PhD
Assistant Professor
The Johns Hopkins University
    School of Nursing
Director of Nursing Research
The Johns Hopkins Oncology
    Center
Baltimore, MD

Joan C. McNally, RN, MSN
Executive Director
Michigan Cancer Foundation
    Services, Inc.
Detroit, MI

Nancy Miller, RN, MS
Assistant Director of Testing
    Services
National Council of State Boards
    of Nursing, Inc.
Chicago, IL

Ida Marie (Ki) Moore, RN, DNS
Assistant Professor
College of Nursing
University of Arizona
Tucson, AZ

Theresa A. Moran, RN, MS
Oncology/AIDS Clinical Nurse
    Specialist
Oncology/AIDS Clinic
San Francisco General Hospital
Assistant Clinical Professor
School of Nursing
University of California
San Francisco, CA

Marian E. Morra, MA
Assistant Director
Yale University Comprehensive
    Cancer Center
New Haven, CT

Lillian M. Nail, RN, PhD
Assistant Professor
University of Rochester School of
    Nursing
Clinician II
University of Rochester Cancer
    Center
Rochester, NY

Susie Lee Nakao, RN, MN
Nurse Manager
Clinical Research Center
Los Angeles County
University of Southern California
Los Angeles, CA

Denise Oleske, RN, DPH
Research Associate
Department of Health Systems
    Management
Department of Preventive
    Medicine
Rush-Presbyterian-St. Luke's
    Medical Center
Assistant Professor
College of Health Systems
    Management
Rush University
Chicago, IL

Sharon Saldin O'Mary, RN, MN
Home Care Coordinator
Stevens Cancer Center
Scripps Memorial Hospital
LaJolla, CA

Edith O'Neil-Page, RN, BSN
Nursing Supervisor
The Kenneth Norris Jr. Hospital
    and Research Institute
Los Angeles, CA

Diane M. Otte, RN, MS, ET
Administrative Director—Cancer
    Program
St. Luke's Hospital Cancer Center
Davenport, IA

Geraldine V. Padilla, PhD
Associate Professor
Associate Dean for Research
School of Nursing
University of California
Los Angeles, CA

Mary Pazdur, RN, MS, OCN
Head Nurse
Discharge Planning
The University of Texas
M.D. Anderson Cancer Center
Houston, TX

Patricia A. Piasecki, RN, MS
Joint Practice
Section of Orthopedic Oncology
Rush-Presbyterian-St. Luke's
    Medical Center
Chicago, IL

Sandra Purl, RN, MS, OCN
Oncology Clinical Nurse Specialist
Section of Medical Oncology
Rush-Presbyterian-St. Luke's
    Medical Center
Instructor
Rush University College of
    Nursing
Chicago, IL

Kathy Ruccione, RN, MPH
Division of Hematology Oncology
Children's Hospital of Los Angeles
Los Angeles, CA

Beth Savela, RN, BSN
Graduate Student
Oncology Clinical Specialist
    Program
School of Nursing
Northern Illinois University
DeKalb, IL

Vivian R. Sheidler, RN, MS
Clinical Nurse Specialist in
    Neuro-Oncology
The Johns Hopkins Oncology
    Center
Baltimore, MD

Joy Stair, RN, MS
Education Specialist
Department of Nursing Education, Quality and Research
Catherine McAuley Health Center
Ann Arbor, MI

Debra K. Sullivan, RD, MS
Research Specialist in Nutrition
Center for Handicapped Children
University of Illinois Hospital
Chicago, IL

Debra J. Szeluga, RD, PhD
Assistant Professor of Clinical
    Nutrition
Assistant Professor of Medicine
Section of Medical Oncology
Co-Director
Nutrition Consultation Service
Rush University
Rush-Presbyterian-St. Luke's
    Medical Center
Chicago, IL

Mary Taverna, RN
Executive Director
Hospice of Marin
Marin County, CA

Claudette G. Varricchio, RN,
    DSN, OCN
Associate Professor
Medical-Surgical Nursing
Niehoff School of Nursing
Loyola University of Chicago
Chicago, IL

JoAnn Wegmann, RN, PhD
Assistant Administrator
Director of Nursing Services
Poway Community Hospital
Poway, CA

Deborah Welch-McCaffrey, RN,
    MSN, OCN
Oncology Clinical Nurse Specialist
Good Samaritan Cancer Center
Phoenix, AZ

Debra Wujcik, RN, MSN, OCN
Oncology Clinical Nurse Specialist
Oncology/Hematology
Vanderbilt University Medical
    Center
Adjunct Instructor of Nursing
Vanderbilt University School of
    Nursing
Nashville, TN

Connie Henke Yarbro, RN, BSN
Clinical Associate Professor
Department of Medicine
University of Missouri-Columbia
Editor, *Seminars in Oncology
    Nursing*
Columbia, MO

J. W. Yarbro, MD, PhD
Professor of Medicine
Director of Hematology and
    Medical Oncology
University of Missouri-Columbia
Columbia, MO

The pace of development in the cancer field and the gratifying assumption of a greater role for nurses in the delivery of cancer care dictates the need for freshness in a modern nursing text on cancer. The second edition of this text provides the opportunity to maintain that freshness. It also provides the opportunity to reflect on where we have been and where we are going. Much of the progress taking place can be described as occurring in two overlapping waves; a breathtaking wave of new technology, developed as a consequence of the biologic revolution, lapping at a wave of significant improvements in technology in existence before 1971. Nineteen seventy-one is a good benchmark year; the key event that year was the passage of the National Cancer Act. The vision of the architects of that Act was prescient. The resources supplied by the US Congress fueled the biologic revolution that is now affecting all of medicine. Before then we had little appreciation of the mechanism of uncontrolled growth we call cancer and how the cell machinery was damaged in the process of carcinogenesis. We knew early diagnosis was useful but not why, and while we had refined methods to control primary tumors with surgery and radiotherapy, more than 65% of the patients died of their disease as a result of micrometastases already present at the time of diagnosis, not included in surgical or radiation treatment fields. To overcome this problem, surgery and radiotherapy had become radicalized, and often mutilating, in an attempt to widen their impact on the illusive cancer cell, which was envisioned as spreading by contiguous involvement of adjacent tissue before entering the blood stream. The use of systemic therapy, concomitant with local treatment, was controversial and of unproven value. Attempts at prevention were almost nonexistent.

In other words, cancer was like a black box. We could remove it or destroy it, when we could identify it; we could examine it, we could measure it, we could weigh it, but we could not out-think it because we could not effectively look inside the cell itself. The biologic revolution wrought by the Cancer Act provided the tools of molecular biology that changed all that.

Now the cancer cell is like a blue print; not only is the machinery of the cancer process exposed for examination and manipulation, but also in this exposure we have uncovered important information in developmental biology—the essence of life itself. We now know that cell growth is controlled by a series of growth regulating genes that operate in a biologic cascade from recessive suppressor genes to dominant genes we know as proto-oncogenes in normal tissue and as oncogenes in cancer tissue, of which there are now more than 40 identified. These genes code for growth factors, their receptors, membrane signal transducing proteins, protein kinases, and DNA binding proteins, all important in signal transmission, which in turn is the way multicellular organisms maintain order in their community of cells. While these genes are involved in normal growth and development, mother nature has wisely provided a means for suppressing their expression in mature organisms since their continued operation would be dangerous. Similarly, the metastatic process is no longer thought to be a random phenomenon tied only to tumor growth but has been found to be an aberration of the process of cell migration in normal development and, like the growth controlling function of oncogenes, subject to manipulation by molecular methods. Cancer can result from damage to any of several of the steps in this genetic cascade. Inherited loss or damage of an allele of a recessive suppressor gene appears to lead to a release of the cascade of oncogenes and uncontrolled expression. Damage to a dominant oncogene can lead to escape from control by suppressor genes. Overproduction of a normal or abnormal protein product of an oncogene can occur due to failure of the cell to respond to "off" signals. The startling advances in molecular technology make it possible to isolate and manipulate the products of these genes with ease and use them as diagnostic and therapeutic targets. This was the promise of the cancer program and this is the payoff.

This new wave is, however, just now reaching the level of practical use. For example, in diagnosis, molecular probes and the extraordinarily sensitive polymerase chain reaction can be used to diagnose gene rearrangements to determine cell lineage in malignancies of lymphoid origin, and specific sequences at break points of nonrandom chromosome translocations can be used to diagnose solid tumors. The polymerase chain reaction can be used as a tool to monitor the effects of treatment by detecting one residual malignant cell out of a million normal cells. A molecular approach to treatment also is surfacing in the form of antisense message compounds, chemically stabilized pieces of DNA complementary for, and inhibitory to, the message strand of the DNA of an operational gene or the message of specific target genes such as oncogenes. An extension of this approach will be the use of analogs of the recently identified products of suppressor genes to attempt to bring the oncogene cascade under control. A crest of this new wave of technology in treatment has reached the clinic in the practical application of the colony-stimulating factors produced through DNA recombinant technology, which is already influencing the use of chemotherapy, and the recombinant-produced interleukins and interferons, which have already produced useful antitumor effects by themselves.

Perhaps the most important and often overlooked implication of the biologic revolution is in its potential to allow meaningful approaches to cancer prevention. One of the main roadblocks to testing new ways to prevent cancer has been the identification of groups of high-risk populations small enough to allow prospective prevention trials to proceed at reasonable costs and with a reasonable prospect of answering important questions in the lifetime of the involved investigators. Genetic analysis of common tumors such as colon, breast, and lung cancers following on the heels of the first work on the identification of deletion of suppressor genes in the rare tumor retinoblastoma indicates that deletions of suppressor genes are common and likely to be tumor specific. These new approaches, when applied to the population at large, should allow us to identify individuals at high risk for getting common cancers. Then and only then can we accurately determine if the many interesting leads in prevention identified in the vast number of epidemiologic studies supported by the cancer program over the last two decades can truly be exploited to prevent common cancers.

This then is the new wave. A simultaneous wave of advancement in existing technology of a more practical nature has occurred in cancer management. The emergence of high-speed computers converted roentgenographic diagnosis and staging from plain film and linear tomography to computerized tomography and made magnetic resonance imaging an indispensable tool. Older, less precise, more morbid methods of diagnosis and staging have slowly, and appropriately, fallen into disuse. In 1971, we had just become aware that drugs could cure some types of advanced cancer, and the exploration of adjuvant chemotherapy had just begun. Now adjuvant drug treatments have proven beneficial in breast, colon, rectal, ovarian, head and neck, bladder, and pediatric tumors and in some kinds of lung cancer and bone and soft tissue sarcoma. Chemotherapy has quietly become the primary treatment for all stages of some types of lymphomas and for some stages of some types of head and neck cancers and bladder cancers. We also have developed a greater appreciation of the reason for treatment failure. A form of multiple drug resistance has been described in common tumors, derived from tissue exposed to the environment, that affects drugs derived from natural sources like some of our best antitumor antibiotics. We are just now begin-

ning to design protocols to circumvent multidrug resistance. The use of bone marrow transplantation to support high doses of chemotherapy has made us acutely aware of past treatment failures due to inadequate dosing that can now be overcome with concomitant use of colony-stimulating factors to promote more rapid recovery of bone marrows. New radiotherapy equipment, coupled with computerized tomography treatment planning, has made radiotherapy less morbid and more acceptable as an alternative to radical surgery.

As a consequence of all this, combined modality treatment is no longer what it was in the early 1970s. It no longer means doing the standard radical surgical procedures, adding the standard extensive and toxic radiation therapy fields, and later the standard drug combination, but instead initial treatment is being offered with a precise design based on the capability of each modality in controlling local tumor and metastases while minimizing toxicity. In other words, cancer management has become a complex medical jigsaw puzzle administered by dedicated professionals, many of whom are nurse practitioners, and almost unnoticed, has become far less morbid. Since cancer treatment is still far too morbid, this latter change has been difficult for many to appreciate. However, those of us who have seen both ends of the spectrum over the past two decades have a greater appreciation of the change in morbidity of treatment than a newcomer. Nowhere is this change more evident than in breast cancer where 15 years ago a radical mastectomy followed by postoperative radiation cured a handful of patients, while leaving the few survivors with the morbid effects of a denuded chest wall and a swollen nonfunctional arm. Now survival is improved with specifically tailored local and systemic treatment with fewer side effects and excellent cosmetic results. Fifteen years ago nausea and vomiting, pain, and marrow suppression were largely uncontrollable side effects, and now all can be managed to a great degree.

Unlike the new wave of advances in molecular biology, which remains to be widely implemented before it will have an impact on cancer mortality, the improvement in current technology has already had an impact on national statistics. In 1971, the relative survival rate for all cancers combined was barely 36%; it has increased to 49% in the last available data ending in 1985. Declines in national mortality, formerly only noted in children under the age of 15, are now apparent in all age groups up to age 65, and if one excludes lung cancer, a largely preventable disease, a decline in national mortality is noted all the way up to age 85.

The challenge before us is to smooth the transition of these successive waves of progress into medical practice. It has never been easy because one must recognize them as they exist, separate and distinct bodies of knowledge, each affecting medical practice in different ways, but waves that will eventually summate. Their combined impact gives us the means to effect a significant reduction in cancer mortality by the year 2000. Successful reduction in cancer mortality, however, depends on a cooperative partnership between the medical profession and the public to use modern information to prevent cancer and to implement newly developed treatment rapidly and effectively nationwide. Aside from lagging support for cancer research, which threatens the momentum of change, the machinery in place to do all this is hampered by outdated regulations, unimaginative reimbursement policies, medical territoriality, and unwarranted pessimism about the prospects for controlling cancer in our lifetime. The prospects have never been better but, as the framers of the National Cancer Act knew, nonscientific reasons and failure of all of us to think about controlling cancer on a national scale are major deterrents to success. Nurses read-

ing this text should keep this in mind because they will play an increasingly important role in the next decade in bridging the various medical specialty interests and the delivery of the new cancer care.

VINCENT T. DEVITA, JR, MD

Physician-in-Chief
Memorial Sloan-Kettering Cancer Center
1275 York Avenue
New York, New York 10021

PREFACE TO THE SECOND EDITION

Our goal in the second edition of *Cancer Nursing: Principles and Practice* is to provide the reader with the most comprehensive information about cancer nursing available in the 1990s. Each of the original 44 chapters in the first edition was thoroughly reviewed and updated. Twenty-five new content areas were added, including Relation of the Immune System to Cancer, Cancer Risk and Assessment, Biotherapy, Bone Marrow Transplantation, AIDS-Related Malignancies, Late Effects of Cancer Treatment, Psychosocial Dimensions: Issues in Survivorship, Sexual and Reproductive Dysfunction, Oncologic Emergencies, Delivery Systems of Cancer Care, Economics of Cancer, Teaching Strategies: The Public, and Teaching Strategies: The Patient. This edition contains 60 comprehensive chapters representing the contributions of over 75 recognized oncology nursing experts.

The exponential increase in information about oncogenes resulting from a massive research effort has provided a greater understanding of the nature of carcinogenesis. This improved understanding is reflected in this second edition and will continue to have a significant impact on the nature of clinical care. Even with this research effort and greater understanding of the nature of carcinogenesis, however, it is unlikely that a magic cure or vaccine for cancer will be available in the near future. There will continue to emerge new approaches to early diagnosis of cancer, new techniques to treat cancer, new measures to ameliorate distressing manifestations of cancer and its treatment, and new approaches to improve the quality of life for cancer survivors. Cancer nurses are integral to these developments. It is to these nurses that this text is dedicated.

The editors wish to gratefully acknowledge the tremendous effort of the contributors who enthusiastically shared their knowledge and expertise and gave their time and energy to this endeavor. We wish to especially acknowledge our husbands Keith, Jim, Larry, and John for their assistance, support, and patience during this mammouth project.

The editors have developed this text to be a comprehensive resource for nurses who provide or manage care for patients in the home, hospital, or community, who teach patients and nurses, and who conduct research to find better approaches to patient care—all of whom contribute to our steady gains in providing quality care to individuals with cancer.

SUSAN L. GROENWALD
MARGARET HANSEN FROGGE
MICHELLE GOODMAN
CONNIE HENKE YARBRO

PREFACE TO THE FIRST EDITION

This text is one I always wished to have. As a graduate student of oncology nursing, and later as an oncology clinical nurse specialist and educator at Rush-Presbyterian St. Luke's Medical Center, I became frustrated by the dearth of texts written at the level of the oncology graduate student or oncology nurse specialist. Oncology nursing texts lack the depth and breadth of scientific information that I believe is an essential element in the armamentarium of the professional nurse; medical literature, while it contains the necessary scientific information, lacks application of scientific principles to the nursing care arena.

In this text, the contributors and I committed ourselves to presenting the reader with the most comprehensive information about oncology nursing available, including relevant science and clinical practice content that addresses both the whys and hows of oncology nursing practice. All chapters cite original published research as the scientific foundation for the application of these findings to clinical practice. All students of oncology nursing— beginning or advanced—will find this book valuable as a text and as a reference for clinical practice.

The disease of cancer in the adult is approached from many angles to address the complex learning needs of the oncology nurse specialist. Part I includes cancer epidemiology and deals with individual and societal attitudes toward cancer and the impact of attitudes on health behaviors. Part II provides the foundation of scientific information about the malignant cell on which all subsequent chapters are built. Concepts such as carcinogenesis, oncogenesis, metastasis, invasion, and contact inhibition are included in Part II, and thorough attention is given to changes that occur in a normal cell and its behavior as it transforms to a malignant cell.

In Part III, the psychosocial dimensions of cancer are approached according to critical phases through which patients, families, and caregivers may pass as they cope with the stressors induced by cancer. Part IV presents a conceptual approach to the most common manifestations of cancer and their effects on the individual with cancer. Each chapter includes pathophysiology, assessment, and medical and nursing therapies. Part V describes each of the major cancer treatment methods, their uses, adverse effects, and nursing care considerations for individuals receiving cancer therapy. Included in this part is a chapter on unproven methods of treatment. Part VI is a comprehensive review of most of the major cancers by body system and the problems experienced by people who live with cancer. (Information pertaining to pediatric malignancies and nursing care of the child with cancer has been omitted. Although pediatric oncology is a critical area of interest for many nurses, it could not be covered in sufficient depth within this text.) Part VII presents continuing-care options for the individual living with the problems imposed by cancer. Part VIII analyzes several issues relevant to the oncology nurse: consumerism, ethics, cancer nursing education, and cancer nursing research. Part IX, which lists oncology resources of many types, is a handy reference tool.

Some of the information presented in this text is out of date even as it is written because of ever-expanding knowledge about cancer and its treatment. As Dr. Vincent DeVita remarked at his swearing-in as Director of the National Cancer Institute (*The Cancer Letter*, 1980:4), "What we now know of the cancerous process and what we do to prevent, diagnose, and treat it will be outmoded and radically different by the end of the 80s." This book is our best effort to put down in writing the science and art of cancer nursing in the 1980s.

SUSAN L. GROENWALD

The Jones and Bartlett Series in Nursing

Basic Steps in Planning Nursing Research, Third Edition
Brink/Wood

Bone Marrow Transplantation
Whedon

Cancer Chemotherapy: A Nursing Process Approach
Burke et al.

Cancer Nursing: Principles and Practice, Second Edition
Groenwald et al.

Chronic Illness: Impact and Intervention, Second Edition
Lubkin

A Clinical Manual for Nursing Assistants
McClelland/Kaspar

Clinical Nursing Procedures
Belland/Wells

Comprehensive Maternity Nursing, Second Edition
Auvenshine/Enriquez

Critical Elements for Nursing Preoperative Practice
Fairchild

Cross Cultural Perspectives in Medical Ethics: Readings
Veatch

Drugs and Society, Second Edition
Witters/Venturelli

Emergency Care of Children
Thompson

First Aid and Emergency Care Workbook
Thygerson

Fundamentals of Nursing with Clinical Procedures, Second Edition
Sundberg

1991-1992 Handbook of Intravenous Medications
Nentwich

Health and Wellness, Third Edition
Edlin/Golanty

Health Assessment in Nursing Practice, Second Edition
Grimes/Burns

Healthy People 2000
U.S. Department of Health & Human Services

Human and Anatomy and Physiology Coloring Workbook and Study Guide
Anderson

Human Development: A Life-Span Approach, Third Edition
Frieberg

Intravenous Therapy
Nentwich

Introduction to the Health Professions
Stanfield

Management and Leadership for Nurse Managers
Swansburg

Management of Spinal Cord Injury, Second Edition
Zejdlik

Medical Ethics
Veatch

Medical Terminology: Principles and Practices
Stanfield

Mental Health and Psychiatric Nursing
Davies/Janosik

The Nation's Health, Third Edition
Lee/Estes

Nursing Assessment, A Multidimensional Approach, Second Edition
Bellack/Bamford

Nursing Diagnosis Care Plans for Diagnosis-Related Groups
Neal/Paquette/Mirch

Nursing Management of Children
Servonsky/Opas

Nursing Research: A Quantitative and Qualitative Approach
Roberts/Burke

Nutrition and Diet Therapy: Self-Instructional Modules
Stanfield

Oncogenes
Cooper

Personal Health Choices
Smith/Smith

A Practical Guide to Breastfeeding
Riordan

Psychiatric Mental Health Nursing, Second Edition
Janosik/Davies

Writing a Successful Grant Application, Second Edition
Reif-Lehrer

CONTENTS

Index

PART VIII

PROFESSIONAL ISSUES FOR THE CANCER NURSE

Chapter 53

Quality of Care

Diane Scott Dorsett, RN, PhD, FAAN

CONCEPTUAL FOUNDATIONS OF QUALITY CARE

Historical Context and Origins

Well over a century ago, Nightingale[1] said that the prime objective in nursing was "to put the patient(s) in the best condition for nature to act." Since then, both conceptually and operationally, care has become the essence of nursing. During the past 10 years, a science of caring has emerged as a discrete theme in the nursing literature,[2-6] but only recently has care been accorded the importance recognized by Nightingale so long ago.

The relevance of care to society's health is becoming increasingly evident as demographic trends, such as an expanding elderly population, accelerate the incidence of chronic disease and as an increasingly advanced treatment technology extends life. Cure, once an important concept in the history of illness, when disease was primarily acute and infectious, has been replaced by the notion of prolonged remission with maximal quality of life. As modern science ushers in a biologic wave of modalities influencing prevention, detection, and treatment, clinical health care providers will continue to face the reality of increasingly rigorous treatments and more critically acute, morbid episodes superimposed on the chronic illness itself. Thus, as Benner[2] eloquently states, "In health care, caring sets up the possibility for cure."

As physicians attempt to master the rapidly changing complexities of cancer treatment in an increasing number of sicker patients, nursing care becomes a central issue. Quality of care is challenged by a health care system that contracts hospital stay time and health care cost coverage and by a health care environment in which large segments of the most vulnerable members of society (nonwhite, poor, less educated), who have greater than average health care needs, also have less than equal access to health care. Furthermore, those disadvantaged who do gain access often receive health care of lower quality—especially when measured in terms of appropriateness, timeliness, comprehensiveness, and continuity.[7] Documented in a publication of the President's Commission for the Study of Ethical Problems in Medicine and Biomedical and Behavioral Research, *Securing Access to Health Care*,[8] cancers of white Americans are detected earlier than those of nonwhites and those of paying patients are found earlier than those of nonpaying ones.

Although the reasons for these trends are complexly interwoven into the social, political, and economic fabric of American society, the outcome places a heavy burden not only on the underserved population but on all other segments of the society as well. Given today's challenges of specialization, complex technology, patterns of chronic illness, and a restrictive health care environment, the quality care of cancer patients and their families demands an interdisciplinary team approach and the extension of the role of nursing in its total management.

By the end of 1988, the Oncology Nursing Society had revised and expanded its scope of practice statement on the basis of a philosophic recognition that persons with cancer and their families need to be fully informed and to participate actively in their care and treatment and, further, that competent, humane care demands a complementary team of specialty practitioners who communicate with one another and augment one another's efforts. Increasingly, the notion of the patient as the owner-manager of his or her total health, with the need for a head coach and a qualified, well-coordinated health care team, has been gaining acceptance.[9]

Recognizing the emerging health care system as possessing an ever-expanding place for the nurse as direct caregiver, educator, administrator, and researcher, the Oncology Nursing Society statement emphasized the importance of the oncology nurse as a *coordinator* of care, collaborating with other health care team members to make the best use of resources available to patients and families and, as their *advocate*, assessing and communicating the uniqueness of each patient's response to cancer, thereby promoting maximum independence and autonomy. In short, oncology nurses, by virtue of their knowledge, skills, and holistic (biopsychosocial) perspective of persons with cancer, are often viewed as the most qualified practitioners to assume the head coach role.

Care and caring

To care is to respond to another in need because of pain, illness, or distress. Caring involves a sense of commitment and responsibility and, when taken to higher levels, can be considered a body of knowledge and skill known tacitly, empirically, or scientifically to accomplish change for the good. Although caring behavior is central to most public and private human activity, when defined for nursing, caring becomes a set of meaning-laden actions.[2,10] To wit, early in the education of most nursing students, Virginia Henderson's classic definition of nursing is introduced:

> Nursing is primarily assisting individuals (sick or well) with those activities contributing to health, or its recovery (or to a peaceful death) that they perform unaided when they have the necessary strength, will or knowledge; nursing also helps individuals carry out prescribed therapy and be independent of assistance as soon as possible.[11]

The definition of nursing as a profession, discipline, and practice, through such theaters of relevance, becomes public domain through the Nurse Practice Act. Nurse practice acts are state determined but are remarkably similar in wording throughout the country. Most legislate nursing as the diagnosis and treatment of human responses in health and illness—a broad definition, further operationalized in the interest of public safety by a regulated and standardized system of education, registration, certification, standards of practice, and quality assurance.

After the broad, formative brushstrokes of Nightingale,[1] who recognized "the fundamental needs of the sick and principles of good care," a concise, comprehensive definition of nursing by Harmer and Henderson,[11] and the more recent revisions that modernized nurse practice acts in this country, nursing began the establishment of a taxonomy of nursing diagnoses.[12-14] Nursing diagnoses operationalize the nurse practice act terminology, "human responses to an actual or potential health problem."[15]

Diagnostic taxonomies generally allow for a clear definition of professional purpose and for faster communication among the practitioners of a discipline, and they become the basis for a profession's research and development activity. As Herberth and Gosnell[13] advise, the next step is the integration of standards of practice and nursing diagnoses (Table 53-1) to foster relevant research,

promote therapeutic interventions, and, ultimately, advance the quality of care.

Caring actions cannot be separated from intent, however, if the outcome is to be effective. It is not enough to practice according to a guiding set of rules and regulations. To achieve even an acceptable level of quality of care, one must have commitment, creativity, and a willingness to innovate at reasonable risk. Knowing one's craft well is not enough. Caring requires knowing our patients and their beliefs, values, and cultural norms and tailoring care accordingly. Thus understanding and defining quality of care in terms of practices that enable health promotion

TABLE 53-1 Functional Health Pattern Categories and Nursing Diagnoses

Health perception–health management pattern

Health maintenance alteration
Health management deficit (total)
Health management deficit (specify)
Health seeking behavior
Noncompliance (specify)
Potential noncompliance (specify)
Potential for infection
Potential for physical injury
Potential for poisoning
Potential for suffocation

Nutritional-metabolic pattern

Alteration in nutrition: potential for more than body requirements or potential obesity
Alteration in nutrition: more than body requirements or exogenous obesity
Alteration in nutrition: less than body requirements or nutritional deficit (specify)
Ineffective breast feeding
Impaired swallowing
Potential for aspiration
Alterations in oral mucous membranes
Potential fluid volume deficit
Fluid volume deficit (actual) (1)
Fluid volume deficit (actual) (2)
Fluid volume excess
Potential or actual impairment of skin integrity or skin breakdown
Decubitus ulcer (specify stage)
Impaired skin or tissue integrity
Altered body temperature
Ineffective thermoregulation
Hyperthermia
Hypothermia

Elimination pattern

Alteration in bowel elimination: constipation or intermittent constipation pattern
Alteration in bowel elimination: diarrhea
Alteration in bowel elimination: incontinence or bowel incontinence
Altered urinary elimination pattern
Urinary incontinence: functional, stress, urge or total
Stress incontinence
Urinary retention

Activity-exercise pattern

Potential activity intolerance
Activity intolerance (specify level)
Fatigue
Impaired physical mobility (specify level)
Potential for disuse syndrome
Total self-care deficit (specify level)
Self-bathing–hygiene deficit (specify level)
Self-dressing–grooming deficit (specify level)
Self-feeding deficit (specify level)
Self-toileting deficit (specify level)
Self-care skills deficit
Diversional activity deficit
Impaired home maintenance management (mild, moderate, severe, potential, chronic)
Potential joint contractures
Ineffective airway clearance
Ineffective breathing pattern
Impaired gas exchange
Decreased cardiac output
Altered tissue perfusion
Dysreflexia
Altered growth and development

Sleep-rest pattern

Sleep-pattern disturbance

Cognitive-perceptual pattern

Pain
Chronic pain
Pain self-management deficit
Uncompensated sensory deficit (specify)
Sensory-perceptual alterations: input deficit or sensory deprivation
Sensory-perceptual alterations: input excess or sensory overload
Unilateral neglect
Knowledge deficit (specify)
Uncompensated short-term memory deficit
Potential cognitive impairment
Impairment thought processes
Decisional conflict (specify)

TABLE 53-1 Functional Health Pattern Categories and Nursing Diagnoses (continued)

Self-perception–self-concept pattern	Altered parenting
	Parental role conflict
Fear (specify focus)	Impaired verbal communication
Anticipatory anxiety (mild, moderate, severe)	Altered growth and development: communication skills
Anxiety	Potential for violence
Mild anxiety	
Moderate anxiety	**Sexuality-reproductive pattern**
Severe anxiety (panic)	
Reactive depression (situational)	Sexual dysfunction
Hopelessness	Altered sexuality patterns
Powerlessness (severe, low, moderate)	Rape trauma syndrome
Self-esteem disturbance	Rape trauma syndrome: compound reaction
Body image disturbance	Rape trauma syndrome: silent reaction
Personal identity confusion	
	Coping–stress tolerance pattern
Role-relationship pattern	
	Coping, ineffective (individual)
Anticipatory grieving	Avoidance coping
Dysfunctional grieving	Defensive coping
Disturbance in role performance	Ineffective denial
Unresolved independence-dependence conflict	Impaired adjustment
Social isolation	Post-trauma response
Social isolation (rejection)	Family coping: potential for growth
Impaired social interaction	Ineffective family coping: compromised
Altered growth and development: social skills (specify)	Ineffective family coping: disabling;
Translocation syndrome	
Altered family process	**Value-belief pattern**
Weak mother-infant attachment or parent-infant attachment	
Potential altered parenting	Spiritual distress (distress of human spirit)

Source: Reproduced by permission from Gordon M: Manual of nursing diagnosis 1988-1989, St. Louis, The CV Mosby Co.

and recovery from illness requires that caring be intrinsic to the process. Leininger[5] defined caring as behavioral attributes characterized by empathy, support, compassion, protection, succor, and education, firmly grounded in a comprehension of the needs, problems, values, and goals of the person or group being assisted.

Quality

The nature of quality is multifaceted and difficult to define, especially in relation to nursing care. Yet quality has emerged as the most important issue in patient care services in the final two decades of the twentieth century. The 1980s witnessed an integration of quality management, control, and assurance in nursing practice. To some observers, this integration has changed practice habits and promoted the individuation of care in innovative ways. These new ways of practice have led to the development of standards of care as the basic unit of analysis in the evaluation of quality in practice.[16]

Quality has become the focus of all cancer service provider groups, including the Commission on Cancer of the American College of Surgeons, the National Cancer Institute, the American Cancer Society, the College of American Pathology, the American College of Radiology, and, in joint affiliation, the American Nurses' Association and the Oncology Nursing Society.[17] Quality was, as Beyers[16]

stated, "the banner of the 1980s" and will be the established base for the next major advance in clinical nursing during the 1990s and beyond.

Quality, by definition, is a set of properties, attributes, and capacities that are essential and unique to the focus of evaluation, be it nursing or a work of art. In a generic sense, quality connotes a degree of excellence as measured by recognized standards. Standards are characterized by utility, durability, stability, flexibility, and aesthetics and, in the health care environment, require the definition of correlates related to both clinical and organizational qualities. Beyers[16] defines these correlates of quality as cost, productivity, and risk.

Historically, approaches to quality management in the United States have gone through several "eras," from inspection and statistical accounting measures (time and motion studies), to quality assurance processes and procedures (chart audit), to the newest era of "strategic quality management."[18] Strategic quality management is based on the realities of market share and fiscal viability since health care is big business and the driving force has become patient satisfaction. The "new" approach to quality recognizes four important factors: (1) recognition of consumer need and response, (2) integrated service teams, (3) standards of practice, organization, and professional performance, and (4) data management systems that document structure, process, and outcome elements.[16]

Beyers[16] views these factors as interactive and as having the potential for a positive effect. When patient needs are understood, recognized, and met by a well-coordinated team of clinicians who are guided by high standards, the associated documentation will allow clinical outcomes to be "known," ultimately modifying patient response for the better.

Thus quality embraces the dimensions of structure (patient and environment norms), process (strategies of quality management), and outcome (documentation of clinical outcomes and patient satisfaction). For many experts, quality is driven by the profit motive. For nursing, quality must be powered both by its value as a public service and by the caring ethic for maximal effect.

The concept of quality of care is grounded in the integration of a sound body of knowledge and skill, standards of practice and performance that promote excellence, a coordinated team approach, and a built-in capacity for innovation (research), with all components fired by a deep sense of caring.

Quality of Care Model

A model of quality of care (Figure 53-1) has been designed to represent the major goals in cancer care and treatment and those structural factors that ensure quality in terms of process and outcomes.

Structure

In the 1980s, several critical components were set in place that allowed for a guiding definition of quality in cancer care. These structural elements include overall *standards for oncology nursing practice and for the professional performance of the nurse* who cares for patients with cancer and their families. These standards are currently undergoing integration with the classification of nursing diagnoses and further categorization into Gordon's 11 functional health pattern categories.[14] Another major structure that promotes quality of care is clinical research and the development of nursing technology to test and improve interventions and maximize positive results. Nursing research in cancer care can be built into every patient care environment on some level. For some, this might mean keeping up with the nursing research literature or participating in a journal club, or it might involve undertaking a small study of one's own or participating in a larger multisite research project. Research allows for the development of nursing technology as well: Audiovisual patient teaching programs, drug dispensers that allow for safer self-administration of the many medications that cancer patients take at home, or measures that aid mobility, protect the skin and mucous membrane, or improve ventilation are examples of methods that achieve practical purposes toward the improvement or refinement of care. As these innovations are developed, they need to be tested and the results shared with others.

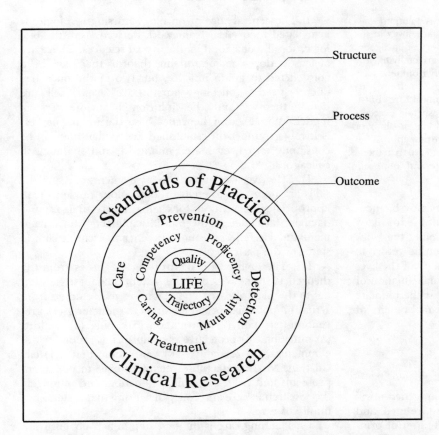

FIGURE 53-1   This model represents the major goals in cancer care and those structural factors that ensure quality of care in terms of process and outcome.

Process

The second dimension of the quality of care model is represented by the process variables of cancer prevention, detection, treatment, and nursing care. This dimension brings together the nursing care–medical treatment complex because the components of this complex are mutually dependent in achieving the desired outcome. More often than not, nursing care revolves around medical treatment but, in the best sense, extends itself beyond the immediate goals of interest to the physician. Cell kill and reduced tumor size are important, but without attention to management of side effects and promotion of functional recovery, the effect is diminished at best and ineffective at worst. In this sense, cure and care are not dichotomous. Care augments and enhances cure and in the process humanizes the total outcome.

Outcome

On a structural bed of sound standards and research innovation, the processes of prevention, detection, treatment, and care lead to patient outcome variables. The objectives of oncology care providers do not stop with the elimination of disease. Given the current status of cancer treatment today, with a documented 50% cure rate in all patients with a diagnosis of cancer,[19,20] Paul Marks, president of Memorial Sloan-Kettering Cancer Center, placed the current climate in perspective:

> The implication of this [sic, cancer biologic revolution] massive research effort is not that cancer will fade away in the next few years, or even decades. The discovery of oncogenes suggests that cancer may be an integral part of living, the result of interaction of our genes with the environment. Certainly, an understanding of the fundamental nature of carcinogenesis will transform the nature of clinical care. But it will not yield a magic bullet to cure the disease, nor a vaccine to prevent it. Cancer will not be eradicated like smallpox or polio. Rather, what seems likely to emerge are new approaches to early diagnosis of cancers and new techniques to treat them, providing steady gains in our ability to cure and, more important, to prevent cancer.[20]

The bottom-line results of 30 years of massive biomedical scientific effort has been an extension of life for many patients with a diagnosis of cancer. Paralleling the work on this frontier, the biopsychosocial scientific effort in nursing has promoted advances in the quality of the lives that medical science has extended. The amalgamation of life extension and quality of life makes clear the ultimate and optimal outcome of cancer care: maximal quality of life for cancer patients and their families.

Standards of Care

Nursing, as a science of caring, is based on a theoretical foundation for practice, continuously tested, refined, and verified by research, and a clearly articulated set of principles guiding that practice. Central to the concept of quality care is a set of standards that exists to guide practice by operationalizing its essence.

The publication of *Outcome Standards for Cancer Nursing Practice*[21] in 1979 and of its integration into the *Standards of Oncology Nursing Practice*[22] in 1987 were joint ventures of the Oncology Nursing Society (ONS) and the American Nurses' Association (ANA). Although the revision, *Standards of Oncology Nursing Practice*,[22] is rooted in the ANA published standards of nursing practice,[23] the former is a separate statement developed in recognition of cancer as a major health problem and of the importance of oncology nursing as a specialty practice devoted to the care of cancer patients and their families.

There are 11 Standards of Oncology Nursing Practice,[22] 6 that address professional practice and 5 that concern professional performance (Table 53-2). Practice standards focus on the process involved in patient care (theory, data collection, diagnosis, planning, intervention, and evaluation), with emphasis on 11 commonly occurring problem areas. Performance standards, in contrast, are criteria for professional development, interdisciplinary collaboration, quality assurance, ethics, and research in nursing as a discipline. To complement practice standards, ONS published *Outcome Standards for Cancer Nursing Education*,[24] *Cancer Patient Education*,[25] and *Public Cancer Education*.[26] A summation of the oncology nursing practice standards follows:

Standards of oncology nursing practice

I. The central core of oncology nursing is a logically articulated theoretical framework derived from the biologic, social, behavioral, and physical sciences. There are at least a dozen major nursing theories that have been constructed to guide practice, but two of the most frequently used in oncology nursing are Orem's self-care deficit theory[27] and the Johnson behavioral system model.[28] With a sound theoretical base, the nursing process is firmly grounded in established knowledge that can be constantly tested, evaluated, modified, and shared with colleagues.

II. Effective communication, assessment, and analytic skills are necessary to enable the oncology nurse to plan appropriate interventions for clients. The result is a sound database, available to the multidisciplinary team, that is maintained to reflect the most current and accurate clinical status of the patient.

III. The ability to make nursing diagnoses from the theoretical framework and the patient's database is essential to the plan of care. The diagnoses may emerge from actual or potential problems in 11 parameters: (1) prevention-detection, (2) information, (3) coping, (4) comfort, (5) nutrition, (6) protective mechanisms, (7) mobility, (8) elimination, (9) sexuality, (10) ventilation, and (11) circulation. Nursing diagnoses enable nurses to document problems and risks, planning, evaluation, and ultimately the research in care and collegial sharing that fosters continuity of care.

IV. Planning care is the first step in actively ensuring quality of care. During the planning process, goals are

TABLE 53-2 Standards of Oncology Nursing Practice

Standards of Professional Practice

I. *Theory:* The oncology nurse applies theoretical concepts as a basis for decisions in practice.

II. *Data collection:* The oncology nurse systematically and continually collects data regarding the health status of the client. The data are recorded, accessible, and communicated to appropriate members of the interdisciplinary team.

III. *Nursing diagnosis:* The oncology nurse analyzes assessment data to formulate nursing diagnoses.

IV. *Planning:* The oncology nurse develops an outcome-oriented care plan that is individualized and holistic. This plan is based on nursing diagnoses and incorporates preventive, therapeutic, rehabilitative, palliative, and comforting nursing actions.

V. *Intervention:* The oncology nurse implements the nursing care plan to achieve the identified outcomes for the client.

VI. *Evaluation:* The oncology nurse regularly and systematically evaluates the client's reponses to interventions in order to determine progress toward achievement of outcomes and to revise the data base, nursing diagnoses, and the plan of care.

Standards of Professional Performance

VII. *Professional development.* The oncology nurse assumes responsibility for professional development and continuing education and contributes to the professional growth of others.

VIII. *Multidisciplinary collaboration:* The oncology nurse collaborates with the multidisciplinary team in assessing, planning, implementing, and evaluating care.

IX. *Quality assurance:* The oncology nurse participates in peer review and interdisciplinary program evaluation to assure that high-quality nursing care is provided to clients.

X. *Ethics:* The oncology nurse uses the *Code for Nurses** and *A Patient's Bill of Rights*† to guide ethical decision making in practice.

XI. *Research:* The oncology nurse contributes to the scientific base of nursing practice and the field of oncology through the review and application of research.

*American Nurses' Association: Code for Nurses with Interpretive Statements. Kansas City, Mo, The Association, 1985.
†American Hospital Association: A Patient's Bill of Rights. Chicago, The Association, 1972.
Source: Reprinted with permission from Standards of Oncology Nursing Practice, © 1987, American Nurses' Association, Kansas City, Mo.

established and methods addressing the above 11 parameters are decided.

V. The implementation of the plan uses independently and interdependently determined actions to achieve its goals. In most cases, however, the nurse should function autonomously but collaboratively with others. Intervention should be flexible, documented, and provide measurable evidence of effect in light of the plan.

VI. Finally, the evaluation of the plan and its outcomes allows for continuous update, revision, improvement, and refinements in the database and diagnoses and for resulting modifications in intervention. This evaluation is done in collaboration with the patient and family and the health care team, is fully documented, and ultimately leads to scholarly, scientific analysis through research.

Standards of professional performance

VII. The first standard for professional performance makes clear (1) that the nurse is accountable for keeping abreast of advances in the field, maintaining current knowledge and skill, and incorporating them into practice and (2) that there is a commitment to the betterment of self, patients, colleagues, and the profession.

VIII. The complexity of cancer care today requires a multidisciplinary approach. Learning how to communicate effectively and to collaborate with team members is another indicator of professional development. There is considerable latitude in this standard in that the nurse may function effectively as participant, coordinator, and leader.

IX. Peer review and program evaluation have become mandated mechanisms in today's health care structure. Actively participating with an open, inquiring, and creative mind maximizes the possibility of quality improvement on individual, unit, and organizational levels.

X. The cancer care experience provides ample opportunity for ethical judgments. The rationale for the ethics standard spells out the profound ethical concerns in oncology nursing: right of self-determination, surrogate decision making, informed consent, treatment options, nontraditional treatment modalities, decisions about quality of life, confidentiality, distribution of resources, and matters of economics and value. Involvement with these issues can be demanding and challenging as well as stressful and exhausting. Continuing education and peer support are important vehicles for professional growth in this area.

XI. The 1970s and 1980s ushered in a new era of research-based practice in nursing. Oncology nursing practice must be kept therapeutically effective through research. The latitude in this performance standard is substantial. Minimally, the practitioner should keep abreast of research-based studies published in the most relevant specialty journals and incorporate findings into practice. Through expanded education, the nurse might ultimately become the principal investigator of his or her own study and might cultivate a scholarly interest in research that becomes a lifelong pursuit and vehicle for the enhancement of quality care.

The most recent 1987 revisions of the *Standards of On-cology Nursing Practice* incorporated the separately published *Outcome Standards for Cancer Nursing Practice* published in 1979. The original outcome standards reflected 10 high-incidence problem areas (Table 53-3) common to cancer as a major chronic disease with "intermittent acute episodes." When integrated with the 1987 revised practice standards concerned with data collection (II), nursing diagnoses (III), planning (IV), and evaluation (VI), the outcome assumes a patient-family-community focus, cuts across all phases of the cancer experience from prediagnosis to death, and recognizes the multiplicity of settings where patients are cared for today. These 10 high-incidence areas provide an essential link between the operating practice standard and quality assurance.

RESEARCH AND EVALUATION IN QUALITY OF CARE

Background and Context

Research-based clinical practice and quality care are the hallmarks of professional nursing. These important processes are based on a theoretical body of knowledge, standards for practice, and valid and reliable measurements that allow for the evaluation of care and the expansion of the scientific foundation of practice.

The nursing literature of the 1970s saw a significant expansion in standardized approaches to measuring the quality of nursing care. As early as 1966, Donabedian[29] identified structure, process, and outcome variables in medicine as the three classic approaches to patient care evaluation.

One of the earliest studies of quality in nursing additionally tested the research tool "Patient Indicators of Nursing Care."[30] Seven physiologic indicators reflecting nursing care–related complications were assessed. This study was a prototype of today's research evaluating patient outcome standards and nursing diagnosis–specific interventions. Majesky et al[30] chose three broad functional categories from Dorothy Johnsons' theoretical framework—infection, immobility, and fluid imbalance—and operationalized them using 27 measurable indicators. The overall goal was to establish a reliable, valid, easy-to-use, clinically useful instrument to evaluate quality of nursing care.

Oncology nursing literature came of age with the beginning publication of two journals, *Cancer Nursing* and *Oncology Nursing Forum*. In a review[31] of research-based articles published in these journals through 1984, a total of 15 were found to evaluate nursing care programs. All interventions tested were educative or of a supportive, counseling nature, perhaps reflecting Herberth and Gosnell's finding[13] that over 40% of diagnoses involve knowledge deficit. Most of the studies did not allow for control group comparisons. Nine articles described tools designed to evaluate patient outcomes. Rarely was care measured

TABLE 53-3 High-Incidence Problems in Cancer Nursing Practice

I. *Prevention and early detection:* Client and family possess adequate information about cancer prevention and detection.

II. *Information:* Client and family possess knowledge about disease and therapy in order to attain self-management, participate in therapy, optimal living and peaceful death.

III. *Coping:* Client and family manage stress optimally according to their individual capacity and in accord with their value system.

IV. *Comfort:* Client and family manage factors that influence comfort.

V. *Nutrition:* Client and family manage nutrition and hydration optimally.

VI. *Protective mechanisms:* Client and family possess knowledge to prevent or manage alterations in protective mechanisms.

VII. *Mobility:* Client and family maintain optimal mobility.

VIII. *Elimination:* Client and family manage problems with elimination.

IX. *Sexuality:* Client and partner can manage threats to sexual function and satisfaction and maintain their sexual identity.

X. *Ventilation:* Client and family can anticipate factors that impair ventilatory function and maintain optimal ventilatory capacity.

Source: Adapted from Oncology Nursing Society. Outcome Standards for Cancer Nursing Practice. Pittsburgh, Pa, The Society, 1979.

directly, and most measures were constructed by the investigator because of the lack of sound instrumentation at that time. Few were tested for accuracy or consistency.

A distinct shift in the cancer nursing literature, noted from 1985 onward, seemed to coincide with the establishment of oncology nursing standards and their clinically useful format (patient outcome standards and functional health classification). Clearly, more authors attempted schema that integrated patients' clinical problems and deficits, nursing diagnoses, assessment parameters, causes, and interventions into plans for care that provided a useful guide for the practicing nurse and a methodical approach for quality assurance programs.

The following review of methods for measuring quality of cancer nursing care recognizes the seminal work of early researchers[32-36] but concentrates on studies published in the cancer nursing literature since 1985 that reflect more recent trends in the field (ie, standards, nursing diagnoses, quality assurance, and measurement methods).

Approaches to Measuring Quality of Care

There are three major approaches to measuring quality of care: (1) quality assurance programs, (2) clinical research that includes both program evaluation and experimental studies of interventions, and (3) measurement tool or instrument development that includes both the construction of quantitative scales, questionnaires, and inventories and qualitative measures that include the establishment of clinical indicators, predictors, and guidelines for assessment.

Quality assurance

The Joint Commission on Accreditation of Health Care Organizations publishes standards used in the accreditation of hospitals and five other types of health care organizations (long-term care, psychiatric care, ambulatory health care, hospice care, and home care organizations) in this country.[37] These standards are concerned with the structures, processes, and outcomes of patient care activities in all services provided by the organization, including nursing services. There are eight standards that address the provision, management, and monitoring of nursing services regardless of location or institutional type. Four of the eight standards are concerned directly with the quality of nursing care: NR3 requires maintenance of established standards of nursing practice; NR5 mandates the use of the nursing process; NR7 delineates written documentation that care reflects optimal standards of practice; and NR8 provides for the monitoring and evaluation of care and the identification and resolution of problems.

The Joint Commission on Accreditation of Health Care Organizations distinguishes between standards of care and standards of practice.[37] Whereas standards of care reflect expected patient outcomes of care activities, standards of practice are concerned with "the structure and process elements used by the nurse and nursing service to provide patient care."[38] Thus a standard of care focuses on the patient, and a standard of practice focuses on the nurse. Patterson[38] differentiates the two concepts further by explaining that a standard of care is what the patient outcome should be and what the patient can expect from nursing service, whereas standards of practice relate to what and how the nurse provides care to achieve the patient outcome. The outcomes of care are generally based on clinical criteria or well-defined indicators that are measurable and that reflect the quality and appropriateness of intervention. Quality, in this sense, depicts the degree of adherence between the standard of care and actual patient outcome, and appropriateness reflects the degree of congruence between what the patient needed to achieve in terms of a desired outcome and what the nurse provided.

Therefore, to operationalize a quality assurance program, the health care institution must maintain a sound system for documentation of nursing care activities and patient outcomes and must establish a system to review and assess regularly both quality and appropriateness. In addition to evaluation, there is need for a system to rectify or resolve problems or breeches of quality in all aspects of care: diagnostic, preventive, therapeutic, rehabilitative, supportive, and palliative.

Depending on the nature and specialization of the nursing care unit, there may be need for a more precise definition of both patient outcomes and nursing practices to achieve those outcomes, or what is known as clinical functions. Oncology nursing is a prime example of the need for care and practice standards to be tailored to the unique needs and problems of the cancer patient and for more precise operationalization of clinical functions such as assessment, evaluation of learning needs, provision of physical care, teaching, goal setting, nursing interventions based on nursing diagnosis, implementation of the medical plan of care and required medications and treatments, and the coordination of nursing goals and plans for care with those of other professional team members.[38]

In these specific cases, both health care institutions and accrediting organizations look to the professional specialty group to establish and promulgate those standards of nursing practice. Quality assurance structures look to organizations such as ONS for current, state-of-the-art research-based standards.[38] On the basis of these published specialty guides, the hospital or agency customizes the standards further to be in line with the nature and character of its own care-giving environment. For example, nursing practice standards at one of the nation's five major cancer centers might differ from those in a small community hospital, where there may or may not be a discrete oncology unit or where there may or may not be a department of nursing research that focuses on oncology care. However, no matter how specialized or how large or small the institution might be, mandated quality assurance accords the *right* to quality of care as defined by the ONS standards of nursing practice to every oncology patient.

The literature is sparse in studies evaluating the quality of cancer nursing care by using patient outcomes as evidence. However, several articles stand out in their effort to improve the quality assurance process. This small body of literature reflects the complexities involved in studying quality and the many dimensions in focus and approach. Five issues important to quality assurance (QA) were examined in nine studies reported in the period from 1985 to 1988: (1) QA audit results for specific areas of care, (2) oncology patient classification systems, (3) Occupational Safety and Health Administration (OSHA) guidelines, (4) clinical database development, and (5) methods to identify and measure oncology nursing competencies and practice proficiency.

Oleske et al[39] conducted a controlled study that measured the effects of both nurse specialist consultation and continuing education on the home care of cancer patients, using an audit measure documenting assessment, intervention, and evidence of outcomes for patients with breast and colon cancers. Findings revealed that improvement in nursing assessment and management performance occurred over time in all three intervention groups. However, only half the criteria for optimal nurse performance were achieved, with little increase in patient outcome scores. The greatest improvements were noted in patients' nutrition, and little improvement was noted overall in the management of pain and physiologic complications. The authors recommend replication and offer the complete set of audit forms on request.

Similarly, Stephany[40] tested the reliability and validity of the Hope Hospice Quality Assurance Tool (HQAT), which assesses physical concerns, patient and caregiver education, and emotional and spiritual support, using operationally defined critera. Test-retest stability and internal consistency of the tool were established. Content, criterion-related, and construct validities were tested and found to be high in the nurse group but only moderate for lay volunteers. The tool was modified, with subsequent improvement in reliability and validity scores. The report provides detailed descriptions of the QA program, standards, and criteria and of the assessment form. The rigor of the study produced an effective audit tool to measure the quality of hospice care.

Arenth[41] developed and validated an acuity classification of oncology patients based on the definition of four categories of emergent status. The system has served as the basis for calculating nursing hours per patient day, patient volumes, nursing utilization or productivity, and variable staffing in a large medical center.

Dudjak[42] described the Radiation Therapy Nursing Care Record, comprising six flowsheets designed to document the nursing care of patients undergoing radiation therapy. The record allows for baseline assessment of risk factors and problems and for nursing practices in assessment, teaching, and other interventions. The record has been used to justify staff needs and cost of nursing care and to establish standards of practice further.

Because safety is a cornerstone of quality assurance for both patients and health care providers, periodic updates such as Gullo's review[43] of safe handling of antineoplastic drugs are essential to the application of the OSHA guidelines to practice. Recommendations for avoiding exposure, for safe disposal, and for health evaluation and monitoring are given clearly according to a well-articulated knowledge framework. Gullo estimated that more than 60% of nurses were not using safe handling techniques, an important factor in quality assurance. Two articles by Williamson et al[44,45] reviewed the occupational risks of infection, musculoskeletal injury, exposure to antineoplastic agents, stress in the work environment, shift work, and reproductive health concerns of nurses. Their articles call for a greater intensity of clinically oriented research efforts in this area.

Two articles suggest methods of establishing a clinical database to provide a structured framework for the collection of critical data with which to formulate nursing diagnoses. Miaskowski and Nielsen[46] developed the Cancer Nursing Assessment Tool to evaluate the integrity of 15 functional systems at high risk because of cancer and its treatment. The assessment included teaching needs and discharge planning. Gray et al[47] published a clinical database that provides description and analysis of age, met-

astatic sites, diagnoses, and associated symptoms of hospitalized patients with advanced cancer. Their study of 1103 patients generated more than 400 variables and provided important information on problem areas related to cancer metastasis. Since symptom management is the "cornerstone of care" in this patient group, the database facilitated the identification of relevant nursing diagnoses and related nursing practices that improved the measurement of quality of care.

On another level, two separate studies by Moore et al[48] and McGee et al[49] sought to establish nurse competencies and to measure proficiency in cancer nursing practice. The Moore team constructed the Appraisal of Practice Behaviors Instrument, based on the five dimensions of the theoretical framework used by ONS to develop the Standards of Oncology Nursing Practice. Three classes enrolled in a master's level oncology nursing graduate program were tested before and after each of the 2 years of their educational program for both frequency and self-assessed proficiency in achieving the ONS outcome standards of oncology practice. The instrument consists of 92 items divided among six subscales. Findings revealed that frequency of practice and proficiency were positively related and that students significantly increased in self-assessed proficiency as their educational program progressed. The investigators suggest further evaluation of the instrument in both academic and clinical settings to expand the database.

In contrast, McGee et al[49] conducted a two-round Delphi survey to identify oncology clinical nurse specialist (OCNS) competencies. The initial pilot study amassed 363 competencies, which the investigators further divided into knowledge, skill, attitude, and human trait categories. Ranking by means for each category revealed that attitude and human traits were ranked highest in importance by the 47 respondents. Attitudes of greatest importance had to do with ethical practice, respect for humanity, responsibility for behavior, and commitment to continued learning. Identifying nursing diagnoses and commitment to cost-effective practices were ranked lowest in the category. The human traits most valued included accountability, common sense, caring, flexibility, and resourcefulness. Of lower importance were sympathy and abstract thinking. The highest number of competencies, 173, were amassed in the "skills" category, and knowledge ranked second in number of competencies, totaling 137. The investigators, in interpreting their results, concluded that attitudes and human traits concerned with caring, commitment, and professionalism were ranked as those most important to OCNS functioning. They considered their results to be consistent with Yasko's survey[50] of 185 OCNSs, who reported a decided "care orientation" described as "keeping the client comfortable, maintaining a therapeutic environment, providing emotional support, personalized care, friendliness, emotional acceptance and ensuring that clients understand their medical problems."

The information generated from these key studies helps to expand and facilitate attempts to improve quality of care. By integrating findings from these and future studies on acuity, audit assessment tools, safety guidelines, clinical databases, and nursing competencies and practice proficiency, quality assurance will move into the era of strategic quality management predicted by Garven[18] and Beyers.[16]

Clinical research

Research offers a means of improving and refining practice to ensure optimal outcomes. The desired result of practice is usually defined as a valuable change in the patient for the better. In most institutional settings, this means cost-effective patient outcomes and consumer satisfaction.

Clinical research, in the context of evaluating quality of care, includes two major categories: (1) experimental studies of nursing interventions and (2) evaluations of programs of care. The program of research in most disciplines is shaped by the intellectual and practical problems and challenges encountered in carrying out its objectives and by the diagnostic and functional categories that constitute its focus. For nursing, these areas for investigation can best be illustrated by the results of two Delphi surveys conducted during the past decade to examine research priorities in cancer nursing.

Oberst[51] polled a group of 575 oncology nurses throughout the United States, asking them what they thought was important to investigate systematically in order to improve their clinical practice. From those nurses giving the most direct care to cancer patients, Oberst's goal was to capture a heuristic force that would have an impact on patient welfare by using the research process as a catalyst. She asked nurses to identify the problems they confront every day in practice, the problems cancer patients have from the time of diagnosis, and how these problems arrange themselves in priority.

The results of Oberst's study determined 10 priorities for cancer nursing research: (1) chemotherapy- or radiation-induced nausea and vomiting, (2) pain, (3) discharge needs, (4) grief, (5) stomatitis, (6) venipuncture in long-term therapy, (7) comfort and dignity of the terminally ill patient, (8) effective analgesia, (9) assistance with providing effective pain management, and (10) understanding the nurses' own attitudes toward pain and how it affects their ability to provide effective pain management. In addition, the oncology nurses responding to Oberst's survey reported that patient- and nurse-related research needs parallel one another. Optimal patient outcomes were inextricably tied to the reduction of deficits in nurse knowledge and skill in the 10 patient-focused research priority areas.

Ten years later, a partial replication of Oberst's work was conducted with 143 practicing oncology nurses from the four western provinces of Canada.[52] Results were similar but were expressed by requests for studies of specific interventions. Of the top 15 research priorities, the following areas emerged as most important: relaxation, imagery, and biofeedback techniques in the reduction of anticipatory nausea and vomiting and other side effects of treatment and in the enhancement of quality of life; ways to increase effectiveness of patient teaching in areas of patient compliance, self-care, and coping; approaches to

improve discharge planning programs; methods of communicating diagnosis and prognosis to patients and families; approaches to strengthen effectiveness in primary care; ways to improve preceptorship programs; and therapeutic approaches to the relief of treatment- and disease-related symptoms and side effects. The emphasis of the Canadian results was clearly on studying nursing practices that improve the patient's condition, rather than on the problem itself. This shift may reflect the result of descriptive nursing research efforts and a more sophisticated practice during the past 10 years after Oberst's survey.[51]

In a review of research-based articles appearing in the cancer nursing literature between 1976 and 1984, Scott[31] found 122 articles representing 25% of all articles published. More than 60% of the studies were published after 1981, most concerned with side effects of treatment (26%) or with oncology nurses themselves (24%). Approximately 15% examined the impact of cancer on the family, and another 16% described phenomena about cancer patients. Only 12% were intervention-management studies, and fewer (7%) offered assessment-measurement approaches to evaluate care.

In a developmental sense, the era before 1985 may be viewed as a descriptive phase when the rich database that exists today was established. Clinical research, comprising both program evaluation and experimental studies of interventions, began slowly between 1980 and 1985, marked by the seminal work of Satterwhite et al,[53] Edlund,[35] Dodd and Mood,[54,55] Johnson,[56] Miller and Nygren,[57] Marty et al,[58] Watson,[59] and Henrich and Schag.[60] Since 1985, there has been an expansion of the cancer research literature addressing the priorities in the two Delphi surveys and testing the therapeutic effect of larger-scale programs of care.

Fourteen experimental studies published since 1984[61-74] (Table 53-4) addressed 3 of the 10 (30%) outcome standards for cancer nursing practice, with more than half testing interventions to promote patient comfort and reduce treatment-related side effects. Five studies (36%) tested interventions to optimize protective mechanisms by preventing infection or reducing skin and mucous membrane integrity deficits. One study (7%) evaluated an educational program to promote early cancer detection practices. As a whole, these studies reflected a growing sophistication in research design and measurement. Most were randomized, controlled investigations of the effect of a clearly defined intervention on a small, homogeneous sample. The instruments employed to measure patient outcomes generally had been tested for reliability and validity or consisted of well-defined clinical indicators rated for construct validity by a panel of experts. All reports discussed study limitations, the generalizability of results, and implications for further research. Moreover, practically all made useful contributions to clinical knowledge.

In the period from 1984 to 1989, a total of 14 program evaluation reports[75-88] (Table 53-5) covering a wider range of outcome standards were published. The largest number (5, or 36%) evaluated programs designed to assist patients and families to cope with cancer. The next largest category (4, or 29%), comfort, described multidisciplinary pain

TABLE 53-4 Experimental Studies of Oncology Nursing Interventions and Patient Outcomes by Functional Pattern Category

Author	Problem	Method	Findings	Implications
I. Prevention and early detection				
Rudolf and Quinn[61]	Education to promote TSE	N = 64 college men; Health Beliefs Survey for Testicular Cancer and Testicular Self-Examination Survey (modified by authors); pretest and posttest; educational program with film and silicone practice model	Subjects lacked knowledge about testicular cancer and TSE Increased perception in benefits and decrease in barriers to TSE resulted Of "never performers," 63% did TSE at least once after program Perception of susceptibility and disease seriousness did not increase	Need for education and for research testing of a variety of educational approaches Nurses should take lead Replication with time between testing and more controlled methods Further testing of instrument
IV. Comfort				
Cotanch et al[62]	Self-hypnosis as antiemetic therapy	N = 20 children, aged 9-18 years, receiving chemotherapy Experimental and control groups Investigator-constructed visual analog scale, self-report, nurse's charting Experimental subjects trained in relaxation and self-hypnosis	Decrease in intensity and severity of nausea and vomiting in experimental group Increased oral intake in experimental group No difference in antiemetic administration between groups	Further research in other age groups
Frank[63]	Music and guided imagery as antiemetic therapy	N = 15 adults on variety of chemotherapy regimens 13 women, 2 men Single group Pretest and posttest STAI Nausea and Vomiting Questionnaire Intervention: musical tapes and poster images during and after chemotherapy	Decreased anxiety (STAI) Decreased intensity of vomiting No difference in perception of nausea, but duration showed nonsignificant downward trend	Test intervention in other stressful, threatening situations (ie, crisis and pain)
Scott et al[64]	Progressive Muscle Relaxation (PMR), guided imagery, and slow-stroke back massage vs drug regimen as antiemetic therapy	N = 17 women with gynecologic cancer receiving chemotherapy Relaxation and drug groups Drug group received high-dose metoclopramide Emetic Process Rating Scale (EPRS) Relaxation group received 1-hour educational program with slide tape and were coached by nurse in relaxation	Relaxation group had reduced total duration Drug group had reduced peak vomiting phase No difference in intensity or amount of emesis between groups Drug group experienced significantly increased diuresis unexplained by intake Content validity of EPRS established Verification of phase periodicity	Testing interventions combining both methods Replication in other populations Continued testing of EPRS Data on norm phase periodicity for other chemotherapy regimens

Cotanch and Strum[65]	PMR as antiemetic therapy	N = 60 Three-group design: experimental, placebo control (music), true control (no intervention) Dukes Descriptive Scale Diary of Food Intake STAI Upper skin-fold size Blood pressure Admission-discharge assessments	PMR most effective in reducing frequency and duration of vomiting, general anxiety, and physiologic arousal and in improving caloric intake in patients 48 hours after chemotherapy	Replication
Parker[66]	Scalp hypothermia to reduce alopecia	N = 12 subjects receiving cyclophosphamide randomly assigned to 2 groups: experimental and control SPENCO Hypothermia Cap Samples of hair loss for 7 days after treatment Scalp photographs	Control subjects have significantly more hair loss than experimental subjects	Clinical use
Dudjak[67]	Mouth care for mucositis therapy	N = 15 subjects receiving radiation therapy to head and neck area Random assignment of experimental and control groups Experimental subjects received hydrogen peroxide solution Control subjects received baking soda and water Oral examination guide Oral Comfort Guide Subjects evaluated 8 times: once before radiation therapy and then once weekly for 5 weeks, at completion, and 1 month after completion	Increase in perceived comfort in experimental group No difference in mouth condition between groups Hydrogen peroxide treatment judged more effective Both groups at lower incidence than published norms Rate of infection equal in both groups	Replication Test other interventions Clinical use

TABLE 53-4   Experimental Studies of Oncology Nursing Interventions and Patient Outcomes by Functional Pattern Category (continued)

Author	Problem	Method	Findings	Implications
Winningham and MacVicar[68]	Aerobic exercise as antiemetic therapy	N = 42 breast cancer patients Matched age and functional capacity Three-group design: experimental (stationary bike), placebo control (mild stretching), control (no treatment) Treatment: supervised 10-week 3-times-per-week aerobic training on cycle ergometer Symptom-Limited Graded Exercise Text (SLGXT) Symptom Checklist 90—Revised Somatization Subscale All tests given before and after treatment	Marked improvement in experimental compared with other groups in patient reports of nausea Increase in somatization scores in experimental groups	Studies of other types of exercise, emetic treatment protocols, and studies to determine difference between exercise and relaxation
Giaccone et al[69]	Scalp hypothermia to reduce alopecia	N = 39 patients receiving doxorubicin Randomly assigned to experimental (scalp hypothermia) or control (no treatment) group SPENCO Hypothermia Evaluations after 2 full chemotherapy cycles Hair loss evaluated by nurse and physician using an operationalized scale	Control subjects (100% alopecia) Experimental subjects, 37% prevention of hair loss No or slight hair loss in 7 of 19 No instances of scalp metastasis in either group	Clinical use
VI. Protective mechanisms Shell et al[70]	Dressings to treat radiation therapy skin reactions	N = 16 patients with moderate to severe radiodermatitis Comparison of moisture-permeable to conventional hydrous lanolin gauze Evaluation of healing time by use of 4 visual inspection parameters in number of days	Healing time for Mvp: 19 days vs 24 days for lanolin gauze	Warrants further study

Study	Purpose	Methods	Findings	Recommendations
Harwood and Bachur[71]	DMSO vs local cooling in extravasation therapy	Animal study using 4 pigs; Posttest control experimental design; Micro measurements by primary investigator; Measured time to healing; DMSO vs local cooling with ice vs no treatment control	Local cooling more highly effective in preventing tissue necrosis after extravasation; No difference between DMSO and control groups; Time to healing increased with DMSO; DMSO not recommended for treatment	More studies to determine optimal schedule of cooling
Jones[72]	Catheter care procedures in central venous catheter infection	Evaluation of 2 catheter care procedures, one using fewer supplies and less time; Assessment of observable evidence of infection, neutrophil count, and blood cultures	No difference; Only common factor connected with likelihood of infection: low neutrophil count at time of positive blood culture	Conduct further studies to refine predictive risk factors
MacGeorge et al[73]	Mixing vs reinfusion methods in drawing blood from Hickman catheter	N = 18 bone marrow transplant patients; Hematocrit (Coulter counter); Visual determination of hemolysis by expert laboratory technician	No statistical difference in accuracy of laboratory values between 2 methods; Mixing has advantage of less infection	Replication in pediatric population with larger sample in variety of clinical settings
Petrosino et al[74]	Dressing to reduce central venous catheter infection	N = 52 patients with central venous catheters; Random assignment to 4 dressing groups: Tegaderm transparent, Op-Site, gauze, no dressing; Observation at 7 and 30 days for 5 indicators: skin culture, oral temperature, erythema, tenderness, drainage	No difference among groups; No dressing option seems simpler and less costly	Further research on skin cleansing techniques

TSE, Testicular self-examination; STAI, State-Trait Anxiety Inventory; PMR, progressive muscle relaxation; DMSO, dimethyl sulfoxide.

TABLE 53-5 Care Program Evaluation Studies

Program	Author	Method	Results
I. Prevention and detection			
Family High Risk Program	Beck et al[75]	Health Family Tree Questionnaire Family health survey to assess satisfaction with program, health practices, health history, and behavior; includes retrospective data	Evaluation ongoing No results as of publication
II. Information			
Patient Education Program	Nieweg et al[76]	Comparison of patient self-care of chemotherapy port infection rates with literature-based norms Weekly clinical assessments No standardized evaluation methods used	Empirically judged effective Takes considerable time Required teaching materials Greater social support involvement Less need for hospitalization Greater patient freedom
III. Coping			
We Can Weekend	Lane and Davis[77]	Postprogram participant evaluation Staff feedback Director-evaluation of training sessions, staff, facilities, schedule, public relations, and supplies	Recommended use of preprogram questionnaires to enable advance custom planning Also use of postprogram questionnaire
Living With Cancer	Fredette and Beattie[78]	Precourse and postcourse knowledge test Precourse and postcourse personal needs assessment Postcourse interviews Written comments of specialist-observer End-of-class and end-of-program evaluations	Coping skills can be taught Profiles "good coper" as one who pursues information and seeks opportunities to learn Adaptive, resilient, optimistic, and assertive Need further exploration into program design for those who desire less or differently structured programs Teaching skills of coping was primary value of program
Cancer Caregivers Program	Cawley and Gerdts[79]	Committee-constructed evaluation tool: evaluates 8 dimensions of care in terms of time, instructor, handouts	Provides steps in establishment of program Evaluation tool developed and provided Ongoing evaluation No results
I Can Cope	Diekmann[80]	Postprogram mail questionnaire	Demographic characteristics Overall evaluation: valuable to help people learn about cancer More research to improve impact on coping
Bereavement Outreach Program	Mosely et al[81]	No formal means of evaluation	Excellent client response Need to tailor program to institution

management programs. The rest were divided among prevention-detection (1, or 7%), information (1, or 7%), nutrition (1, or 7%), and two economic feasibility studies (14%) of an adult day care hospital and a home transfusion program.

The therapeutic programs generally were well defined, as was the patient population. Most were service innovations based on the institution's database of patient needs and problems. In a majority of these studies, evaluation methods proved to be the weakest component. Although all programs were judged as valuable by the investigators, only half employed evaluation criteria developed before program initiation. Some measured quality by the number of clients seen or by unsolicited patient feedback. Others, however, made use of standardized surveys, questionnaires, interviews, and preprogram and postprogram

TABLE 53-5   Care Program Evaluation Studies (continued)

Program	Author	Method	Results
IV. Comfort			
Home Pain Management Program	Coyle et al[82]	Evaluated 123 patients with advanced disease for pain management at home	Nurse becomes primary liaison Successful pain management at home with use of analgesic and behavioral modes Team as expert information resource in community
Continuous SC Infusion Pain Management Program	Coyle et al[83]	Evaluated 15 patients for quality of pain management	Avoids repeated injection, need for intravenous access, analgesia delay, pain breakthrough
Pain Management Team	Ferrell et al[84]	No evaluation of effect of interventions on pain	Patient visits: 7500 (750 patients) over course of 5 years Community presentations: 300
Patient-controlled Analgesia (PCA) Service	Kane et al[85]	Patient questionnaire on discharge Nurse evaluation of two pumps re safety, ease of use, saving of time Bedside flow sheets to rate pain and sedation Daily patient evaluation by PCA team	Use of pump gives excellent control of pain in postsurgical patients, has few problems, and frees nurse to care for patient Further studies in chronic pain populations needed Choice of one pump over another
V. Nutrition			
Home Parenteral Nutrition Program	Konstantinides[86]	Patient teaching flow sheet No formal evaluation methods presented	Cost estimated between $55,000 and $70,000 for nutritional solutions, supplies, home visits, clinic follow-up, and laboratory costs Guides for patient teaching, discharge planning, laboratory monitoring, and follow-up given
VI. General Focus			
Day Hospital for Cancer Patients	Clark[87]	Economic feasibility measures	One-year pilot project Ongoing as of publication
Home Care Transfusion Program	Pluth[88]	Cost comparisons with patients receiving transfusions in different settings Client satisfaction Difficulties in implementation	Cost-effective and beneficial to patients' quality of life

comparisons of knowledge tests or needs assessments with baseline findings. Almost all investigative teams communicated willingness to share their programs with others but advised tailoring them to the unique needs of the institution and their patient populations. Most suggested the need for further study and program modifications or refinements.

Although the program evaluations reflected significant effort in planning and execution by hardworking teams, it must be remembered that program evaluation is a mature methodology, generally requiring an expert team of outside investigators to conduct the study. Two noteworthy examples include the Brown University evaluation of the Adult Day Care Hospital, Memorial Sloan-Kettering Cancer Center[89] and the as yet unpublished University of

Washington study of the effect of the Planetree Unit, a primary-nursing, family-centered care facility at Pacific Presbyterian Medical Center, San Francisco.

The overall picture of 28 studies published over a 4-year period suggests the beginning establishment of a clinical scientific base for practice. Clearly, much more research is needed in all standards-of-practice domains. Research that replicates or builds on the work of others and that refines established interventions may be the most economic ventures. However, to address meaningfully the issue of quality of care, longitudinal studies expanding the clinical database and testing effects of nursing intervention over time are critically needed. The oncology nursing research program, to have an impact on quality of care, will need not only to continue building the growing knowledge base in symptom management and patient education but also to turn attention to the issues of quality of life, recovery, transition, and the effect of a host of new modalities on patients' lives and health.

Measurement tool development: Quantitative

As psychometric theory advances and the results of nursing research build over time, better methods for measuring quality of care will emerge. Hartshorn.[90] Duffy,[91] and Lynn[92] emphasize the importance of using reliable and valid instruments in clinical research. Duffy said that research-based practice should be precise enough to be replicable and to produce predictable patient outcomes. Hartshorn warned that results from studies employing poor instruments cannot be accepted or implemented. Indeed, many nursing studies that have required considerable time and effort conclude with a long list of limitations to the generalizability of their findings and with an underdeveloped interpretation of important data because of faulty design, inadequate sampling technique, and use of untested measurement tools.

The basic ingredients of sound quantitative measurement techniques include adequate reliability and validity of the instrument. Reliability tests both the stability (test-retest correlations) and the internal consistency (intercorrelations among items or alpha coefficient) of an instrument. Correlations of at least 0.8 in internal consistency and test-retest correlations ensure that the instrument is reliably measuring the construct it purports to measure and is stable in its ability to reproduce results in repeated testing of the sample. A third type of reliability, interrater reliability, is also important to ensure that all persons using a set of evaluation criteria have closely correlated results.[93]

Validity testing offers a way to assess the ability of the instrument to measure the construct of interest accurately and objectively. The three most important types of validity include construct, content, and criterion related (predictive or concurrent).[90,93] One of the most definitive signs of increasingly improved and sophisticated cancer nursing research is growing evidence that reliable and valid instruments were used.

Table 53-6 provides a partial list of cancer nursing measurement tools* grouped by functional category, including the construct measured and whether evidence of reliability and validity testing are given.[94-114] Note that most of these instruments quantify patient attributes. The aim is to establish further a normative database or to measure the qualitative outcomes of nursing practice, or both.

Measurement tool development: Qualitative

During the past few years, an increasing interest in qualitative methods of research has become evident in the nursing literature. Measuring quality of care quantitatively

*For a current, inclusive discussion of clinical research tools in nursing, consult Frank-Stromborg's *Instruments for Clinical Nursing Research.*[94]

does not readily capture the contextual nature and natural richness of the situational and interpersonal data that compose the nursing care environment.

Nursing literature generally reflects attempts at establishing patient databases composed of qualitative sets of indicators, predictors, and assessment parameters that form the etiologic foundations of patient concerns and nursing practices. For example, if we review the available quantitative tools, most are based on the identification of indicators grouped to facilitate diagnostic reasoning. However, less precision is found in scoring instrument results. Few scoring systems are based on large amounts of normative data, particularly those established in healthy populations that allow clear comparisons and interpretation of new data.

The most recognized qualitative approaches include case study, grounded theory, phenomenology, and ethnography, among others (Ammon-Gaberson and Piantanida.)[115] Qualitative research begins with carefully conceptualized and clearly articulated research questions to guide data collection and later interpretation. The motive is to understand an aspect of human experience and to shape a representation of it from the data. The results of the qualitative method may include (1) operationalizing a single concept, (2) developing a conceptual framework, (3) establishing guidelines for practice, (4) creating portraits, paradigm cases, or typologies, and (5) forming theory.

Although reliability testing and validity testing in the conventional sense do not have a place in the qualitative process, there are sound principles and methods to guide study design, data gathering, data analysis and management, data interpretation, and paradigm construction. These processes are no less rigorous than those of the quantitative approach. In many areas of quality of care research, the qualitative paradigm or a combination of the qualitative and quantitative paradigms may be the best approach.

The qualitative cancer nursing research literature represents a mixed bag of clinically relevant information that, for the purposes of a quality-of-care discussion, may be categorized according to format and content considerations. The research articles have been grouped as either indicators, predictors, or guidelines for care.

Indicators are sets of variables that describe empirically an important clinical manifestation. These sets are derived generally from a review of published work on the subject or a descriptive exploratory or qualitative study, or both. For example, Saunders and Valente's article[116] on suicide in cancer patients brings together their wealth of empirical knowledge as well as general information about depression and suicide. One outcome is a useful "Brief Suicide Assessment Guide" for practitioners. In contrast, Thorne[117] reported the results of her phenomenologic study of the family cancer experience, providing important insights into family perceptions and coping strategies when a member has cancer. Therefore information in a wide variety of content areas produced sets of clues to facilitate better understanding of many common clinical issues.

Predictors are variables that have been tested to deter-

TABLE 53-6   Tools to Measure Patient Outcomes

Tool	Author	Construct	Findings	Implications
Quality of Life Index (QLI)	Ferrans and Powers[95]	Quality of life	Likert scales (2) to determine importance and satisfaction in 18 life areas: life goals, general satisfaction, stress, physical health; reliability established; validity established; versions for normal, healthy adults and for kidney transplant, heart transplant, kidney dialysis, and cancer patients	Establishing norms in different populations
Cancer Malaise Scale	Kobashi-Schoot et al[96]	Physical fatigue, mental fatigue, malaise, psychologic complaints in radiotherapy cancer patients; validity established	Malaise increased during course of treatment; physical symptoms increased late in course of treatment; malaise correlates with "feeling ill" or "not well"	Further correlation stratified by treatment level of radiation exposure
Quality of Life Index (QLI)	Padilla and Grant[97]	Linear analog; psychologic well-being, physical well-being, symptom control; 14 items; reliability established; validity established		Further testing in variety of subject populations; use to test intervention effectiveness
Information Preference Questionnaire (IPQ)	Hopkins[98]	Information seeking; 5-point scale measuring preference for treatment information	Information seeking negatively related to age and severity of disease; reliability established; validity established	Needs additional testing to establish criterion and construct validities
Emetic Process Rating Scale (EPRS)	Scott et al[64]	Analog scale: nausea, retching, vomiting, intake, output, vital signs, treatment; validity established	Evaluated antiemetic effect of clinical relaxation vs drug intervention; scale found clinically useful	Further reliability and validity testing
Sexual Adjustment Questionnaire (SAQ)	Waterhouse and Metcalf[99]	Desire, activity level, relationship, arousal, techniques, orgasm	Persons with cancer significantly reduced scores on activity level, relationships, and techniques	Continued refinement and larger sample testing
Derdiarian Informational Needs Assessment (DINA)	Derdiarian[100]	Informational needs related to disease: personal, family, and social parameters		Further instrument assessment and use in patient referral and follow-up
Patient Care Needs Survey	Fleming et al[101]	Comfort needs in advanced cancer patients: physiologic, spiritual, psychosocial, patients' rights, dignity, self-worth	Identified 7 themes of comfort; decreased with severity of illness; calls for social support approach, including multidisciplinary	Further development and testing
Human Needs Assessment Scale	Lilley[102]	Likert scale of 35 human needs based on work by Yura and Walsh; modified to a 4-point scale; reliability established; evaluates importance of need	Instrument easy to use; nurses perceived patients' human needs similarly to patients' own assessment	Suggest development of nursing diagnosis and evaluation of nursing care to be based on this Human Need Model
Quality of Life Questionnaire (QLQ)	Young-Graham and Longman[103]	Likert-type brief scale: social dependency, symptom distress, behavior-morale, direction of life change; reliability established	Pilot study of patients with melanoma to test model of major hypothesized factors in quality of life	Further use in other populations; internal consistency confirmed

TABLE 53-6 Tools to Measure Patient Outcomes (continued)

Tool	Author	Construct	Findings	Implications
Derogatis Sexual Functioning Inventory (DSFI) (modified)	Blackmore[104]	Affect, body image, symptoms, drive, satisfaction, activity	Reduction in sexual activity postoperatively in orchidectomy cancer group	More research on sexuality of cancer patients
McGill Pain Questionnaire	Camp[105]	Location, quality, pattern, increase, intensity, verbal-nonverbal symptoms; reliability established; validity established	Compared patient perceptions and nurse documentation; less than 50% of patients' pain perceptions were documented	Replication and assessment of pain management protocols
Hypercalcemia Knowledge Questionnaire (HKQ)	Coward[106]	Hypercalcemia risk factors and knowledge		Need for educational program to evaluate
Derdiarian Behavioral System Model	Derdiarian[107]	Achievement, affiliation, aggressive-protective, dependence, elimination, ingestion, restoration, sexuality; based on Johnson Behavioral Symptom Model; reliability established; validity established	Defines imbalance in behavioral subsystems caused by illness; predicts direction and quality of change; sensitive to age, site of cancer, and stage of cancer	Further studies in larger samples
Oral Assessment Guide	Eilers et al[108]	Stomatitis or oral mucositis and mucosal changes in radiotherapy and chemotherapy patients: voice, swallow, lips, tongue, saliva, mucous membranes, gingivae, teeth and dentures	Clinical guide to evaluate oral care protocols and toxic effects of treatment protocols and persons at risk	Further clinical use
Breast Self-examination (BSE) Belief and Attitude Questionnaire	Lauver[109]	Remembering, competence, comfort, interference, efficacy; reliability established	Positive relationship between frequency of BSE and competence, remembering, and comfort	Replication in larger, heterogeneous population with test-retest reliability; further testing for methods to promote competence and remembering
Pain Assessment Tool (PAT) and Pain Flow Sheet (PFS)	McMillan and Williams[110]	Ongoing assessment of pain and its management	Pain intensity and level of sedation documented in two-group study	Further research with both tools
Self-care and Symptom Report Interview	Rhodes et al[111]	Symptom distress, self-care activities, coping strategies regarding fatigue and weakness; based on Orem's self-care deficit theory	Lays foundation for tool to measure symptom occurrence and distress and to assess self-care efficacy	Ongoing development and testing
Linear Analogue Modification (LAM) of Profile of Mood States (POMS)	Sutherland et al[112]	Emotional distress: fatigue, anxiety, confusion, depression, energy, anger	Significant correlation between LAM and POMS in 29 subjects	To evaluate patients' ongoing emotional status as base for psychosocial interventions over time
Cancer Knowledge Test	Weinrich and Weinrich[113]	Belief in cancer myths, recall of American Cancer Society 7 warning signals, recognition of disease symptoms	Overall significant difference in cancer knowledge based on race, education, and income	Evaluation of health teaching on elderly, less educated, and low-income black persons
Champion's Instrument and Williams' Breast Inventory	Williams[114]	Likert scale of 5 constructs of Health Belief Model, health history, and personal knowledge	Health motivation represents 18% of variance; barriers, 8%; age differences	Further testing of variables

mine their ability to predict a future event with some degree of accuracy. Predictors are critical to nursing's role in health promotion and prevention. For example, Hays' article[118] on predictors of hospice utilization identified specific patient and family parameters that, when taken into consideration early enough in the nursing plan of care, have a good chance of strengthening the family unit so that the patient can be maintained at home under quality care conditions for longer periods. Another illustration of the establishment of predictors is the research that has identified clusters of variables predicting the occurrence of anticipatory nausea and vomiting.[119,120]

Guidelines for care are organized, integrated schemata for practice. These presentations are readily identifiable by title descriptors such as nursing care, nursing interventions, nursing implications, the nursing role, nursing assessments, nursing management, and nursing plans for a variety of patient problems, specialized treatments, or situations. In most cases, guidelines are in tabular format, resembling the traditional nursing care plan (problem,

care, scientific rationale) with updated language such as nursing diagnoses, nursing etiology, nursing interventions, and nursing evaluations by outcome criteria.

Table 53-7 provides a list of indicators, predictors, and assessment guidelines used in recent studies addressing quality of care.[121-153] These articles report studies of cancer-related disease and treatment problems, psychosocial adjustment, risk factors, and family response and coping.

QUALITY IN PERFORMANCE: APPLICATIONS IN PRACTICE

No discussion of care is complete without a look at process—the performance of nursing care and its meaning for both patient and nurse. Although patient outcome has become the basis for care evaluation, the multiple forces impinging on a patient's condition often make this method

TABLE 53-7   Indicators, Predictors, and Guidelines for Quality of Care

Indicators

Fever patterns in neutropenic patients (Henschel[121])

Psychologic model of adjustment in gynecologic cancer patients (Krouse[122])

Family cancer experience (Thorne[117])

Sexual and reproductive issues for women with Hodgkin's disease (Cooley and Cobb[123,124])

Cancer-induced hypercalcemia (Coward[125])

Primary caregiver's perception of the dying trajectory (Holing[126])

Alterations in taste during cancer treatment (Huldij et al[127])

Family responses to cancer hospitalization (Lovejoy[128])

Characteristics of pain in hospitalized cancer patients (Donovan[129])

Sexual changes after gynecologic cancer treatment (Jenkins[130])

Cisplatin-related peripheral neuropathy (Ostchega et al[131])

Weakness, fatigue, and self-care abilities (Rhodes et al[111])

Suicide in cancer patients (Saunders and Valente[116])

Cancer pain control behavior (Wilkie et al[132])

Predictors

Patterns of lung cancer dyspnea (Brown et al[133])

Anticipatory nausea and vomiting associated with cancer chemotherapy (Duigon[119])

Patterns of hospice utilization (Hays[118])

Radiotherapy symptom profile (King et al[134])

Carotid artery rupture (Lesage[135])

Colorectal cancer (Messner et al[136])

Glucocorticosteroid-induced depression (Post-White[137])

Needs of family members of cancer patients (Tringali[138])

Anticipatory nausea and vomiting (Coons et al[120])

Patterns of nausea, vomiting, and distress with antineoplastic drug protocols (Rhodes et al[139])

Guidelines for Care

Prevention of chemotherapy-associated pneumonia in non-Hodgkin's lymphoma (Foote[140])

Primary, secondary, and tertiary interventions for lymphedema (Getz[141])

Management of disseminated intravascular coagulation (Rooney and Haviley[142])

Care of patients treated with intrapleural tetracycline for malignant pleural effusion (Rossetti[143])

The compromised host (Gurevich and Tafuro[144])

Management of venous access ports (Moore et al[145])

Morphine infusion for intractable cancer pain by implanted pump (Paice[146])

Care of head and neck cancer patients receiving myocutaneous flap reconstructive surgery (Rodzwic and Donnard[147])

Care of patients receiving radiation therapy for rectal cancer (Hassay[148])

Care of patients receiving third-generation cephalosporins (Link[149])

Assessment of gynecology patients (Moreland[150])

Needs of the spouse of the patient with advanced cancer (Stetz[151])

Care of the family with cancer (Lewandowski and Jones[152])

Skin care during radiotherapy (Strohl[153])

partially precise at best. Outcomes are relative and frequently are only partly related to the quality of nurse performance. More often, quality is deeply embedded in the rich mutual interpretations of care and caring that constitute the nurse-patient bond. Measuring quality of care by documented patient outcome is only one aspect of the multipronged approach demanded, an important indication that evaluation must go beyond the standard.

Determining the quality of a process is tricky and yet critical to the search for excellence. There are four important patterns to the process of giving and receiving care. The first is *mutuality*. Care behavior and the caring attitude forge a mutuality of response between two people that is characterized by reciprocity and complementarity. The experience is shared and cooperative, and the roles of caregiver and care receiver are complementary in that there is a degree of dissimilarity in the nature of the role relationship that works in a nondissonant way, allowing for harmony. However, the degree of dissimilarity is important in that the effect of care can be compromised if patient-nurse perceptions are either too much alike or radically different.

The nature of the mutual experience of caregiver and care receiver and their interacting perceptions are central to the quality of care. A growing literature focused on the congruity of nurse and patient perceptions reflects this phenomenon. In an early study by Jennings and Muhlenkamp,[154] caregivers' perceptions of their patients' affective states and the patients' self-reports of their anxiety, hostility, and depression were significantly different. Caregivers (eg, physicians, nurses, nursing assistants) assessed patients as feeling significantly worse than patients reported feeling. Findings were interpreted in light of "Wright's requirement-of-mourning hypothesis" that caregivers may perceive patients as having negative feelings so that the caregivers' own value systems, which place emphasis on health, will be supported."[155]

In 1987, Verron et al[156] hypothesized that attitudes of health care providers, grounded in their values, influence the quality of patient care. The authors cited work linking learning, experience, and consequent changes in attitude with positively modified behavior that endured for long periods.[157] Further, they attempted to identify and measure attitude themes pertinent to caring for oncology patients. The "Ideas About Oncology Patient Care Scale" (IAOPC) resulted, generating four attitude-related factors: therapy, future outlook, terminality, and drug use. Through repeated instrument testing, the attitudes were found to be multidimensional, another indication of the complexities of measuring human responses to caregiving and care receiving.

Larson[3,158,159] laid a foundation for unraveling the intricacies involved in giving and receiving care. She interviewed two separate samples of patients and nurses to determine what nurse behaviors were most and least important in making cancer patients feel "cared for." Her assumption was that the optimal expectation of nursing care is for patients to feel cared for as a result of nursing actions. Feeling cared for was defined as a sensation of well-being and safety linked to the behavior of the nurse.

Nurses and patients were asked to rank, in order of importance, 50 nurse caring behaviors categorized by six action themes: anticipation, accessibility, explanation-facilitation, provision of comfort, establishment of trust, and monitoring with follow-through. Findings revealed that patients and nurses held very divergent opinions of what was most important. The highest-ranked behaviors reported by patients were those demonstrating competency, actions mostly concerned with monitoring and follow-through and with accessibility. Actions rated highest by nurses were more focused on meeting comfort and psychosocial needs such as listening and touch. In an examination of the top 10 responses of both groups, however, several mutual choices appeared: being quickly accessible, giving good physical care, putting the patient first, and listening. These choices indicated several important shared values.

Mayer[160] replicated Larson's study and found similar results. There was 100% agreement between samples of nurses in both studies regarding the most and least important caring behaviors. Comparisons of the two patient groups revealed 40% agreement for the most important behaviors and 80% for the least important. Across both studies and all samples, conventions of professional etiquette such as appearance, cheerfulness, and polite social behavior were viewed as least important. In Mayer's study, listening was again rated highest by nurses, and knowing how to give injections and intravenous infusions, and managing technical equipment remained most important to patients. Mayer concluded that patients seem to value the instrumental, technical caring skills and that nurses are more attuned to expressive caring behaviors.

These results might reflect understandable differences in perception between the two groups. Patients seemed to value those competencies and skills most concretely apparent and directly linked to their welfare. Nurses, on the other hand, may have perceived expressive and instrumental dimensions of care as inextricably connected, similar to the mutuality of care and cure. Who can deny the effect when patient preparation, technical skill, and gentleness are integrated during administration of an uncomfortable, intrusive procedure? To emphasize one aspect without the others decontextualizes care and strips it of its healing quality.

Several other comparison reports have documented discrepancies between patients' self-reports and their nurses' knowledge and understanding of patients' needs. Sodestrom and Martinson[161] found that 76% of a sample of nurses caring for hospitalized terminally ill patients considered spiritual needs low on the list of priorities because of the lack of time to incorporate spiritual assessment into care. Although the nurses correctly identified the meaning and purpose of their patient's relationship with God and the patient-nurse definitions of the term *spiritual* did not differ significantly, the nurses in this study did not view themselves as essential in meeting the spiritual needs of their terminally ill patients.

As the location of cancer care increasingly moves into the home, the concept of caregiver expands to include family members and others in charge of the patient's welfare. In light of this trend, congruence between caregiver and care recipient perceptions of quality of life was examined in 23 care dyads in a home hospice program (Curtis and Fernsler[162]). The overall trend, although not statistically significant, was for patients to report a higher quality of life for themselves in comparison with their caregivers' assessments. Patients reported better sleeping and pain control than did caregivers, but much less fun and sexual satisfaction. Thus nurse caregivers are not alone in their struggle to interpret the patient's situation accurately.

The needs of family members as they care for their loved ones with cancer are emerging as an important dimension in quality of care. Dyck and Wright[163] found that almost half of their sample of next-of-kin said that nurses did not do anything for them as family members, nor did they expect anything. Their expectation, however, seemed to be a function of limitations in their knowledge of the role of the nurse and what was thought to be the appropriate focus—the patient. If the patient was competently cared for and the nurse kept the family accurately informed, families said they could not expect more. Yet, a parallel analysis of their needs documented acceptance, support, and comfort as being very important to them. Furthermore, their rank-order of traits looked for in nurses differed depending on the stage of the patient's illness. Competence was number one in the early diagnostic stage, friendliness when the disease recurred, and compassion during the terminal stage. The authors concluded that appropriate emphasis of a trait is contextually determined and a significant way that nurses may express "caring for" patients.

The second major pattern in the caregiving and care-receiving process is *contextuality*. The contextual aspects of care have been highlighted repeatedly in these studies, with location of care and phase of illness emerging as two important determinants of the most appropriate clinical approach. Often, phenomenologic studies provide the best look at contextuality.

For example, Thorne,[117] in studying helpful and unhelpful communications in care, refers to cancer as "a modern metaphor for human confrontation with existential uncertainty." She found that communication is important in shaping the illness experience. Patients in Thorne's study were able to recall communication with health care providers during their illness and distinguish between styles that were more and less helpful. She found that the more uncertain a patient's situation, the greater was the vulnerability to communication characterized by lack of concern. On the other hand, the providers' feelings of failure, vulnerability, and hopelessness were part of the total picture as well. Nurses did not figure prominently into this compilation of opinions about helpful and unhelpful communicators, although study subjects reported that physicians communicated more about the disease and nurses provided advice about treatment and the illness. More often, a communication was perceived to be helpful if it was thought to be intentionally supportive. The most frequent unhelpful type was described as advice that was intentionally unhelpful, when the person withheld information or abused his power. Moreover, most important to the caring process was content, style, and a manner perceived by the patient as intentionally designed to be useful, encouraging, and supportive.

As a unit, these studies highlight the importance of mutuality and contextuality in determining the quality of nursing care performance. Yet, two other patterns have emerged as major influences on quality of performance; these patterns are so mutually dependent that they must be considered as one: *competence and proficiency*.

Benner[164,165] says that the practical knowledge embedded in expert nursing needs to be understood and yet has not been fully elucidated. Since clinical practice involves constant interpretation and prediction based on complex, contextual information, expertise increases as the nurse becomes intuitively able to read the situation as a whole as a result of past experience. The experience of the nurse is central to proficiency, which Benner views as having five levels: novice, advanced beginner, competent nurse, proficient nurse, and expert. Experience is the vehicle by which the nurse passes through these phases.

Progress in the movement from novice to expert is reflected by three gradual changes in performance. Initially, rather than relying solely on abstract principles and procedures to guide nursing practice, the nurse acquires a personal knowledge rich in "paradigms" of various care issues. The paradigms emerge from past experience that not only challenges previously held perceptions but is powerful enough to change and refine those preconceptions and understandings. Later, as the nurse gains experience, situations are viewed holistically, with the nurse focusing only on the most relevant elements and having a deep sense of confidence in intuitive interpretations. Finally, there is full involvement in the situation as a confident, effective performer.

The fourth major pattern of the care process is *intentionality of caring*. Intentionality of caring represents the connecting pattern or matrix holding together mutuality, contextuality, and competence with proficiency. Intentionality of caring requires awareness and a determined effort to provide quality care in any setting or to facilitate others as they provide care for cancer patients. Intentionality of caring serves to enhance quality in practice by the following:

- Recognizing that care is mutual—a cooperative venture between two human beings, based on a balanced complement of perceptions

- Considering the context of the care environment on the basis of an understanding of the shared meaning of the circumstances

- Encouraging pride in one's acquired competencies (knowledge, skills, attitudes, and traits) and having a desire to increase proficiency and become expert

Overall, intentionality of caring links the science and art of nursing knowledge and skill. Its most overt manifestation in practice is known as clinical judgment.

CONCLUSION

Every health care provider group today is struggling with the definition, provision, and evaluation of quality care. Nursing comes to the task from a long tradition of empirically established caring skills and a more recent scientific knowledge based on clinical research.

For two decades, experts in the quality assurance field have advocated a three-dimensional approach to the quality question based on structure, process, and outcome variables and their relatedness (see Figure 53-1). Structural elements are those grounding fundamentals that provide a sense of shared purpose and criteria against which effect can be measured. The structural elements include nursing's direction, definition, education, legislation, diagnostic taxonomy, standards of practice, research and technology, and programs of peer review and quality assurance.

Process is a much more elusive phenomenon in that it represents the individualized enactment of competencies characterized by knowledge, skills, human traits, and attitudes[49] under diverse and unique environmental conditions (contextuality) where the mutuality of caregiver and care receiver is central. Process is most manifest in the intentionality of caring of the care provider and in the proficiency with which competencies are revealed. Therefore process is much more difficult to evaluate in comparison with the components of structure and outcome.

Oncology nursing has come closest to evaluating the process dimension by defining standards of performance that recognize several critical determinants of quality: continuously working to perfect the art, science, and skill of practice; participating as a contributing, valued member of the health care team; utilizing the problem-solving process in the planning, organization, and execution of care and in its evaluation through the conduct or utilization of research; and providing a health care service to patients on the basis of a host of both independent and interdependent interventions conducted in an autonomous way. The measurement of process is based generally on written documentation and periodic peer evaluation. Some attempts have been made to categorize[164] and to measure[48] proficiency, and the literature on caring as a science is expanding rapidly.

Outcome criteria have been defined in terms of patient outcomes, quality of life, and, for nursing to some degree, maximum life extension. These criteria are best represented by patient outcome standards and by a burgeoning literature focused on the quality of life of the person with cancer and his or her family. As we gain knowledge about the quality of life, the purpose of nursing as a science of caring will more clearly be understood, and will further enable us to foster, nurture, and strengthen its quality.

REFERENCES

1. Nightingale F: Notes on Nursing. New York, Appleton-Century-Crofts, 1859.
2. Benner P: Nursing as a caring profession. Working paper for the Academy of Nursing Annual Meeting, October 16-18, 1988, Kansas City, Mo.
3. Larson P: Cancer nurses' perceptions of caring. Cancer Nurs 9(2):86-92, 1986.
4. Gaut DA: A philosophic orientation to caring, in Leininger MM (ed): Care: The Essence of Nursing and Health. Thorofare, NJ, Slack, 1984, pp 17-26.
5. Leininger MM: Care: The Essence of Nursing. Thorofare, NJ, Slack, 1984.
6. Watson J: Nursing: The Philosophy and Science of Caring. Boston, Little, Brown, 1979.
7. Dougherty CJ: American Health Care: Realities, Rights, and Reforms. New York, Oxford University Press, 1988.
8. President's Commission for the Study of Ethical Problems in Medicine and Biomedical and Behavioral Research: Securing Access to Health Care, vol I. Washington, DC, US Government Printing Office, 1983.
9. Oncology Nursing Society: Board approves revised scope of practice statement. ONS News 3(6):1-2, 1988.
10. Taylor C: Philosophic Papers, vols I and II. Cambridge, Cambridge University Press, 1985.
11. Harmer C, Henderson V: Principles and Practices of Nursing. New York, Macmillan, 1956.
12. Mundinger L: Nursing diagnoses for cancer patients. Cancer Nurs 1:221-226, 1978.
13. Herberth L, Gosnell DJ: Nursing diagnosis for oncology nursing practice. Cancer Nurs 10(1):41-51, 1987.
14. Gordon M: Nursing Diagnoses: Process and Application. New York, McGraw-Hill, 1982.
15. American Nurses' Association: Nursing: A Social Policy Statement. Kansas City, Mo, The Association, 1980.
16. Beyers M: Quality: The banner of the 1980s. Nurs Clin North Am 23:617-623, 1988.
17. Winchester DP: The assurance of quality for the cancer patient. Paper presented at the American Cancer Society Symposium on Advances in Cancer Management, Hilton Towers, Los Angeles, Calif, December 1988.
18. Garven DA: Managing Quality: The Strategic and Competitive Edge. New York, The Free Press, 1988.
19. National Cancer Institute: Five-year survival rates. SEER Program. Washington, DC, US Government Printing Office, 1983.
20. Henderson M: Introduction, in Roberts L (ed): Cancer Today: Origins, Prevention, and Treatment. Washington, DC, National Academy of Sciences Press, 1984.
21. Oncology Nursing Society: Outcome Standards for Cancer Nursing Practice. Pittsburgh, Pa, The Society, 1979.
22. Oncology Nursing Society and American Nurses' Association: Standards of Oncology Nursing Practice. Kansas City, Mo, The Association, 1987.
23. American Nurses' Association: A Plan for Implementation of Standards of Nursing Practice. Kansas City, Mo, The Association, 1979.
24. Oncology Nursing Society: Outcome Standards for Cancer Nursing Education. Pittsburgh, Pa, The Society, 1982.
25. Oncology Nursing Society: Cancer Patient Education. Pittsburgh, Pa, The Society, 1982.

26. Oncology Nursing Society: Public Cancer Education. Pittsburgh, Pa, The Society, 1983.

27. Orem DE: Nursing Concepts of Practice. New York, McGraw-Hill, 1987.

28. Johnson DE: The behavioral system model for nursing, in Riehl JP, Roy C (eds): Conceptual Model for Nursing Practice (2nd ed). New York, Appleton-Century-Crofts, 1980.

29. Donabedian A: Structure, process and outcome standards. Am J Public Health 59:1833, 1969.

30. Majesky SJ, Brester MH, Nishio KT: Development of a research tool: Patient indicators of nursing care. Nurs Res 27:365-371, 1978.

31. Scott DW: The Research Connection: Practice, Research, Theory. Keynote Address: American Cancer Society Nursing Research Conference, Honolulu, Hawaii, June 1985. Proceedings. Denver, American Cancer Society, 1986.

32. Brown MH, Kiss ME: Cancer audit. Cancer Nurs 2:1-6, 1979.

33. Legge JS, Reilly BJ: Assessing the outcomes of cancer patients in a home nursing program. Cancer Nurs 3:357, 1980.

34. Valencius JC, Packard R, Widiss T: The ONS-ANA Outcome Standards for Cancer Nursing Practice: Two models for implementation—Implementation of the Nutrition Standard at City of Hope National Medical Center. Oncol Nurs Forum, 7:137-140, 1980.

35. Edlund BJ: Patient education: Determining the effectiveness of an ostomy care guide in facilitating comprehensive patient care. Oncol Nurs Forum, 8(3):43-46, 1981.

36. Wood HA, Ellerhorst JM: Using site-specific nursing algorithms as an adjunct to oncology nursing guidelines. Oncol Nurs Forum 10(3):22-27, 1983.

37. Joint Commission on the Accreditation of Hospitals: Accreditation Manual for Hospitals (AMH/88). Chicago, The Commission, 1987.

38. Patterson CH: Standards of patient care: The Joint Commission focus on nursing quality assurance. Nurs Clin North Am 23:625-638, 1988.

39. Oleske DM, Otte DM, Heinze S: Development and evaluation of a system for monitoring the quality of oncology nursing care in the home setting. Cancer Nurs 10:190-198, 1987.

40. Stephany TM: Quality assurance for hospice programs. Oncol Nurs Forum, 12(3):33-40, 1985.

41. Arenth LM: The development and validation of an Oncology Patient Classification System. Oncol Nurs Forum, 12(6):17-27, 1985.

42. Dudjak LA: Radiation Therapy Nursing Care Record: A tool for documentation. Oncol Nurs Forum 15:763-777, 1988.

43. Gullo SM: Safe handling of antineoplastic drugs. Translating the recommendations into practice. Oncol Nurs Forum 15:595-601, 1988.

44. Williamson KM, Selleck CS, Turner JC, et al: Occupational health hazards for nurses: Infection. Image 20:48-53, 1988.

45. Williamson KM, Turner JG, Brown KC, et al: Occupational health hazards for nurses. Part II. Image 20:162-168, 1988.

46. Miaskowski CA, Nielsen B: A cancer nursing assessment tool. Oncol Nurs Forum 12(6):37-42, 1985.

47. Gray G, Adler D, Fleming C, et al: A clinical data base for advanced cancer patients: Implications for nursing. Cancer Nurs 11(2):77-83, 1988.

48. Moore IM, Piper B, Dodd MJ, et al: Measuring oncology nursing practice: Results from one graduate program. Oncol Nurs Forum 14(1):45-49, 1987.

49. McGee RF, Powell ML, Broadwell DC, et al: A Delphi survey of oncology nurse specialist competencies. Oncol Nurs Forum, 14(2):29-34, 1987.

50. Yasko JM: A survey of oncology clinical nursing specialists. Oncol Nurs Forum 10(1):25-30, 1983.

51. Oberst MT: Priorities in cancer nursing research. Cancer Nurs 1:281-290, 1978.

52. Western Consortium for Cancer Nursing Research: Priorities for cancer nursing research. Cancer Nurs 10:319-326, 1987.

53. Satterwhite BA, Pryor AS, Harris MB: Development and evaluation of chemotherapy fact sheets. Cancer Nurs 3:277-284, 1980.

54. Dodd MJ, Mood DW: Chemotherapy: Helping patients to know the drugs they are receiving and their possible side effects. Cancer Nurs 4:311-318, 1981.

55. Dodd MJ: Self-care for side effects in cancer chemotherapy: An assessment of nursing interventions. Part II. Cancer Nurs 6:63-67, 1983.

56. Johnson J: The effects of a patient education course on persons with a chronic illness. Cancer Nurs 5:117-123, 1982.

57. Miller MW, Nygren C: Living with cancer: Coping behaviors. Cancer Nurs 1:297-302, 1978.

58. Marty PJ, McDermott RJ, Gold RS: An assessment of three alternative formats for promoting breast self-examination. Cancer Nurs 6:207-211, 1983.

59. Watson PJ: The effects of short-term postoperative counseling on cancer/ostomy patients. Cancer Nurs 6:21-29, 1985.

60. Heinrich RL, Schag CC: A behavioral medicine approach to coping with cancer: A case report. Cancer Nurs 7:243-247, 1984.

61. Rudolf VM, Quinn KL McE: The practice of TSE among college men: Effectiveness of an educational program. Oncol Nurs Forum 15:45-48, 1988.

62. Cotanch P, Hockenberry M, Herman S: Self-hypnosis as antiemetic therapy in children receiving chemotherapy. Oncol Nurs Forum 12(4):41-46, 1985.

63. Frank JM: The effects of music therapy and guided visual imagery on chemotherapy-induced nausea and vomiting. Oncol Nurs Forum, 12(5):47-52, 1985.

64. Scott DW, Donahue DC, Mastrovito RC, et al: Comparative trial of clinical relaxation and an antiemetic drug regimen in reducing chemotherapy-related nausea and vomiting. Cancer Nurs 9:178-187, 1986.

65. Cotanch P, Strum S: Progressive muscle relaxation as antiemetic therapy for cancer patients. Oncol Nurs Forum 14(1):33-37, 1987.

66. Parker R: The effectiveness of scalp hypothermia in preventing cyclophosphamide-induced alopecia. Oncology Nurs Forum 14(6):49-53, 1987.

67. Dudjak LA: Mouth care for mucositis due to radiation therapy. Cancer Nurs 10:131-140, 1987.

68. Winningham ML, MacVicar MG: The effect of aerobic exercise on patient reports of nausea. Oncol Nurs Forum 15:447-450, 1988.

69. Giaccone G, DiGuilio F, Morandini MP, et al: Scalp hypothermia in the prevention of doxorubicin-induced hair loss. Cancer Nurs 11:170-173, 1988.

70. Shell JA, Stanutz F, Grimm J: Comparison of moisture vapor permeable (MVP) dressings to conventional dressings for management of radiation skin reactions. Oncol Nurs Forum 13(1):11-16, 1986.

71. Harwood KVS, Bachur N: Evaluation of dimethylsulfoxide and local cooling as antidotes for doxorubicin extravasation in a pig model. Oncol Nurs Forum 14(1):39-44, 1987.

72. Jones PM: Indwelling central venous catheter–related infections and two different procedures of catheter care. Cancer Nurs 10:123-130, 1987.

73. MacGeorge L, Steeves L, Steeves RH: Comparison of the mixing and reinfusion methods of drawing blood from a Hickman catheter. Oncol Nurs Forum 15:335-338, 1988.

74. Petrosino B, Becker H, Christian B: Infection rates in central venous catheter dressings. Oncol Nurs Forum 15:709-717, 1988.

75. Beck S, Breckenridge-Patter S, Wallace S, et al: The Family High-Risk Program: Targeted cancer prevention. Oncol Nurs Forum 15:301-306, 1988.

76. Nieweg R, Greidanus J, deVries EGE: A patient education program for a continuous infusion regimen on an outpatient basis. Cancer Nurs 10:177-182, 1987.

77. Lane CA, Davis AW: Implementation: We Can Weekend in the rural setting. Cancer Nurs 8:323-328, 1985.

78. Fredette S, La F, Beattie HM: Living with cancer: A patient education program. Cancer Nurs 9:308-316, 1986.

79. Cawley MM, Gerdts EK: Establishing a cancer caregiver's program: An interdisciplinary approach. Cancer Nurs 11:266-273, 1988.

80. Diekmann JM: An evaluation of selected "I Can Cope" programs by registered participants. Cancer Nurs 11:274-282, 1988.

81. Mosely JR, Logan SJ, Tolle SW, et al: Developing a bereavement program in a university hospital setting. Oncol Nurs Forum 15:151-155, 1988.

82. Coyle N, Monzillo E, Loscalzo M, et al: A model for continuity of care for cancer patients with pain and neuro-oncologic complications. Cancer Nurs 8:111-119, 1985.

83. Coyle N, Mauskop A, Maggard J, et al: Continuous SC infusions of opiates for cancer patients with pain. Oncol Nurs Forum, 13(4):53-57, 1986.

84. Ferrell BR, Wenzl C, Wisdom C: Evolution and evaluation of a pain management team. Oncol Nurs Forum 15:285-289, 1988.

85. Kane NE, Lehman ME, Drugger R, et al: Use of patient-controlled anesthesia in surgical oncology patients. Oncol Nurs Forum 15:29-32, 1988.

86. Konstantinides NI: Home parenteral nutrition: A viable alternative for patients with cancer. Oncol Nurs Forum 12(1):23-29, 1985.

87. Clark M: A day hospital for cancer patients: Clinical and economic feasibility. Oncol Nurs Forum 13(6):41-45, 1986.

88. Pluth NM: A home transfusion program. Oncol Nurs Forum 14(5):43-46, 1987.

89. Lewis PM: Implementing practice and organizational models. Cancer Nurs 8:75-78, 1985 (suppl 1).

90. Hartshorn JC: Research-based practice: The need for, use and reporting of instrument reliability and validity. Heart Lung 16:100-101, 1987.

91. Duffy ME: Research in practice: The time has come. Nurs Health Care 6:127, 1985.

92. Lynn MR: Reliability estimates: Use and disuse. Nurs Res 34:254-256, 1985.

93. Nunally JC: Psychometric Theory. New York: McGraw-Hill, 1978.

94. Frank-Stromborg M (ed): Instruments for Clinical Nursing Research. Norwalk, Conn, Appleton & Lange, 1988.

95. Ferrans C, Powers M: Quality of Life Index: Development and psychometric properties. Adv Nurs Sci 8(1):15, 1985.

96. Kobashi-Shoot JAM, Gerrit JFPH, Frits SAM et al: Assessment of malaise in cancer patients treated with radiotherapy. Cancer Nurs 8:306-313, 1985.

97. Padilla G, Grant M: Quality of life as a cancer nursing outcome variable. Adv Nurs Sci 8(1):45, 1985.

98. Hopkins MB: Information seeking and adaptational outcomes in women receiving chemotherapy for breast cancer. Cancer Nurs 9:256-262, 1986.

99. Waterhouse J, Metcalf MC: Development of the sexual adjustment questionnaire. Oncol Nurs Forum 13(3):53-59, 1986.

100. Derdiarian AK: Informational needs of recently diagnosed cancer patients. Cancer Nurs 10:156-163, 1987.

101. Fleming C, Scanlon C, D'Agostino NS: Patient care needs survey. Cancer Nurs 10:237-243, 1987.

102. Lilley LL: Human need fulfillment alteration in the client with uterine cancer: The registered nurse's perception versus the client's perception. Cancer Nurs 10:327-337, 1987.

103. Young-Graham K, Longman AJ: Quality of life and persons with melanoma: Preliminary model testing. Cancer Nurs 10:338-346, 1987.

104. Blackmore C: The impact of orchidectomy upon the sexuality of the man with testicular cancer. Cancer Nurs 11:33-40, 1988.

105. Camp LD: A comparison of nurses' recorded assessments of pain with perceptions of pain as described by cancer patients. Cancer Nurs 11:237-243, 1988.

106. Coward DD: Hypercalcemia knowledge assessment in patients at risk of developing cancer-induced hypercalcemia. Oncol Nurs Forum 15:471-476, 1988.

107. Derdiarian AK: Derdiarian Behavioral System Model (DBSM). Scholarly Inquiry for Nursing Practice, 2(2):103-121, 1988.

108. Eilers J, Berger AM, Petersen MC: Development, testing and application of the oral assessment guide. Oncol Nurs Forum 15:325-330, 1988.

109. Lauver D: Development of a questionnaire to measure beliefs and attitudes about breast self-examination. Cancer Nurs 11:51-57, 1988.

110. McMillan SC, Williams FA, Chatfield R, et al: A validity and reliability study of two tools for assessing and managing cancer pain. Oncol Nurs Forum 15:735-741, 1988.

111. Rhodes VA, Watson PM, Hanson BM: Patients' descriptions of the influence of tiredness and weakness on self-care abilities. Cancer Nurs 11:186-194, 1988.

112. Sutherland HJ, Walker P, Till JE: The development of a method for determining oncology patients' emotional distress using linear analogue scales. Cancer Nurs 11:303-308, 1988.

113. Weinrich SP, Weinrich MC: Cancer knowledge among elderly individuals. Cancer Nurs 9:301-307, 1987.

114. Williams RD: Factors affecting practice of BSE in older women. Oncol Nurs Forum 15:611-616, 1988.

115. Ammon-Gaberson KB, Piantanida M: Generating results from qualitative data. Image 20:159-161, 1988.

116. Saunders JM, Valente SM: Cancer and suicide. Oncol Nurs Forum 15:575-581, 1988.

117. Thorne SE: Helpful and unhelpful communications in cancer care: The patient perspective. Oncol Nurs Forum 15:167-172, 1988.

118. Hays JC: Patient symptoms and family coping. Cancer Nurs 9:317-325, 1986.

119. Duigon A: Anticipatory nausea and vomiting associated with cancer chemotherapy. Oncol Nurs Forum 13(1):35-40, 1986.

120. Coons HL, Leventhal H, Nerenz DR, et al: Anticipatory nausea and emotional distress in patients receiving cisplatin-based chemotherapy. Oncol Nurs Forum 14(3):31-35, 1987.

121. Henschel L: Fever patterns in the neutropenic patient. Cancer Nurs 8:301-305, 1985.

122. Krouse HJ: A psychological model of adjustment in gynecologic cancer patients. Oncol Nurs Forum 12(6):45-49, 1985.

123. Cooley ME, Cobb SC: Sexual and reproductive issues for women with Hodgkin's disease. I. Overview of issues. Cancer Nurs 9:188-193, 1986.

124. Cooley ME, Yeoman AC, Cobb SC: Sexual and reproductive issues for women with Hodgkin's disease: Application of PLISSIT Model. Cancer Nurs 9:248-255, 1986.

125. Coward DD: Cancer-induced hypercalcemia. Cancer Nurs 9:125-132, 1986.

126. Holing EV: The primary caregiver's perception of the dying trajectory: An exploratory study. Cancer Nurs 9:29-37, 1986.

127. Huldij A, Giesbers A, Poelhuis EHK, et al: Alterations in taste appreciation in cancer patients during treatment. Cancer Nurs 9:38-42, 1986.

128. Lovejoy N: Family responses to cancer hospitalization. Oncol Nurs Forum 13(2):33-37, 1986.

129. Donovan MI, Dillon P: Incidence and characteristics of pain in a sample of hospitalized cancer patients. Cancer Nurs 10:85-92, 1987.

130. Jenkins B: Patients' reports of sexual changes after treatment for gynecological cancer. Oncol Nurs Forum 15:349-354, 1988.

131. Ostchega Y, Donahue M, Fox N: High-dose cisplatin-related peripheral neuropathy. Cancer Nurs 11:23-32, 1988.

132. Wilkie D, Lovejoy N, Dodd M, et al: Cancer pain control behaviors: Description and correlation with pain intensity. Oncol Nurs Forum 15:723-731, 1988.

133. Brown ML, Carrieri V, Janson-Bjerklie S, et al: Lung cancer and dyspnea: The patient's perception. Oncol Nurs Forum 13(5):19-24, 1986.

134. King KB, Nail LM, Kreamer K, et al: Patients' descriptions of the experience of receiving radiotherapy. Oncol Nurs Forum 12(4):55-61, 1986.

135. Lesage C: Carotid artery rupture: Prediction, prevention, preparation. Cancer Nurs 9:1-7, 1986.

136. Messner RL, Gardner SS, Webb DD: Early detection: The priority in colorectal cancer. Cancer Nurs 9:8-14, 1986.

137. Post-White J: Glucocorticosteroid-induced depression in the patient with leukemia or lymphoma. Cancer Nurs 9:15-22, 1986.

138. Tringali CA: The needs of family members of cancer patients. Oncol Nurs Forum 13(4):65-70, 1986.

139. Rhodes VA, Watson PM, Johnson MH, et al: Patterns of nausea, vomiting and distress in patients receiving antineoplastic drug protocols. Oncol Nurs Forum 14(4):35-44, 1987.

140. Foote M: Nursing care of the patient with non-Hodgkin's lymphoma: Prevention of pneumonia associated with combination chemotherapy. Cancer Nurs 8:263-271, 1985.

141. Getz DH: The primary, secondary and tertiary nursing interventions of lymphedema. Cancer Nurs 8:177-184, 1985.

142. Rooney A, Haviley C: Nursing management of disseminated intravascular coagulation. Oncol Nurs Forum 121(1):15-22, 1985.

143. Rossetti AC: Nursing care of patients treated with intrapleural tetracycline for control of malignant pleural effusion. Cancer Nurs 8:103-109, 1985.

144. Gurevich I, Tafuro P: The compromised host: Deficit-specific infection in the spectrum of prevention. Cancer Nurs 9:263-275, 1986.

145. Moore CL, Erickson KA, Yanes LB, et al: Nursing care and management of venous access ports. Oncol Nurs Forum 13(3):35-39, 1986.

146. Paice JA: Intrathecal morphine infusion for intractable cancer pain: A new use for implanted pumps. Oncol Nurs Forum 13(3):41-47, 1986.

147. Rodzwic D, Donnard J: The use of myocutaneous flaps in reconstructive surgery for head and neck cancer: Guidelines for nursing care. Oncol Nurs Forum, 13(3):29, 1986.

148. Hassay KM: Radiation therapy for rectal cancer and the implications for nursing. Cancer Nurs 10:311-318, 1987.

149. Link DL: Antibiotic therapy in the cancer patient: Focus on third generation cephalosporins. Oncol Nurs Forum 14(5):35-41, 1987.

150. Moreland BJ: A nursing form for gynecology patient assessment. Oncol Nurs Forum 14(2):19-23, 1987.

151. Stetz KM: Caregiving demands during advanced cancer: The spouse's needs. Cancer Nurs 10:260-268, 1987.

152. Lewandowski W, Jones SL: The family with cancer: Nursing intervention throughout the course of living with cancer. Cancer Nurs 11:313-321, 1988.

153. Strohl RA: The nursing role in radiation oncology: Symptom management of acute and chronic reactions. Oncol Nurs Forum 15:429-434, 1988.

154. Jennings BM, Muhlenkamp AF: Systematic misperception: Oncology patients' self-reported affective states and their care-givers' perceptions. Cancer Nursing 4:485-489, 1981.

155. Wright BA: Physical Disability: A Psychological Approach. New York, Harper & Row, 1960.

156. Verron JA, Longman A, Clark M: Development of a scale to measure undergraduate students' attitudes about caring for patients with cancer. Oncol Nurs Forum 14(5):51-55, 1987.

157. Robb S: Attitudes and intentions of baccalaureate nursing students toward the elderly. Nurs Res 28(1):43-50, 1979.

158. Larson P: Important nurse caring behaviors perceived by patients with cancer. Oncol Nurs Forum 11(6):46-50, 1984.

159. Larson P: Comparison of cancer patients' and professional nurses' perceptions of important nurse caring behaviors. Heart Lung 16:187-192, 1987.

160. Mayer DK: Oncology nurses' versus cancer patients' perceptions of nursing care behaviors: A replication study. Oncol Nurs Forum 14(3):48-52, 1987.

161. Sodestrom KE, Martinson IM: Patients' spiritual coping strategies: A study of nurse and patient perspectives. Oncol Nurs Forum 14(2):41-46, 1987.

162. Curtis AE, Fernsler JI: Quality of life of oncology hospice patients: A comparison of patient and primary caregiver reports. Oncol Nurs Forum 16:49-53, 1989.

163. Dyck S, Wright K: Family perceptions: The role of the nurse throughout an adults' cancer experience. Oncol Nurs Forum 12(5):53-56, 1985.

164. Benner P: From Novice to Expert: Excellence and Power in Clinical Nursing Practice. Menlo Park, Calif, Addison-Wesley, 1984.

165. Benner P, Wrubel J: The Primacy of Caring: Stress and Coping in Health and Illness. Menlo Park, Calif, Addison-Wesley, 1989.

Chapter 54

Economics of Cancer

Arlene E. Fleck, RN, MNEd

INTRODUCTION

In the past, the ability to apply clinical expertise to solve patient care problems was the major concern of the cancer nurse specialist. However, in today's health care arena the challenge is to integrate this clinical expertise and apply it in a cost-effective manner. A cost-effective approach is one that emphasizes balancing cost requirements and standards of excellence.

Cancer care is changing rapidly because of new technology, innovative therapy, and current economic and health care policy issues. Nurses specializing in oncology must be prepared to adapt to this constant change. This chapter will explore the economic environment, which is a major influencing factor in the practice of oncology nursing. The discussion begins with a review of basic economic theory and the historical and current issues that have an impact on health care economics. The remainder of this chapter will emphasize how these economic changes are affecting cancer care.

SCOPE OF THE PROBLEM

Since the early 1980s, revolutionary changes have occurred in the health care economics of this country. Before that time, the word "economics" did not have the strong association with health care that it does today. In today's health care environment, nurses are exposed to new phrases: "cost justification," "more does not mean better," "quality versus cost," and "lack of resources," to name just a few. These phrases represent dramatic changes that were introduced when expenditures for health care reached 9.4% of the US gross national product (GNP), or $147 billion, in 1982; this figure was a sharp contrast to the 1960 statistics, in which health care expenditures were only 4.5% of the GNP. It has been estimated that by the turn of the century, health care will account for 15% of the GNP. These rising figures have waved red flags in front of government officials who continually are trying to trim the federal budget. The rise in health care costs is being scrutinized not only by politicians but by business leaders and consumers as well. Pressure by these groups has been applied to constrain the use of health care resources. To accomplish this task, nurses and other health care professionals must continue to deliver patient care in sufficient quantities and of acceptable quality to meet public demands—in other words, to do more with less.

ECONOMICS THEORY

Historically, economics has not been a popular elective course among student nurses, nor has there been a demand for the ability to apply economic principles to the health care field. However, with the current major emphasis on the high costs of health care and national health policy changes, an introduction to economics could become not only interesting but also beneficial. An ability to analyze economic issues can provide important insights into the operation of health care systems and the evaluation of health care policies.

Economics is the science that deals with the production, distribution, and consumption of wealth, or resources. The economy is the management of the production, allocation, and consumption of resources in this country. In simple words, it is the study of supply and demand. Figure 54-1 illustrates a normal, or balanced, economic environment.[1] Two parties are involved in the exchange of money. One party is the supplier, who provides the goods or services to the other party, the consumer. The consumer is responsible for the demand of the goods or services. Pricing is established to balance the supply and demand of goods and services. This pricing establishes an important equilibrium:

$$Supply = Demand$$
$$and$$
$$Demand = Supply$$

The ability of price to act as a balance point between the supply and demand of a good or service is referred to as the concept of *price elasticity* or *price sensitivity*. This concept is illustrated in Figure 54-2. It can be predicted that when the price of a good or service falls, the quantity demanded will rise. The significance of this concept is readily apparent in health care provided during the late 1960s and early 1970s. For most Americans, health care had no price; it was essentially free. Health insurance coverage was a standard part of virtually every employee benefit package. Most Americans believed health care services

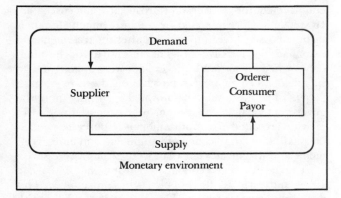

FIGURE 54-1 Normal economic environment. In a normal economic environment, there are essentially two parties—supplier and consumer (also referred to as payor and orderer). The former supplies goods and services, and the latter demands goods and services. Money, or the promise of it, is exchanged between the two parties, thus establishing a market price for the goods and services. (Source: Ward WJ Jr: An Introduction to Health Care Financial Management. Owings Mills, Md, Rynd Communication, 1988, p 5.)

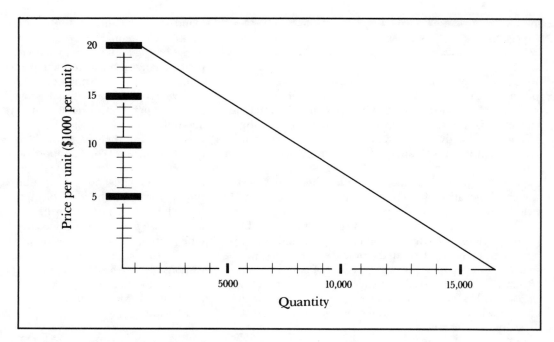

FIGURE 54-2   Price sensitivity. As the price goes down, the demand for the goods and services goes up.

to be their "right"—not a privilege. The cost of any health care was never an issue because only insurance companies, rarely the consumer, saw the bill or charges. The ready access to health care coverage as an employee benefit often encouraged indiscriminate use of high-cost services. The prevailing attitude was that of obtaining the best and most sophisticated care regardless of cost. This health care behavior caused costs to spiral.

Persons who were unemployed or retired, and who did not have health care insurance coverage provided by an employer, were often eligible for federal health insurance programs (ie, Medicare or Medicaid). The method of federal payment for services was retrospective and cost based. Hospitals were reimbursed by the government for their incurred costs of treating patients after the treatment and care had been delivered. The incentive for hospitals (where 70% of all Medicare dollars were spent[2]) was to spend as much money as possible on the care of each patient. The more money a hospital spent, the more the government paid. This system of payment for services provided resulted in overutilization of resources, extended hospitalization, duplication of equipment, and more treatments and diagnostic tests than were actually necessary.

The health care economic environment of the late 1960s and early 1970s is depicted in Figure 54-3.[1] This diagram illustrates why problems arose in the US health care economic system.[1] Because neither the consumer, physician, or health care professional was concerned with the price of the goods or services, the demands became unlimited. Consumers came to expect a health care system that provided everything possible. Physicians, nurses, and other health care professionals continued to use all available technology and resources to care for the patient, often in excess of what was required. The increased number of

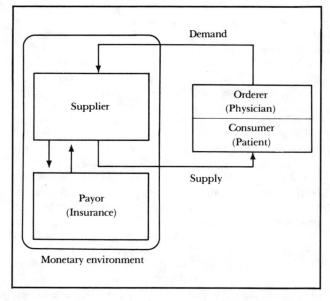

FIGURE 54-3   Health care economic environment. The economic environment as applied to health care is significantly different. Note that there are now four parties instead of two and that the supply of and demand for health care services no longer include the payor for those services. Because the monetary environment does not include the orderer, or consumer, price is unable to establish a balance between supply and demand. (Source: Ward WJ Jr: An Introduction to Health Care Financial Management. Owings Mills, Md, Rynd Communication, 1988, p 8.)

malpractice lawsuits caused physicians to practice defensive medicine, ordering more tests than usual and thereby driving costs upward. Moreover, costs rose because people were living longer and thus contributing to the increasing number of elderly citizens, many of whom have chronic health care needs. Thus, in the 1980s, there was a resultant demand for more available health care resources than could be satisfied. To address and sustain these increasing demands, the Ninety-seventh Congress passed the Tax Equity and Fiscal Responsibility Act (TEFRA) in August 1982. This payment system changed the method of providing inpatient services for Medicare and Medicaid beneficiaries from a retrospective, cost-based payment system to a prospective payment system.

PROSPECTIVE PAYMENT SYSTEM

History

The prospective payment system (PPS) was signed into Public Law 98-21 as part of the Social Security Amendment of 1983. This system reimburses hospitals with a fixed payment that is based on the complexity of the problems that precipitated during the patient's hospitalization. The exact amount is determined by using one or more of the 477* diagnosis related groups (DRGs). Each DRG is assigned a specific, fixed rate of payment for which the hospital is reimbursed regardless of the actual cost of the patient's care. The individual DRGs originally were developed by a group of researchers at Yale University as a hospital management tool; they were adapted for use as a federal payment system, after being field-tested in New Jersey. In the pilot study, the major factor observed was the number of days that a patient stayed in the hospital.[3] It was believed that if the number of days a patient stayed in the hospital could be decreased, the overall hospital bill would also be decreased. By 1982, all acute care hospitals in New Jersey were reimbursed according to the PPS; a 6% reduction in comparison with national hospital costs was observed.[4]

To help standardize hospital costs throughout the country, researchers assigned a specific weight to each DRG. This weighting factor reflects the estimated relative costs of hospital resources used (ie, laboratory tests, medications, medical and surgical supplies, room, ancillary services) per patient discharge. The principal sources of data to compile the cost weights originally were based on the Medicare cost reports for 1981 and on a national representative sample of inpatient Medicare claims.

The Health Care Financing Administration (HCFA) agency of the federal government now assigns the appropriate weighting factor for each DRG. An average standardized cost for each of the original 468 DRGs was developed from the cost data received; the statistical method of regression was used to establish a variance for each DRG. It can be estimated statistically that 95% of the patients assigned to a specific DRG actually will incur the cost allocated within the parameter of the DRG.[5]

This system was integrated gradually over the first five years of its inception (1983-1987); hospitals were reimbursed at a prospective payment rate for each discharge that was a blend of national and regional data and the respective hospital's historic cost per case. Effective Aug. 21, 1988, the method to determine payment rates was adjusted and was based only on national/regional standardized information. The individual hospital's costs were no longer recognized as a factor.

Calculation

An example of a 1989 prospective payment calculation is shown in Figure 54-4. An understanding of how a payment is calculated for a hospital is important for nurses because it provides a basis for understanding many of the current and future trends of health care economics. For a more extensive history on the DRGs or calculation details, see references 6, 7, 8, 9, and 10.

Exemptions

All hospitals that participate in the Medicare system are reimbursed by the PPS with the exception of the following:

1. **Long-term hospitals:** average length of inpatient stay more than 25 days.
2. **Psychiatric hospitals and units:** primarily engage in treatment of mentally ill persons.
3. **Rehabilitation hospitals and units:** meet federally established criteria for a rehabilitation center.
4. **Children's hospitals.**
5. **Hospitals located in states with state-regulated PPS plans (Maryland, New Jersey).**
6. **Veterans Administration hospitals.**
7. **Cancer hospitals:** those recognized by the National Cancer Institute (NCI) as comprehensive cancer centers or as clinical cancer research centers. The entire facility must be organized primarily for the treatment of, and research on, cancer. As of 1989, the hospitals recognized under this exemption included MD Anderson Cancer Center, Houston, Tex; Fox Chase Cancer Center, Philadelphia, Pa; Kenneth Norris, Jr., Cancer Center, University of Southern California, Los Angeles, Calif; City of Hope National Medical Center, Duarte, Calif; Fred Hutchinson Cancer Center, Seattle, Wash; Memorial Sloan-Kettering Cancer Center, New York, NY; Roswell Park Memorial Institute, Buffalo, NY; and Dana-Farber Cancer Institute, Boston, Mass.

DRGs were developed with a primary orientation toward the short-term, acute care hospitals. Their applicability in specialty (exempt) hospitals is limited.

*In 1982, when DRGs were first used in the hospitals, there were 470 of them. As the need for other DRGs was established, the number increased. In 1989 there were 477 DRGs.

Baseline Data

1. Fiscal Year 1989
2. 300-bed acute care hospital (urban)
3. Census Region 2
4. Principal diagnosis example: DRG 82, Respiratory Neoplasms

Formula

$$\left[\begin{array}{c} \text{Adjusted labor component =} \\ \text{Labor component} \times \text{Wage index} \\ \$2,374.22 \times 1.0206 = \\ \$2,423.13 \end{array} \right]^1 + \begin{array}{c} \text{Nonlabor component}^2 \\ \$840.95 \end{array} \times \begin{array}{c} \text{DRG weight}^3 \\ 1.2367 \end{array} = \$4,036.69$$

Payment rate to hospital = $4,036.69
Hospital costs for patient "A" = <u>3,200.00</u>

Profit for hospital $ 836.69

¹*Adjusted labor component* is determined by the mean urban or rural cost per discharge and is then adjusted to reflect regional differences in hospital wages. This figure is derived from regional and national aggregate data of cost reports submitted by hospitals and reflects labor-intensive costs (ie, wages, salaries, employee benefits, professional fees).

²*Nonlabor component* is adjusted to the appropriate regional or national standardized figure. The geographic location and the urban or rural designation of the hospital is also considered. This figure accounts for all other resource consumption for patient care.

³*DRG weights* are based on a nationwide random sample study. The variables reviewed in hospitals to arrive at a cost-reimbursement figure per case includes length of stay, per diem cost in routine and special care, estimated cost of ancillary services (eg, laboratory work, radiography, drugs, medical supplies). From these reports, each DRG is assigned a relative weight that reflects the resources needed to care for a patient with a specific diagnosis. PROPAC annually recommends to the secretary of the US Department of Health and Human Services the appropriate annual percentage change in payment for hospital inpatient discharges. This report is due by March 1 of each year.

FIGURE 54-4   Prospective payment calculation. Specific details for calculating a prospective payment reimbursement are outlined. Although there is no need to memorize this calculation, it is important to understand which components are used to compute the reimbursement. This knowledge will help the student to understand many of the dilemmas encountered by the prospective payment system.

Hospital Cost-Per-Case Comparisons

To establish a set price per DRG for every acute care hospital in the United States is virtually impossible. A variety of variables can cause fluctuations in the federal payment amount. The variables that are used to compare one hospital's cost per case to another's include the case mix (a classification by diagnosis of a hospital's caseload or patient population), labor costs, urban or rural location, and teaching intensity. These adjustment factors, which were incorporated into the PPS system, explain an estimated 65% of the variation in the average cost per case.[11] The teaching-intensity variable was originally a "pass-through" reimbursement (the costs of education were reimbursed). However, in the past several years the system has been adjusted in such a manner that only a percentage of teaching costs are reimbursed.

The current PPS assumes that variations in cost per case that are not accounted for by the above-described adjustment factors are due to differences in hospital efficiency. As hospitals become more efficient (ie, produce targeted health care outcomes with the least costly input), these additional variations in costs will be significantly reduced.[12]

Monitoring Activities

The PPS legislation requires close monitoring of costs. Each hospital is required to contract with a peer review organization (PRO) established by the US Department of Health and Human Services. The purpose of the PROs is to conduct required medical reviews to ensure that quality patient care is provided and maintained and that the duration of hospital stay is appropriate to the level of required care. The Health Care Financing Administration (HCFA) also will review periodically the records of each hospital for compliance with the PPS regulations and will deny payment if the regulations are not followed.

To update and maintain the new Medicare payment system, Congress established the Prospective Payment Assessment Commission (PROPAC).* A 15-member commission of experts was appointed by the Office of Technology Assessment (OTA)† in 1983.[13] The PPS law mandates that PROPAC make recommendations annually to the secretary of the US Department of Health and Human Services and to Congress in two primary areas[14]: the annual percentage increase in Medicare expenditures on a per-case basis (the update factor) and the DRG patient classification categories and weights. In recent years, PROPAC has been reviewing several other areas: the hospital market-basket structure (a figure used to estimate inflation rates in the price of patient-utilized goods and services purchased by hospitals); improvements in the case-mix measurement (measurement of a hospital's inpatient population and its severity of illness or resource needs); capital expenditure policy (outlay made by a hospital to the purchase of a fixed asset such as a piece of equipment for a period greater than a year[1]); and the effects of PPS on rural hospitals.

Impact of PPS

The change in hospital reimbursement from costs incurred to fixed rates has caused drastic restructuring of health care incentives. If the actual cost of a patient's care is less than the fixed or assigned DRG rate, the hospital retains the excess amount. These DRGs are known as "winners." If the hospital's costs exceed the fixed payment scale, the hospital must absorb the excess costs. These DRGs are known as "losers." Hospitals are striving to reduce costs to an efficient and effective level. Adaptation to prospective reimbursement has caused changes in the health care environment. The following section will discuss several key trends that have resulted from the implementation of PPS; the decrease in the length of stay in the hospital, the restraint of technologic advancement, and the limitation of access to health care. Each trend will be discussed in terms of its history or development, its relation to current issues, and its impact on nursing.

Decrease in length of stay

History The original studies at Yale University that provided the methodology for the DRGs used length of stay (LOS) as the dependent variable. This variable was chosen because the initial purpose of developing DRGs was to improve utilization review activities, which consisted of reviewing the appropriateness of patient care services

by a single-diagnosis method.[3] Before the Yale study, a single-diagnosis patient classification system (the International Classification of Diseases, Adapted, Eighth Revision [ICDA-8]) was used for the review of patient care. This scheme was limited to classifying patients only by similar ailments. Yale researchers adjusted the classification system by adding the LOS variable. After the Yale researchers reviewed the results of their work, they concluded that the LOS variable was not entirely appropriate, because variations were too wide. They therefore found it necessary to consider several other classification factors in addition to ICDA-8 codes and LOS. The revisions included classifying diseases on the basis of 23 major diagnostic categories (MDCs) based on human anatomy. These 23 MDCs are divided further by factors that have an impact on the patient's LOS: the patient's age, the presence of comorbidities (ie, the presence of diseases or conditions concurrently with the patient's principal condition), disease complications, and the use of surgical procedures (Figure 54-5). These additional factors still are not an inclusive list for determining a patient's LOS. The assumed homogeneity* of each particular DRG needs to be examined critically because many other factors can contribute to variations in a patient's LOS. Some of these factors are listed below:

1. The severity index reflects the stage of the patient's illness within each DRG, which significantly influences the extent of resource consumption. As an example, a patient with cancer who has just been informed of disease progression is undergoing 5 days of inpatient chemotherapy. The patient has a vascular access device that is malfunctioning. Chemotherapy based on DRG 410 is used. This classification gives no consideration to special services such as patient teaching for chemotherapy side effects, adjustment of procedures because of a malfunctioning vascular access device, or increased psychologic support needed because of disease metastasis.
2. The socioeconomic status of the patient is a concern, because the disadvantaged patient may require more resources (such as nursing care, education, discharge planning, and social service) than others with similar diagnoses.
3. Hospitals that care for patients with severe and complex cases will likely be underpaid relative to hospitals who have less complex cases.
4. A physician's or surgeon's practice that is unique may affect the patient resource consumption. As an example, reconstructive surgery after mastectomy may require an extra 5 days in the hospital.

Current trends A great emphasis in hospital care management is to decrease the number of hospital days, which strongly affects the utilization of resources. Consequently, there is a powerful incentive to discharge patients earlier

---

*A person interested in keeping abreast of PROPAC's latest recommendations, as reported to the secretary of the US Department of Health and Human Services, can be added to the mailing list to receive these reports by calling the PROPAC office at (202)453-3986.
†The OTA was created in 1972 as an analytic arm of Congress. OTA's basic function is to help legislative policy makers anticipate and plan for the consequences of technologic changes. OTA provides Congress with independent and timely information about the potential effects of the changes. The board is composed of the OTA director and members of the US House of Representatives and US Senate.

---

*Homogeneity is defined as the expectation that the variances in cases classified under the same DRG are equal.

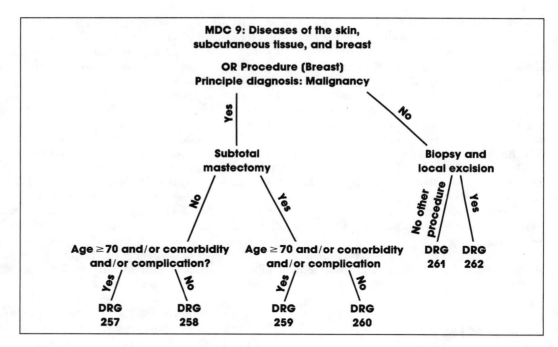

FIGURE 54-5 Algorithm for DRGs. This illustration is an example of the splitting process for a major diagnostic category, MDC 9. This decision tree, or algorithm, helps the medical records department to classify a patient's discharge status under a particular DRG category. The criteria or splitting process used to select the appropriate DRGs includes the use of an operating room (OR procedure), the principal diagnosis, the type of OR procedure, the age of the patient, and the type or severity of complication or comorbidity.

than before. During the past several years, Medicare's reimbursed LOS has progressively decreased. Since 1984 the average decrease for each year has been 2.1%; in 1989 the average LOS was 8.8 days.[15] Of greatest concern is the pressure for inappropriately shortening the LOS, especially for the elderly patient. The job of the PROs is to monitor this factor carefully.

Greater responsibility has been given to the hospital's medical records department for providing data for current and retrospective patient care studies. These studies can be used to document the complex care required by patients with cancer.

Nursing implications Nurses have a greater need than ever before to increase patients' self-care knowledge and skills. Teaching self-care is not a specific intervention but, rather, is an attempt to provide a model of care. The emphasis is on managed care throughout a lifetime.[16]

Coordinating discharge planning is a vital role for the nurse. Continuity of care between the hospital and home must be ensured. Because patients are leaving the hospital setting sooner, home care agencies have grown, increasing the need for home care nurses, especially those with acute care experience.

Nursing case management models have been developed to maximize resources and expertise needed in the care of hospitalized patients who have similar diagnoses. An example of a case management model is that of the New England Medical Center Department of Nursing. A strategy was initiated that formally joins a specific group of nurses together into a group practice. This group nursing practice is then linked to a specific physician. Together the nurses and physicians care for patients throughout the continuum of hospitalization. Case management assignments may be aligned with caseloads in a variety of ways; for example, a nurse may be assigned to a physician and all his or her patients, assigned to manage cases within a geographic unit, or assigned to cases on the basis of diagnosis. Collectively, the nurses and physicians are responsible for developing standards, management tools, and designs for delivery of care.[17] This plan can be very effective because nurses and physicians together are responsible for more than 80% of all the resources expended during each hospitalization.[15] A case management plan at the New England Medical Center is used to discuss possible cause-and-effect relationships in commonly encountered patient problems. The plan also results in the development of intermediate patient goals that outline appropriate nursing and physician interventions needed to achieve the specific desired clinical outcomes. The entire plan is designed to function within the DRG LOS framework.[18] Through these strategies, this center was able to reduce the LOS for patients undergoing induction therapy for leukemia from 48 to 32 days.[18] Case management requires the nurse to be prepared at a bachelor's or master's degree level of education, because nurses in this role must define and facilitate clinical and financial outcomes.[15]

Restraint of technologic advancement

History   With the birth of the PPS, new terminology has evolved in health care agencies. Words such as cost-effectiveness, cost efficiency, cost saving, competition, and feasibility echo in the administrative offices. When a request is made for an item that uses new technology, administrators want documentation or a feasibility report before approving the purchase. Items using new technology include drugs, devices, diagnostic equipment, and any equipment needed for medical and surgical procedures that prevent, diagnose, and treat disease. It is estimated that 20% to 50% of the growth in health care costs can be attributed to new technology.[12] Initially, under the PPS, capital expenditures were reimbursed on the basis of the actual costs, a "pass-through." The initial cost of the purchase was not the major concern; rather, the indirect costs of operation, maintenance, and salary for trained personnel were the issues. These indirect costs are accounted for in the DRG calculation under the labor and nonlabor components. If a hospital's indirect figures are not in line with the standard DRG calculation, the hospital loses money for the specific DRG.

Not only are the indirect costs a concern, but Congress continues to mandate percentage reductions in hospital capital payments. In fiscal year 1989, hospitals received only 85% of Medicare's share of allowable capital-related costs.[12]

The government uses different avenues to influence the development and utilization of technology. The following are some of these avenues[12]:

- National Institutes of Health: supplies financial support for both basic and applied research related to the development of new medical technologies.

- Food and Drug Administration (FDA): reviews the safety and efficacy of new medical technologies, drugs, and medical devices.

- State government: regulates, in many states, the purchase of new equipment through a certificate of need (CON) program.

- Medicare and Medicaid: influence indirectly the availability of new technology through decisions regarding reimbursement.

- Office of Health Technology Assessment (OHTA): evaluates safety and efficacy of new technology and recommends for or against Medicaid coverage.

- Patent laws: provide manufacturers with a monopoly for a period of several years.

Current trends   In addition to the federal government's historic involvement, third-party payers (insurance companies) have developed techniques to control costs. This involvement is in response to the soaring health care costs, high insurance premiums, and the introduction of the PPS. Some of the techniques are as follows[12]:

- Technologic assessment. Many third-party payers have established formal processes for evaluating the clinical and economic effects of new technology.

- Utilization review. Insurers are constantly reviewing the course of treatment provided and establishing protocols for appropriate treatment. If their protocols are not followed, payment is not given.

- Case management. Insurers are using case management techniques to direct patients to efficient providers.

- Selective contracting and price discounting. Some health care systems have developed contracting mechanisms with suppliers of drugs, medical supplies, and equipment. These mechanisms provide patient care at a fixed, discounted price.

Several major concerns regarding the PPS have been raised in regard to technologic advancement. Some of the concerns that have been discussed in the literature include the incentives provided to hospitals for restricting the adoption of new technology; the access to purchasing new technology, which may be given only to those hospitals that have proven cost reductions in the DRG categories utilizing the technology; the possibility that new technologies that increase costs of treatment within specified DRGs may not be readily adopted, even if they can effect an improvement in patient care; the restrictions in state-of-the-art medical care for hospitalized Medicare recipients; and the possible reduction of expenditures by manufacturers of technologic equipment for research and development, as a response to cost-cutting policies. Although there are no data to confirm the occurrence of these phenomena, the concerns are realistic.

In 1989, consideration was given to a proposal that would give the US Department of Health and Human Services the authority to evaluate new medical technology and to judge its cost-effectiveness for patient care.[19] Moreover, several years ago, Project Hope, under contract to PROPAC, began studies to investigate which technologies would significantly increase inpatient operating costs and which would decrease costs. Some examples from Project Hope of cost-increasing technologies estimated for fiscal year 1990 were implantable infusion pumps, magnetic resonance imaging, and monoclonal antibodies used as diagnostic agents.[20] Among those technologies estimated to be cost decreasing were endoscopic lasers, gallstone lithotripsy, and peripheral vascular angioplasty.[20]

Updating the current reimbursement system is an omnibus job, but it must be done on a routine, consistent, scientific basis. Many of the technologic advancement issues relate directly to the care of patients with cancer. These issues will be explored in a later section of this chapter.

Nursing implications   No longer is it appropriate for nurses to base decisions regarding patient care on the assumption that resources are unlimited. In any economy or organization, resources are scarce relative to demands.

There will always be more demands on available resources than can be satisfied. As a result of these demands, output must be rationed. The objective of rationing is to use available resources to maximize social welfare or institutional well-being.[21] As health care expenditures continue to take a large share of our society's total resources, pressure will continue to increase on the industry to justify outcomes relative to their costs.

Nurses must be able to justify the resources that are needed for improving patient care. This goal can be accomplished through the use of financial management tools or techniques. Some examples of these techniques include feasibility studies and cost analysis studies.

A feasibility study is a documentation process to determine whether a new program should be developed and implemented in a health care agency.[22] These studies provide a comprehensive economic and financial forecast for a new idea or program.

The basic steps of a feasibility study include the following:

- Define objectives: List the goals that the study is to achieve.

- List assumptions: Discuss the existing conditions that the reader of the feasibility study would otherwise not be familiar with if he or she had not read it. This section allows the reader to understand the writer's global perspective of the situation or problem.

- Describe the current situation: Answer the question, Why is this project possible? Then present relevant background data on the project, list who or what is in competition, and discuss the macroenvironment (eg, government, legal issues).

- Develop a plan of action: List what will be done, assign a person or persons to act, provide a time line or framework, and document the cost.

- Record the projected profit and loss: Discuss the expected financial gains or losses of the project.

- Enlist the assistance of the institution's finance department for the coordination of this section.

- Describe controls: Present a plan for monitoring the study.

- Prepare an executive summary: Write an abbreviated overview of the proposed plan. This section of the proposal is usually the one that most decision makers on the management team will review. It should therefore be as brief and concise as possible—usually one page. The executive summary is the first section of the feasibility study.

Cost-analysis techniques generally are classified as one of two types: cost-benefit analysis (CBA) or cost-effective analysis (CEA). Larson and Peters[23] define each of these techniques: "Cost-benefit analysis assigns monetary value to all costs and benefits of a potential program, practice or product, resulting in a cost-benefit ratio" (eg, a decision needs to be made on whether an outpatient oncology unit will be designed or on whether an outpatient department will be expanded). Cost-effective analysis is defined as follows: "All the costs measured in dollars necessary to achieve a certain effect (benefit) are calculated and expressed as cost/unit of effectiveness."[23] This technique is used to compare relative costs of several alternatives. All the alternatives are designed to have the same outcomes (eg, inserting an indwelling catheter for a chemotherapy regimen versus administering individual doses via venipuncture). Steps used in conducting either analysis also have been delineated by the Office of Technology Assessment (OTA). Larson and Peters[23] reviewed the OTA analysis steps as follows:

1. Define the problem.
2. State objective of the proposed program, practice change, or product.
3. Identify alternatives.
4. Define the perspective of the analysis. (For example, does it represent costs and benefits to the patient or to employees? If it represents more than one viewpoint, each should be analyzed separately.)
5. Analyze costs (include both direct and indirect costs).
6. Evaluate benefits (in dollars for CBA, in effects for CEA).
7. Determine the present value of any future costs and benefits by calculating a discount. This is called discounting. Formula: Present value = Future value (1 + Interest rate) interval in years
8. Analyze uncertainties. Substitute different values from within the range of possible values for costs and benefits calculated to determine whether changes in the values will alter the conclusions of the analysis. (This is called a sensitivity analysis.)
9. Address ethical issues (ie, the appropriate distribution of limited resources in the population, the accessibility of programs and resources, the extent to which the analysis can be influenced by bias).
10. Interpret results.

Another important contribution that nurses can make in an evaluation of new technology is to organize a product evaluation committee (PEC) or to serve as a member of the committee. The PEC is responsible for controlling which product or service will be used in a health care agency. Larson and Maciorowski[24] describe a four-step process to be utilized by a PEC:

- Step 1: All requests for new products or changes in the use of existing products are directed to the PEC.

- Step 2: Product options are explored in depth by potential users and by the PEC.

- Step 3: Product options are carefully evaluated on the basis of a review of the literature (historical and research perspectives), consultation with other experts, and field testing of products. Methods of field testing should be consistent for everyone involved. The PEC should use objective criteria (eg, quality of product compared with that of others, safety, serviceability, cost, standardization, prevention of duplication of products).

- Step 4: Summarize findings in a comparison chart.

When nurses increase their understanding and utilization of these processes, cost-effectiveness will no longer be a "buzz word" but, rather, a significant approach for the justification of resources needed to care for patients and their families.

Limitation of access to health care

History   "Access to care" refers to a person's ability to pay for the health care services provided. Before the early 1980s, few patients had financial burdens from medical expenses; their health care insurance carrier paid any bills, and the burden of health care expenses was therefore on the third-party payer. With the implementation of the PPS, the issue of access to care has gained prominence.

A brief history of health care coverage in the United States is helpful in gaining a perspective on this issue[25]:

- Before the 1930s: Ninety percent of the money spent on medical bills came directly from the patient's own pocket.

- During the great depression, beginning in 1929: The cost of medical care rose sharply, and people had less money to spend on medical bills. Doctors were collecting only 40% of the fees they charged.

- 1935: The American Hospital Association, which represented hospitals throughout the United States, promoted Blue Cross insurance to pay for hospital stays.

- During World War II, beginning in 1941: Although the federal government halted price and wage increases, health insurance was not counted as a wage. This enabled labor unions to negotiate for better health care coverage.

- 1950: The high cost of national health care was beginning to gain attention by the politicians. The cost per person was $80.

- 1965: Medicare and Medicaid federal health insurance programs started. Medicare is a program for people 65 years of age or older and for certain disabled people; Medicaid is a program for people with very low income (federal regulations mandate that each state be responsible for administering the program and establishing income levels for cash assistance). Health insurance coverage became a common employee benefit. Federal and state governments paid about 26% of all monies spent for health care in the United States. National health care costs rose to $141 per person.

- 1970: Medical costs went up faster than the general rate of inflation. In this era of explosive growth for medical technologies and services, intensive care units became very popular. The cost of national health care continued to climb, until it reached $340 per person.

- 1980: The early 1980s were regarded as a time of economic recession. The government's share of the national medical bill rose to 43%, and national health care costs rose to $1054 per person. Health care costs consumed one fourth of the corporate profits left after paying taxes. As a result government and industry (the employers) started paying closer attention to the health benefit package.

- 1983: TEFRA was passed. Prospective reimbursement was implemented for the national Medicare program; however, each state had the responsibility for establishing its own reimbursement process for the Medicaid program.

Throughout the 50-year period from the 1930s to the 1980s, many uninsured, indigent Americans were not eligible for employee or government-assistance benefits. Hospitals provided charity care to these patients by shifting costs. Cost shifting is the practice of charging higher rates to those patients whose care is paid through an insurance plan and then using the extra income to compensate for the cost of care for those patients who are unable to pay their bills. As a result of this cost-shifting practice, insurance premiums rose. For example, in some states the cost of insuring a family of four rose about 400% between 1980 and 1989.[26] With these enormous increases, corporations reduced their health care benefits. Today it is becoming more difficult, with cutbacks by both the government and big business, for hospitals to afford to provide uncompensated care to the 37 million uninsured Americans.[12] To do so would require an increase in a hospital's gross revenue, which is not the focus of cost-containment efforts.[27]

Current trends   The demand for charity care is steadily increasing at a time when many hospitals have negative operating margins. (A 1988 American Hospital Association report indicated that about half of all hospitals had lost money and were concerned about their financial failure[28]; about 200 hospitals have closed since the PPS began in 1983.[7]) A significant reason for the increased need for charity care is the number of persons who are in the active work force but who do not receive health insurance as an employee benefit. Approximately 90% of uninsured persons are employed in companies or businesses that do not offer employee health insurance.[12] These small companies cannot afford to offer health coverage benefits. As our nation continues the transition from a manufacturing to a service economy, this category of uninsured persons will increase. Service companies are usually small and nonunionized, and both of these characteristics are associated with limited employer-sponsored insurance plans. Almost half of uninsured persons are under 25 years of age, and one third of this group are children or other dependents.[12]

Many employers are changing their traditional health insurance benefits, in which the worker chooses his own physician and receives reimbursement for all or part of the incurred expenses. Instead, they are adopting programs that restrict both the extent of coverage and physician selection. As recently as 1984, a total of 96% of insured workers were covered by the traditional plan, compared with the current 28% of workers enjoying such plans in 1989.[26] Newly organized care delivery systems have been introduced.

Alternative care delivery systems   An array of acronyms such as HMO, IPA, and PPO (see below) have emerged in the literature. They represent models of health care coverage in which companies offer employee health benefits and at the same time monitor and evaluate the "appropriateness" of medical care prescribed by physicians. A term that may be used to summarize this activity is "managed care."

One of the most popular alternatives is the *health maintenance organization* (HMO). HMOs are membership organizations that provide health care ranging from prevention to treatment for a prenegotiated price during a fixed period. Members may solicit care from only those doctors and hospitals designated by the HMO. This type of alternative care delivery system is the oldest alternative to the traditional health insurance plan. Prepaid group practices, as they were first called, started in farming communities in the 1800s.[25] In the 1940s, Henry Kaiser, an industrialist, founded the HMO known as Kaiser-Permanente. He believed in the "preventive" approach to medicine, rather than the "curing the sick" approach.[29] He encouraged persons to visit a physician before illness developed—preventive health maintenance. These visits were paid for by the HMO and was a distinctly different approach from traditional health care benefits (eg, Medicare, Blue Shield), which would only pay if the patient had a problem that needed treatment. Today, Kaiser-Permanente represents one of the biggest corporation-backed HMO chains in the United States. HMOs first gained national prominence in the 1970s under President Nixon's Administration. During that time, Congress passed the Health Maintenance Organization Act, which created a national policy designed to control escalating health care costs. Federal loans and other incentives were provided to increase HMO growth. HMOs provide corporations with the financial advantage of fixed rates of reimbursement, rather than steadily increasing health insurance premiums. Under this plan, physicians are salaried employees of the HMO.

The *individual practice association* (IPA) is a type of HMO in which the participating physician accepts patients who are HMO members and those who are "fee for service" patients. The physician is reimbursed for care provided to the HMO patients according to a set fee schedule. This fee includes the cost of diagnostic tests and the fee for a referral to a specialist if needed. The physician who does not spend all the allotted money received from the set fee schedule may keep some portion or all of the balance. However, if costs exceed the predetermined rates, the physician must pay the difference.

A *preferred provider organization* (PPO) is another alternative plan for health care coverage. This is a negotiated business arrangement between an industry or business (the buyer) and a hospital or physician (the seller). A limited number of physicians and hospitals join a network and offer a discounted fee for service. In PPO plans, members pay a reduced fee or nothing at all when they are seen by a PPO physician. The physicians and hospitals in the PPO are able to discount their fees in return for a guaranteed volume of patients. The PPO offers the employer cost-controlling mechanisms through a claims review process. This process provides for prospective review of recommended diagnostic tests, surgery, and hospitalizations. Any care that is considered unnecessary is not approved. The PPOs usually offer a wider selection of physicians and hospitals than HMOs offer.

It is estimated that before the year 2000, up to 80% of the insured population will be enrolled in HMOs or PPOs.[26] The greatest controversy surrounding these alternative health care systems is in the implications of the strong incentive to reduce overall spending. Some persons believe that these delivery systems result in fewer tests and procedures or in delays in their being prescribed, to the detriment of the patient's health. Moreover, strong ethical concerns are raised when physicians have the authority to approve or disapprove patient referrals to specialists and at the same time are permitted to keep a percentage of the money they save by not referring patients to specialists. One questions whether such a system can produce unbiased judgment. There are few data available to confirm or deny this phenomenon.

In defense of the alternative care delivery system, the results of two studies showed that there were no statistical differences between the HMO population and the fee-for-service population in the care provided for the diagnosis and treatment of patients with breast cancer or colorectal cancer.[30,31] Variables analyzed for these studies included the mean age of diagnosis, the duration of symptoms before diagnosis, the number of physician visits for symptoms due to cancer before diagnosis, the stage of disease at which diagnosis was made, the methods of diagnosis and treatment, the length of hospital stay, the severity and type of complications, and survival rates. Further research is needed to explore the pros and cons of managed care and validate data and conclusions.

National health care   Many Americans have been "spoiled" by the fact that they have been able to receive immediate access to almost any kind of medical treatment. However, health care is not a constitutional right, a fact that has become more apparent as the impact of the PPS continues to be felt. The news media have covered numerous stories about the state and federal funding cutbacks that are causing important public health programs, clinics, and county hospitals to close. Even television entertainment has portrayed persons going to an emergency department and being denied care because they do not have health insurance. A county in the San Francisco Bay area even hired bioethics consultants to help them decide priorities for emergency care.[32] Oregon was one of the first states to ration health care for the poor. In June 1987 the Oregon legislature voted to stop using Medicaid funds to pay for heart, liver, bone marrow, and pancreas transplants.[33] In December 1987 a 7-year-old leukemia patient from Portland, Oregon, whose mother was on welfare, died after the state refused to pay for a bone marrow transplant.

In addition to poor persons, elderly persons, who generate 29% of this nation's health care expenses, are suffering.[33] Physicians who care for frail elderly persons are penalized for having patients who require longer hospitalization. Proposed legislation such as the Catastrophic Health Care Act were attempts to assist the elderly, but at the current time little has been accomplished to help this struggling segment of the population.

Another startling fact that has an impact on the care of elderly persons is that $50 billion a year is spent on patients during the last 6 months of life.[33] This fact has raised questions about the rationing of medical care for persons with a limited life expectancy (ie, elderly persons). For example, should an elderly person with a diagnosis of incurable adenocarcinoma of the lung be given chemotherapy, and if so, for how long?

A growing number of persons in this country are arguing that the American health care system has failed and that the nation needs some kind of nationalized health insurance system. A 1989 poll showed that 89% of Americans believed that fundamental changes are needed.[34] In the past, physicians have strongly opposed the idea of a nationalized health insurance system; however, proposals are being developed, such as the one outlined by Hummelstein and Woolhandler,[35] in which the government would fund all health care but would leave the existing private delivery structure intact; hospitals would not be owned, nor would physicians be employed, by the government.

The United States is one of the few remaining industrial nations that does not have some kind of national health financing program. In the United States, the per capita health care cost is 41% higher than in Canada, 61% higher than in Sweden, 85% higher than in France, 131% higher than in Japan, and an astounding 171% higher than in Great Britain.[36]

An organization that compares the health care of 24 wealthy countries is the Organization for Economic Cooperation and Development (OECD). The OECD reveals that medical practice is similar everywhere and that physicians are quick to learn about the medical advances in other countries; however, the biggest difference between wealthy countries and poorer ones is in the organization and financing of health care in the former.[37] The OECD has also addressed the phenomenon that although countries have much different health care systems, their problems are the same: how to financially restrict the practices of hospitals and physicians, how to secure adequate treatment for poor and elderly persons, and how to control an apparently infinite demand for health care.[37]

The next logical question that comes to mind is, Is the quality of care in the United States better than in other countries? When quality indicators such as life expectancy and infant mortality rates are considered, the United States ranks low. However, in the United States, rationing of medical care through waiting lists (as in countries with nationalized health care systems) is not yet the norm. In Great Britain, waiting lists for elective procedures such as hip replacements or cataract surgery can stretch up to 2 years.[29] Moreover, kidney dialysis ordinarily is not provided for anyone more than 55 years of age,[33] whereas in the United States, this procedure is available to anyone. The fact that the United States does have the highest

health care costs but produces the most sophisticated care is an outcome that must not be dismissed.

Our country is pondering the idea of a nationalized health care plan. The time for radical reform is fast approaching as the health care budget continues to soar. Corporate business leaders believe that many Americans are demanding more health care than is needed.[36] However, concern regarding the assessment and definition of quality care is an even bigger issue for many Americans. Reports such as "Quality of Medical Care: Information for Consumers"* have been prepared by the OTA for Congressional review. Paul M. Elwood, Jr, MD, founder of InterStudy, a Minnesota-based health-care-policy think tank, is generally credited with coining the term "health maintenance organization." He is investigating a new theory known as outcome management, in which a collection of objective criteria would help providers, payers, and purchasers to define the relationship between medical interventions and health outcomes.[38] For collection of these data, a quality-of-life scale has been designed and tested. It is based on a 5-minute test, self-administered by patients, that measures their ability to function.[38] This tool is now in the testing stage.

In the 1990s, cost-effective quality care will be a dominant theme. Keeping abreast of the latest information and research is imperative for health care professionals.

Nursing implications There has not been a more important period than the present for nurses to become proactively involved in helping to formulate our nation's health care policies in relation to access to care. A variety of directions can be taken:

- Initiate an educational program to increase the knowledge and skills of the public in regard to decision-making ability, balancing quality with cost. According to competitive theory, the cost and quality of care will be guided by the consumers who weigh price and quality levels in the selection of health insurance and medical care providers.[12]

- Develop clinical nursing research methods that investigate strategies to reduce health care costs without compromising care. According to Fuch,[39] "10% of delivered care may be considered harmful and another 10% is delivered with marginal benefits. If funding cuts were concentrated on this 20% the overall negative effect on health care would be minimal." The results from nursing research can be presented to legislators to assist them in making decisions about cutbacks. Nursing research can answer questions about which cutbacks have serious health implications versus those that will not have any adverse clinical affects.

- Engage in political activities. As drastic changes continue to appear on the horizon, nurses must take a proactive stance in health care decisions, rather than being reactive and merely trying to justify or rectify

*A copy of this report can be purchased through the Superintendent of Documents, US Government Printing Office, Washington, DC (GPO stock no. 052-003-01114).

the current changes. There is a political movement in this country for organizing grass-roots health care organizations. To date, 10 states have organized groups of concerned citizens who tell their legislators how they want their tax dollars spent on health care issues such as rationing and biomedical ethics. (See the Yellow Pages for information regarding this organization.)

• Nurses are advocates of patient care and should assist consumers in the decision-making process of selecting the alternative care system that is the best for their needs. Millensen[25] identified several questions to help people who are considering health care provided by an HMO or PPO:

1. What do comments from friends or acquaintances indicate about the reputation of the physicians and hospitals that belong to the HMO?

2. How are the HMO physicians paid? Is there a financial incentive to withhold certain kinds of services or specialist referrals?

3. What happens if a person becomes sick away from home or outside his HMO service area? Does the HMO pay for care provided elsewhere?

4. Can consumers choose their primary physician, or are they assigned?

5. Are all the physicians who are listed as members of the HMO actually available? (Sometimes a popular physician is unable to accept referrals for new patients.)

6. What are the benefits of the particular HMO? For example, are home prescription drugs and home care visits available?

For those consumers considering a PPO, it is appropriate to consider the following questions:

1. Do the participating physicians and hospitals meet the consumer's specific needs for medical care? For example, are specialized services for certain illnesses or treatments, pediatric facilities, maternal care, prescriptions, and home care available?

2. How much will the PPO pay toward the care provided by a physician who is not participating in the discounted fee arrangement?

3. Are financial incentives given to physicians that might motivate them to increase the number of office visits and prescribed tests to make up for discounted fees?

4. Will the PPO pay for a second opinion if it is sought before consumers undergo any tests or treatments that might not be warranted?

• Develop mechanisms to document, in financial terms, the nursing care needed to care for indigent patients. Reports show that the acuity level of the indigent patient is higher.[40,41] This information should be directed to members of PROPAC and Congress—the persons who are responsible for recommending reimbursement figures for indigent care.

• Read *In Search of Excellence*, by Peters and Waterman.[42] This book provides insight into how companies have arrived at strategies for cost savings, cost-effectiveness, and quality services and thus offers the nurse an added perspective on how to influence such changes in the future. A major theme of the book, which can serve as a caution for the hospital industry, is that low-cost providers are not winners over the long term.

• Keep abreast of agenda of the Joint Commission on Accreditation of Healthcare Organizations (the agency responsible for accrediting health care organizations) for the study of change. This study is a major research and development project that is intended to improve the Joint Commission's ability to evaluate health care organizations and generate greater attention to the quality of patient care. Clinical indicators will be used to evaluate specific areas of patient care (eg, obstetrics, oncology). The Association of Community Cancer Centers (ACCC) is developing a multistep method for validating clinical indicators in cancer care. Organizations such as the American College of Surgeons, the ACCC, the American Society of Clinical Oncology, and the Oncology Nursing Society usually provide updated reports on the status of this study.

SPECIFIC ECONOMIC ISSUES IN CANCER CARE

Economics has a major effect on the outcome and delivery of today's patient care. Unfortunately, the specialty of oncology did not escape the PPS regulations. During the 1970s and early 1980s, cancer care has had a "sacred cow" reputation with an "ask and you shall receive" attitude. However, this honeymoon phase is coming to an end in the eyes of today's insurance providers and federal officials. The specialty must now begin to justify all its resource costs. For some hospitals and administrators, cancer is not seen as a "winner" from a cost perspective; consequently, resources such as specialized personnel and state-of-the-art technology are scarce. In this section of the chapter, current issues imposing threats to the specialty of oncology will be addressed.

Oncology as a specialty embodies several unfavorable economic conditions: trend of increasing patient volume; hospital intensive, high acuity care needs; chronicity; a need for intensive monitoring throughout treatment; and the abundant need for psychologic interventions. The specific details of the problems change frequently, but the overall picture of cancer care is that it is expensive, in need of budgetary cuts and under the scrutiny of the legislators.

Cancer-Specific DRGs

The ACCC has been the leader in reporting information specific to cancer DRGs. In the past several years, this organization has gathered information from 90 of its affiliated hospitals. Information of interest from the compilation and analysis of these data includes the following[43]:

- There are 76 cancer or cancer-related DRGs. Forty-four DRGs, or 9.2% of all DRGs are designated as "pure" cancer DRGs for their title includes the presence of the word cancer. These are indicated in Table 54-1 by a "P."

- The 15 DRGs with the highest total gross reimbursement or relative income for each cancer DRG have been identified by calculating the total gross reimbursement, or overall income, for each of the specified cancer or cancer-related DRGs in the 90 institutions surveyed by the ACCC[44] (Table 54-2). Please note that these high-gross-reimbursement DRGs do not necessarily constitute "winning DRGs" for hospitals. In fact, many of the DRGs that have the highest gross reimbursement are "losers"—unprofitable for hospitals. For example, the type of cancer with the highest incidence in this country is lung cancer; thus the highest number of cancer patients are categorized under DRG

TABLE 54-1 Cancer and Cancer-related DRGs

DRG No.	DRG Title	DRG No.	DRG Title
"P" 10	Nervous System Neoplasms, Age ≥70 and/or Complications	"P" 203	Malignancy of Hepatobiliary System or Pancreas
"P" 11	Nervous System Neoplasms, Age <70 W/O Complications	"P" 239	Pathologic Fractures and Musculoskeletal and Connective Tissue Malignancy
46	Other Disorders of the Eye, Age ≥18 W/Complications	256	Other Diagnoses of Musculoskeletal System and Connective Tissue
47	Other Disorders of the Eye, Age ≥18 W/O Complications	"P" 257	Total Mastectomy for Malignancy, Age ≥70 and/or Complications
48	Other Disorders of the Eye, Age to 17	"P" 258	Total Mastectomy for Malignancy, Age 70 W/O Complications
"P" 64	Ear, Nose, and Throat Malignancy	"P" 259	Subtotal Mastectomy for Malignancy, Age >70 and/or Complications
73	Other Ear, Nose, and Throat Diagnoses, Age ≥18	"P" 260	Subtotal Mastectomy for Malignancy, Age <70
"P" 82	Respiratory Neoplasms	261	Breast Procedure for Nonmalignancy Except Biopsy and Local Excision
145	Other Circulatory Diagnoses W/O Complications	262	Breast Biopsy and Local Excision for Nonmalignancy
164	Appendectomy W/Complicated Principal Diagnosis, W/Complications	272	Major Skin Disorders, Age ≥70 and/or Complications
165	Appendectomy W/Complicated Principal Diagnosis, W/O Complications	273	Major Skin Disorders, Age <70 W/O Complications
"P" 172	Digestive Malignancy, Age ≥70 and/or Complications	"P" 274	Malignant Breast Disorders, Age >70 and/or Complications
"P" 173	Digestive Malignancy, Age <70 W/O Complications	"P" 275	Malignant Breast Disorders, Age <70 W/O Complications
185	Dental and Oral Disease Excluding Extraction and Restoration, Age ≥18	276	Nonmalignant Breast Disorders
187	Dental Extractions and Restorations	284	Minor Skin Disorders, Age <70 W/O Complications
188	Other Digestive System Diagnoses, Age ≥70 and/or Complications	300	Endocrine Disorders, Age ≥70 and/or Complications
189	Other Digestive Diagnoses, Age 18 to 69 W/O Complications	301	Endocrine Disorders, Age <70 W/O Complications
190	Other Digestive System Diagnoses, Age to 17	"P" 303	Kidney, Ureter, and Major Bladder Procedure for Neoplasm
"P" 199	Hepatobiliary Diagnostic Procedure for Malignancy		

TABLE 54-1 Cancer and Cancer-related DRGs (continued)

DRG No.	DRG Title	DEG No.	DRG Title
"P" 318	Kidney, Urinary Tract Neoplasms, Age ≥70 and/or Complications	399	Reticuloendothelial and Immunity Disorders, Age <70 W/O Complications
"P" 319	Kidney and Urinary Tract Neoplasm, Age <70 W/O Complications	"P" 400	Lymphoma or Leukemia W/Major OR Procedure
334	Major Male Pelvic Procedures W/O Complications	"P" 401	Lymphoma or Leukemia W/Minor OR Procedure, Age ≥70 and/or Complications
"P" 336	Transurethral Prostatectomy, Age ≥70 and/or Complications	"P" 402	Lymphoma or Leukemia W/Minor OR Procedure, Age <70 W/O Complications
"P" 338	Testes Procedure for Malignancy	"P" 403	Lymphoma or Leukemia, Age ≥70 and/or Complications
"P" 344	Other Male Reproductive System OR Procedure for Malignancy	"P" 404	Lymphoma or Leukemia, Age 15 to 69 W/O Complications
345	Other Male Reproductive System OR Procedure Except for Malignancy	"P" 405	Lymphoma or Leukemia, Age to 17
"P" 346	Malignancy, Male Reproductive System, Age ≥70 and/or Complications	"P" 406	Myeloproliferative Disorder or Poorly Differentiated Neoplasm W/Major OR Procedure and Complications
"P" 347	Malignancy, Male Reproductive System, Age <70 W/O Complications	"P" 407	Myeloproliferative Disorder or Poorly Differentiated Neoplasm W/Major OR Procedure W/O Complications
352	Other Male Reproductive System Diagnoses	"P" 408	Myeloproliferative Disorder or Poorly Differentiated Neoplasm W/Minor OR Procedure
"P" 353	Pelvic Evisceration, Radical Hysterectomy and Radical Vulvectomy	"P" 409	Radiotherapy
"P" 357	Uterus and Adenexal Procedures for Malignancy and/or Complications	"P" 410	Chemotherapy
"P" 363	Conization and Radioimplant for Malignancy	"P" 411	History of Malignancy W/O Endoscopy
"P" 366	Malignancy, Female Reproductive System, Age ≥70 and/or Complications	"P" 412	History of Malignancy W/Endoscopy
"P" 367	Malignancy, Female Reproductive System, Age <70 W/O Complications	"P" 413	Other Myeloproliferative Disorder or Poorly Differentiated Neoplasm, Age ≥70 and/or Complications
368	Infections, Female Reproductive System	"P" 414	Other Myeloproliferative Disorder or Poorly Differentiated Neoplasm, Age <70 W/O Complications
369	Menstrual and Other Female Reproductive System Disorders	"P" 465	Aftercare W/History of Malignancy as Secondary Diagnosis
395	Red Blood Cell Disorders, Age ≥18	467	Other Factors Influencing Health Status
396	Red Blood Cell Disorders, Age to 17	"P" 473	Acute Leukemia W/O Major OR Procedure, Age >17
398	Reticuloendothelial and Immunity, Disorders, Age ≥70 and/or Complications		

OR, Operating room; "P", "pure" cancer DRGs; W/, with; W/O, without.

82 (respiratory neoplasms). Hospital care for these patients is usually more expensive than the allowed DRG reimbursement. If a hospital's largest number of cancer patients are in the DRG 82 category, its highest gross reimbursement will be from this DRG. However, each time a hospital seeks reimbursement through Medicare for patients with lung cancer, they lose money, making this DRG unprofitable for the hospital.

• Variations in cancer DRG profits and losses are also related to regional location. Patterns of care vary

TABLE 54-2   Fifteen Cancer or Cancer-Related DRGs with the Highest Total Gross Reimbursement

	DRG Title		DRG Title
DRG 188	Other Digestive System Diagnoses, Age ≥70 and/or Complications	DRG 172	Digestive Malignancy, Age ≥70 and/or Complications
DRG 400	Lymphoma or Leukemia W/Major OR Procedure	DRG 257	Total Mastectomy for Malignancy, Age >70 and/or Complications
DRG 401	Lymphoma or Leukemia W/Minor OR Procedure, Age ≥70 and/or Complications	DRG 82	Respiratory Neoplasms
DRG 303	Kidney, Ureter, and Major Bladder Procedure for Neoplasm	DRG 203	Malignancy of Hepatobiliary System or Pancreas
DRG 10	Nervous System Neoplasms, Age ≥70 and/or Complications	DRG 395	Red Blood Cell Disorders Age ≥18
		DRG 239	Pathologic Fractures and Musculoskeletal and Connective Tissue Malignancy
DRG 403	Lymphoma or Leukemia, Age ≥70 and/or Complications	DRG 409	Radiotherapy
DRG 408	Myeloproliferative Disorder or Poorly Differentiated Neoplasm W/Minor OR Procedure	DRG 410	Chemotherapy

OR, Operating room; *W/*, with
Source: Adapted from Mortenson LE, Young JL Jr, Ney MS: Variations in cancer DRG profit and loss by hospital size and region of the nation. Oncol Issues 3(4):19, 1988.

throughout the United States and include recommended types of treatment and average length of stay in a hospital setting. In a 1988 ACCC study, 4 of the 15 cancer DRGs with the highest total gross reimbursement in Table 54-2 were selected for review (Table 54-3). Twelve hospitals from the Northeast and Mid-Atlantic areas, 9 hospitals in the Southeast, 14 hospitals in the Midwest, 3 hospitals in the Southwest, and 9 hospitals in the West participated in the study. If a hospital is located in a high-cost region for the DRG chemotherapy category, such as in the Midwest (see Table 54-3), the hospital will probably lose money on this DRG.[44] On the other hand, hospitals located in the southeastern region of the United States will probably make money on this DRG. (Note that the financial figures for the northeastern region in the chemotherapy category listed in Table 54-3 are also a good example of high gross reimbursement for a DRG but a "loser" for hospitals.) Examples of other DRG variations by regional location can also be seen in Table 54-3.[44]

A copy of similar reports may be requested from a hospital's finance department. An oncology clinical nursing specialist (OCNS) should examine this institutional list to identify which DRGs are "winners" and which are "losers." Individual hospitals can compare their data with those of national studies such as the one completed by the ACCC. If there is a negative difference between a hospital's financial DRG data compared with the regional data, measures to improve this status should be investigated. (For example, can length of stay be decreased? Are

procedures such as intravenous chemotherapy administration, dressing changes, mouth care protocols, and antibiotic protocols too costly?) If there is a significant difference between the hospital's DRG data and the regional data, this information should be shared with other OCNSs.

When an institution's profit-loss DRG list is reviewed, the variability of volume must be considered. It is important to ensure that those DRGs with the highest volume are monitored to produce "winning" DRGs for the hospital. If a DRG is a "loser," the hospital, with the assistance of an OCNS, must find ways to improve profit margins with such strategies as reducing the length of inpatient stay; by reviewing the necessity and appropriateness of tests, procedures, and drugs that are prescribed; and by determining other variable costs that might be financially draining factors.

In an analysis of the profit-and-loss nature of a cancer program, it is important to avoid two major pitfalls. First, the patient with cancer should not be used as the unit of analysis. This practice ignores the importance of multiple admissions for patients with cancer. Instead, the unit of analysis should be the cancer admissions. A report from the ACCC data revealed that half of all cancer patients' admissions are generated by one fourth of the cancer patients.[45] Second, a limit should not be set on the number of DRGs analyzed for the entire oncology product line. For example, if one is interested in assessing the hospital's profitability in the treatment of lung cancer, data from numerous DRGs (eg, numbers 82, 75, and 76, or a total of 26 others) should be used to analyze profitability, rather than limiting the data to only DRG 82 (Respiratory Neo-

TABLE 54-3 National Regional Variations in DRG Profits and Losses

Region	No. of Discharges	Average Profit/Loss	Average Reimbursement	Average Cost	Total Reimbursement
DRG 82: Respiratory neoplasm					
NE	812	$(517)	$4536	$5054	$3,683,491
SE	633	284	3665	3950	2,820,120
MW	939	645	4505	3860	4,230,550
SW	176	339	5042	4703	887,413
WEST	431	(287)	4531	4818	1,953,049
DRG 257: Total mastectomy for malignancy, age ≥70 and/or complications					
NE	257	$ 403	$3725	$3322	$ 845,559
SE	248	(109)	3277	3387	812,754
MW	290	547	4102	3556	1,189,650
SW	82	443	3603	3159	295,434
WEST	262	810	4110	3300	1,076,926
DRG 409: Radiation therapy					
NE	275	$(1416)	$4978	$6394	$1,368,964
SE	45	1101	3318	2216	149,293
MW	76	(481)	3733	4214	283,718
SW	10	235	3554	3319	35,537
WEST	55	(28)	3501	3529	192,551
DRG 410: Chemotherapy					
NE	1831	$ (53)	$1486	$1539	$2,720,180
SE	854	93	1346	1252	1,149,567
MW	851	(302)	1714	2016	1,458,328
SW	388	(76)	1472	1548	571,101
WEST	1057	(73)	1654	1727	1,748,484

NE, Northeast and Mid-Atlantic; *SE*, Southeast; *MW*, Midwest; *SW*, Southwest.

Source: Adapted from Mortenson LE, Young JL Jr, Ney MS: Variations in cancer DRG profit and loss by hospital size and region of the nation. Oncol Issues 3(4):17-18, 1988.

plasms). The combined DRG list best reflects the true profit or loss figure. If these two mistakes are made, a significant portion (up to 40%) of the cancer program revenues are likely to be missed.[45]

Clinical Trials

The future of clinical trials has been a major concern since the inception of DRGs. In 1983 a study was done to illustrate that the cost of conducting clinical research was too great. The results of this New Jersey–based study concluded that the average loss for each patient in a clinical trial was $1057, or 30 times greater than the loss for patients not in a clinical trial.[46] Additional costs for clinical trials occur because of the increased use of laboratory and radiology tests, the need for an environment conducive to safe, high-quality care (eg, a special unit, an educated interdisciplinary team, higher staff/patient ratios, nutritional support) and data management. The HCFA's response to this inflated figure was that "the Medicare program has always been prohibited from paying the research costs and for items or services that are either experimental

in nature or that are paid for by another government entity."[47] The HCFA also commented "that there is substantial federal support through NCI's programs."[47]

This issue became most problematic as a result of work done by researchers at Yale University in assigning weights to the cancer-related DRGs. Patients in clinical trials were not differentiated from others. Thus, when hospitals conducting research (eg, in community clinical oncology programs [CCOPs]) were reimbursed under the PPS, they lost money. Ironically, before the PPS, Medicare did pay for the costs of research, such as the patient's care on specialized oncology units, services provided by the interdisciplinary team, and laboratory and radiology services.[10]

One potential solution to this problem was the suggestion by the ACCC to create "DRG 471" for patients in clinical trials. This strategy was initially rejected by the HCFA. In the spring of 1983, an amendment was passed to provide exemption or adjustment for hospitals involved in providing cancer treatments or engaged in cancer research. Congress limited the amendment by including only three comprehensive cancer centers: MD Anderson Cancer Hospital, Fox Chase Cancer Center, and City of Hope National Medical Center. Since then, five more hospitals were added (refer to DRG cancer hospital exemptions on page 1181). This amendment, however, still did not solve all the problems. Thus many patients who were eligible to receive investigational drugs through clinical trials (eg, patients whose cancer is refractory to all known forms of standard therapy) would not be covered because they were receiving care in a hospital that was not exempt. Thus the cost of receiving investigational drugs was prohibitive for such patients.

To intensify the problem, many insurance companies are following the HCFA's policy. An NCI report to the U S Senate, "Remedies and Cost of Difficulties Hampering Clinical Research," noted that Medicare policy excludes coverage for investigational therapy because treatment with agents not yet approved by the FDA does not satisfy the "reasonable and necessary" criteria included in the legislative language relating to Medicare.[48] In addition, this same report pointed out that many third-party insurance contracts are excluding payments for patient care costs associated with investigational drugs. Although this exclusion has been a part of most insurance contracts for many years, it was not enforced until recently because of the growing emphasis on cost containment. Thus some insurance companies are denying claims whenever an investigational agent is clearly a part of the therapy. Claims that are denied may include the entire cost of hospitalization regardless of what the cost would be without the investigational treatment.[48] The NCI and other health-related organizations are attempting to convince third-party carriers that the treatment received by patients in clinical trials represents the best approach medically that can be offered.[48]

To draw the attention of Congress to the need for change in this reimbursement trend, factual data documenting the scope of the problem must be presented. The National Center for Health Services Research and the NCI are conducting a retrospective research study entitled the Hospital Cost and Clinical Research Project (HCCRP). The principal objectives of the study are (1) to determine whether there are cost differences between protocol and nonprotocol patients and (2) to estimate the extent to which incentives for hospitals to participate in clinical trials may have changed after the implementation of the PPS.[49]

The most frightening concern expressed occasionally by third-party payers is that living longer can waste resources because new technology does not prevent or cure disease but, rather, prolongs the course of illness, especially for patients who are near death. This disturbing concept surfaces at times when budget problems in health care are being discussed. Treating cancer patients with stage III or stage IV disease is viewed by some as a financially ineffective use of national resources. Reese[50] discussed the cost-effectiveness of cancer treatment in the United Kingdom, which has a national health program, and reported that patients with cancer are being denied the best treatment available because of the spending limits imposed by the National Health Service. For example, treatment to reduce pain and improve the quality of life were not always available, and some hospitals could not afford to give chemotherapy because of the costs. Costs

were determined by dividing a measure of the effectiveness of intervention in avoiding death or long-term disability into the cost of treatment for one patient.[50] A maximum of 17,000 francs (approximately $25,000) was documented as the amount available to save a life or avoid severe disability (a high-dose methotrexate chemotherapy regimen would exceed this figure). Fortunately, these cost-assessment procedures are not the primary sources for decision making about care to be provided. The thought of calculating the worth of a person's life by a formula is astounding. Yet Reese[50] concludes that the rationing of resources for cancer patients is inevitable and that cost assessment is a means of enabling hospitals and physicians to make optimal use of resources.

Changes in reimbursement policies occur on an almost daily basis. Medicare, Medicaid, and private insurers presently handle reimbursement on a case-by-case basis and usually require a written narrative (a preauthorization) of the patient's diagnosis, prognosis, treatment plan, effectiveness of prior treatment, and supporting data on the efficacy of the drugs to be used.[51] Policies and regulations vary from one state to another.

Funds are available for clinical trials from the NCI. However, the designated budget is not adequate to support the current explosion in scientific discovery and biotechnology. For example, President Bush's budget request in 1989 for the NCI was $1.6 billion; an additional $90 million was needed to sustain the existing level of services.[48]

Pharmaceutical companies often assist in funding clinical trials because the trials provide a means of testing their products. Companies usually pay an agreed-on dollar figure per accrued patient, with funding for laboratory tests, clinical coordination, data management, and physician fees, but rarely does the budget allocate money for the cost of routine patient care and clinical management, including the cost of hospitalization.[51]

To add further confusion to the reimbursement scenario, new institutions or corporations are being developed outside the auspices of the NCI to deliver advanced technologic care to patients whose cancer is refractory to standard therapy. An example of such an institution was the Biologic Therapy Institute, Biotherapeutics, Inc, of Franklin, Tennessee where patients paid their own medical expenses to receive experimental therapy. Unfortunately, financial difficulties caused Biotherapeutics, Inc, to close. Such delivery systems are called patient sponsored and promulgate the notion that care is available for those who can pay. In addition, we live in the era of the "baby boom" generation, when consumers are willing to pay extra for high-quality services.[52] The future for patient-sponsored research is not well defined, but already the National Academy of Sciences Institute of Medicine is proposing guidelines for responsible behavior in research.[53]

Through self-education, patients, legislators, and nurses can have an impact on the issue of reimbursement for clinical trials. Barbara Hoffman, JD, vice-president of the National Coalition for Cancer Survivorship, summarizes the predicament of clinical trials[54]:

The current lack of adequate health insurance coverage for experimental clinical trials and newly developed treatment bodes poorly for improving cure rates in the near future. The costs that society is paying now for cancer treatments is slight when compared with the cost of productive lives lost to oncology care that is dictated by M.B.A.s rather than M.D.s.

Unlabeled Use of FDA-Approved Chemotherapy Drugs

The government and insurance companies began in the late 1980s to deny reimbursement for drugs used for indications that do not fall within the package-insert guidelines approved by the FDA (unlabeled drugs). Some insurers (in northern California and Michigan) are denying reimbursement for unlabeled indications of chemotherapy, calling the use of such drugs experimental.[55]

The ACCC conducted an audit of 3500 patients' records from 1986 in 165 oncologists' offices. The audit concluded that of the eight most frequently used chemotherapy drugs, 46% were being used for unlabeled indications[56] (Table 54-4). The impact of this conclusion for the third-party payers who can deny payment is an annual savings of $150 to $200 million; for patients with cancer, it means that 372,000 were denied treatment with vincristine, 218,000 were denied treatment with cyclophosphamide, 88,000 were denied treatment with cisplatin, and 121,000 were denied treatment with methotrexate.[55] All these treatments are considered standard medical practice. In addition, approximately 90% of chemotherapy is given in standard combination regimens, and none of these combinations have ever had FDA approval.[55]

Insurers are asking drug manufacturers to obtain FDA approval for indications not listed on the label. Pharmaceutical representatives say that this process of supplemental application is a very time-consuming and costly endeavor, ranging from $500,000 to $5 million.[57] In addition, the burden on the FDA would be astronomic! However, "under Section 502 of the Federal Drug and Cosmetic Act, the FDA must support the policy that an approved drug must be labeled, promoted and administered only for uses for which its safety and efficacy have been established."[57] This guideline has not always been followed, however. In the past, the package inserts were mainly used only as a guide for physicians.

As the reader can surmise, we are just beginning to see cost-cutting warfare. Nurses must keep abreast of the most current information for creating profitable strategies for oncology programs. Keeping well informed will also enable nurses to react quickly as advocates for patients who are being denied payment for their health care.

Outpatient Oncology Care

Implementation of the PPS caused a major shift in the treatment environment, from inpatient to outpatient care. Patients who were receiving treatment for cancer, especially chemotherapy, felt the impact most heavily. The

TABLE 54-4 Eight Chemotherapy Agents with High Frequencies of Unlabeled Uses

Agent	Unlabeled Diagnoses
Adriamycin	GI/digestive cancers Other malignancies
Cytoxan	GI/digestive cancers Lung cancers Other malignancies
Fluorouracil	Lung cancers Metastatic adenocarcinoma Metastatic prostate cancer
Methotrexate	GI/digestive cancers Ovarian cancers Other malignancies
Mutamycin	Rectal cancers Lung cancers Breast cancers Ovarian cancers Other malignancies
Oncovin	GI/digestive cancers Breast cancers Lung cancers Other malignancies
Platinol	GI/digestive cancers Lung cancers Metastatic thyroid cancer Malignant melanoma Metastatic uterine cancer Other malignancies
Vepesid	GI/digestive cancers Ovarian cancers Brain cancer Hematologic malignancies

Source: Mortenson LE: Audit indicated half of current chemotherapy uses lack FDA approval. Oncol Issues 3(1):22, 1988.

DRG limit for reimbursement, pressure for early patient discharge, and patient preference have been strong incentives for the accelerated growth of outpatient cancer care facilities. The delivery of quality outpatient care has quickly become possible through advanced technologic support (eg, vascular access devices, ambulatory infusion pumps), the results of pharmacology research (eg, oral chemotherapeutic agents), and the specialized knowledge and skills of oncology nurses and physicians. Management of toxic effects has become possible on an outpatient basis by increasing the education and responsibility of patients and their families. Moreover, triage by telephone has become an important monitoring modality in outpatient cancer care (see Chapter 50, Ambulatory Care).

Shifting chemotherapy to the outpatient setting has not sheltered it from the scrutiny of insurance coverage, however. The HCFA received an allocation of $70,000 in 1988 to study the reasonableness of current Medicare payment levels for outpatient chemotherapy.[58] Recommendations based on the study will be made to Congress.

To ensure payment from an insurance company, the health care provider should contact the company to determine whether it will pay for outpatient treatment, which billing codes should be used, and which limitations are applicable to a particular patient. In 1989 a group practice of oncologists working in a hospital outreach clinic was ordered to return $75,000 in chemotherapy supervision fees charged during the prior 2½ years.[59] The ruling was based on a long-standing Medicare regulation whereby only the entity that owns or leases the space in which outpatient chemotherapy is delivered and that pays the employees can charge for the office visit, drug charges, and administration and supervision for chemotherapy.[59]

Preventive Cancer Care

The concept of wellness has been part of nursing and medicine for years and is reflected in the axiom "An ounce of prevention is worth a pound of cure." However, not until the medical world convinced the industrial world, through profitable financial data reports, did industry understand that this concept was both medically and economically sound. A report from the National Cancer Health Statistics indicates that $10.3 million was spent for medical care for cancer in 1985.[60] Care for male patients with lung cancer accounted for $1 million of this figure (48% of these patients were younger than 62 years of age, and 52% were 65 and older); $0.9 million was spent on female lung cancer patients (74% were less than 65 years of age and 26% were 65 and older). The investment in smoking cessation programs has the potential to effect great savings for industry. Another federal study demonstrated that hospital care expenditures account for roughly 60% to 75% of the total direct cost of cancer, compared with about 35% to 50% spent on hospital care for all other diseases.[61] The American Cancer Society estimates the average cost of treating a malignancy to be $60,000.[62] At the time of publication, more current information had not been compiled. One study at the University of Pennsylvania's Wharton School, Institute of Health Economics, found that companies can save more than 40% in hospitalization costs by implementing wellness programs for employees.[26] Wellness programs are increasingly popular; two of every three firms with 50 employees or more now offer some health promotion activity.[26] Worried about the skyrocketing costs of caring for employees with cancer, industry has also started cancer screening programs. Lately, more insurance providers are investigating mammography screening. However, a discouraging report in *Newsweek* noted that the expense to insurers would be about $5 billion if a third of the nation's women had screening mammograms annually, rather than $2 billion per year to treat cancer.[29] Such calculations can have only a negative impact on reimbursement. On the positive side, legislators are taking actions to ensure that mammograms will be covered for Medicare beneficiaries. Also, close to half of the states in the nation have laws requiring that third-party insurers pay for screening mammography. For changes in the future of cancer prevention and screening to be positive, many cost-benefit studies must be initiated and must produce evidence of overall cost savings.

THE FUTURE OF NURSING IN THE ECONOMICS OF HEALTH CARE

Changes in health care policy and economics are not new. In each decade there has been a different reason—the 1960s access to care, the 1970s technologic advancements, the 1980s cost containment, and the 1990s cost containment with quality care. The birth of the prospective payment system has offered nursing the chance to turn from a reactionary, follow-the-textbook, nostalgic approach and to become a proactive, creative, open-minded, economically aware profession. It is important to retain the successes and values that nursing has obtained throughout the years while also being ready to advance to a new era of influence and power.[2]

An initial impact of the PPS on nursing was to uncouple nursing services from hospital per diem charges along with charges for housekeeping, dietary, and laundry services. The effort to make this change began in 1977 when the New Jersey Health Department initiated the development of a nursing allocation-of-resources model that was DRG specific; the model was called relative intensity measures (RIMs) of nursing.[10] The RIMs have been criticized for methodologic failure; the necessary time for planning care, obtaining the resources needed for patient care, and evaluating the care was not allocated.[10,63] These daily nursing activities are often more time-consuming than nursing assessments or interventions. However, in the RIMs study, emphasis was given to these components of assessment and intervention. Also criticized was the assumption that care delivered equals care required.[64]

Various other schemes have been used to determine the cost of nursing services or to estimate nursing resource utilization. In 1985 a report from the American Nurse's Association Center for Research,[65] entitled "DRGs and Nursing Care," was submitted to the HCFA. The project was funded through an HCFA grant. The pilot study examined the relationship between DRGs and both nursing resource utilization and nursing costs. This report noted that the DRGs were developed without explicit attention to nursing resource use or nursing costs in hospitals, which is a significant component of overall hospital activities and costs. Data from the study consisted of approximately 1600 patient records from two hospitals in Wisconsin. Twenty-one DRGs, selected in relationship to high frequency with which they were encountered among the hospitalized Medicare beneficiaries, were examined for this study. The principal findings outlined in the study were as follows:

- DRG relative cost weights generally appear to reflect differences in nursing resource requirements among the DRGs in the study.

- Some DRGs in the study are interpretable groupings of patients, both in terms of total hours of nursing care by DRG and in terms of the daily pattern of nursing resource consumption during the course of hospitalization.

- Even though nursing care was not given explicit attention when the prospective pricing was developed, nursing costs as defined in the study have been shown to account for between 20% and 28% of hospital costs for two thirds of the DRGs in the study.

- Sufficient variations in nursing resources utilization patterns and in nursing costs were found to suggest further study in the refinement of prospective pricing. This study clearly defines the need for nursing to be identified in prospective pricing. However, to date, the Prospective Payment Assessment Commission has not acknowledged this fact. The only concern related to nursing that the Commission discussed in its June 1989 report to Congress was the shortage of registered nurses.[66]

Although there has been great interest and concern about determining nursing care costs for separate billing in the past several years, rapid movement in that direction has been limited because of the lack of financial and hospital administration support. Unfortunately, some of the nursing literature even suggests that such cost assessments may not be helpful and may not be effective unless the professional nursing staff is salaried.[63] Even with these restraints, success has been achieved in many hospitals toward the goal of billing patients directly for nursing costs. Hospitals in Arizona, Connecticut, New York, and Miami have been noted for their achievement in this area.[2]

CONCLUSION

The PPS will not be static: changes will occur over time and will further restrict health care payments. A significant opportunity for nurses will be to conduct or participate in the clinical research needed to determine which nursing interventions are most beneficial from a cost-benefit perspective. Although nurses have traditionally developed a variety of interventions to manage patient care problems, there has been minimal research to determine which approaches produce the best results. It is important to determine not only which approaches are the best but also which are the best at the lowest possible cost. When nurses collaborate in this type of research, they will have an impact on the cost of health care and consequently will gain recognition by health care and policy leaders. Seldom are nurses appointed to advisory committees that are involved in research studies with a direct influence on changing our

nation's health policy. The nursing profession must strive for this recognition.

Perhaps the greatest impact of the DRGs on nursing is in delivery systems for nursing care, which often have not kept pace with the rapid and complex changes in health care.[16] A current popular nursing delivery system is primary nursing. This delivery system is being monitored by nursing executives not only for its quality but for its patient care costs. However, newer changes in nursing care delivery systems are on the horizon. O'Malley et al[16] note that these delivery systems will have to be redesigned to (1) integrate with hospital business plans, (2) be consumer driven, outcome focused, and flexible, and (3) define more clearly the practice of professional nursing, which requires an advanced level of clinical and management skills at the bedside. One example of a redesigned system that was discussed earlier in this chapter is case management.

In the decade of the 1990s, the profession of nursing should continue to pursue recognition by health care leaders as the most vital link in successfully managing quality patient care at low cost. By unifying the large number of nurses in this country through professional nursing organizations, nurses can become a strong and powerful voice in the health care arena.

The role of the clinical nurse specialist (CNS) will be a pivotal position in the nursing organization structure. Yasko and Fleck[10] state:

> The CNS, with emphasis on the word nursing as the focus of their practice, will be needed to ensure the implementation of sophisticated patient care, which includes: the development, implementation, and evaluation of standards of care; systematic early discharge programs; methods to document accurately the delivery of nursing care; systems to determine the cost/benefit [ratio] of new supplies and equipment; methods to more effectively and efficiently teach patients and significant others self care; and systems to determine the cost of planning, implementing and evaluating nursing care.

REFERENCES

1. Ward W: An Introduction to Health Care Financial Management. Owings Mills, Md, National Health Publishing, 1988.
2. Davis CK: Health care economic issues: Projection for oncology nurses. Oncol Nurs Forum 12(4):17-22, 1985.
3. Diagnosis Related Groups: Their Evolution. Current Applications and Future Implications. (Executive Series No. J58341.) Cleveland, Ernst and Whinney, 1980.
4. Bird S, Mailhot C: DRGs: A new way to reimburse hospital costs. AORN J 38:773-777, 1983.
5. Joel L: DRGs: The state of the art of reimbursement for nursing services. Nurs Health Care 4:560-563, 1983.
6. Medicare program: Proposed rules. Federal Registry 54(87):19663, May 1989.
7. Hunt K: DRG: What it is, how it works and why it will hurt. Med Econ Sept 5, 1983, pp 262-272.
8. Shaffer F: DRGs: History and overview. Nurs Health Care 4:389-396, 1983.

9. Vladek BC: Medicare hospital payment by diagnosis related groups. Ann Intern Med 100:576-591, 1984.

10. Yasko JM, Fleck AE: Prospective payment (DRGs): What will be the impact on cancer care? Oncol Nurs Forum 11(3):63-72, 1984.

11. US Department of Health and Human Services: Report to Congress: DRG refinement: Outliers, severity of illness and intensity of care. Washington, DC, The Department, 1987.

12. National Committee for Quality Health Care: An American health strategy: Ensuring the availability of quality health care. Washington, DC, The Committee, 1988.

13. Young D: Prospective Payment Assessment Commission: Mandate, structure and relationships. Nurs Econ 2:309-311, 1984.

14. Young D: PROPAC: Future directions. Nurs Econ 4:12-15, 1986.

15. Tokarski C: Hospital inflation: A recurring problem. Mod Healthc 18(45):38-43, 1988.

16. O'Malley J, Loveridge C, Cummings S: The new nursing organization. Nurs Manage 20(2):29-33, 1989.

17. Definition. The Center for Nursing Case Management, New England Medical Center 3:1-3, 1988.

18. Definition. The Center for Nursing Care Management, New England Medical Center 2:1-4, 1987.

19. Tokarski C: Group hit government plan to access technology coverage. Mod Healthc 19(14):21, 1989.

20. Prospective Payment Commission: Report and recommendations to the Secretary, US Department of Health and Human Services. Washington, DC, The Commission, March 1989.

21. Hicks L: Using benefit cost and cost-effectiveness analysis in health care resource allocation. Nurs Econ 3(2):78-84, 1985.

22. Hochhauser M: A format for health care feasibility studies. Health Mark Q 4(2):35-41, 1986.

23. Larson E, Peters D: Integrating cost analysis in quality assurance. J Nurs Quality Assurance 1(1):1-7, 1986.

24. Larson E, Maciorowski L: Rational product evaluation. J Nurs Adm 16(7,8):31-36, 1986.

25. Millenson M: New options in health insurance, in Zeleny RO (ed): The World Book Health and Medical Annual. Chicago, World Book, 1988, pp 99-107.

26. Miller A, Bradburn E, Hager M, et al: Can you afford to get sick? Newsweek 113(5):45-51, 1989.

27. Murphy E: Health care: Right or privilege? Nurs Econ 4(2):66-68, 1986.

28. Wagner L, Toakrski C: Speculation begins. Mod Healthc 19(3):24-31, 1989.

29. Easterbrook G: The revolution in medicine. Newsweek 109(4):40-74, 1987.

30. Hughes J, Heckel V, Vernon S, et al: HMO versus FFS practice: A four-year retrospective analysis of colorectal cancer diagnosis and treatment—is there a difference in quality of care? Quality versus reimbursement and other conundrums. Proceedings of the 15th National Association of Community Cancer Care, 1989 (abstr).

31. Kulkarni PR, Vernon SW, Jackson GL, et al: Stage at diagnosis of breast cancer, comparison in a fee-for-service and health maintenance organization practice. Med Care 27:608-621, 1989.

32. Hilton B: Time for hard choices in health care. Pittsburgh Press, section 1B, p 3, March 15, 1989.

33. Robinson D: Who should receive medical aid. Parade Magazine, pp 4-5, May 28, 1989.

34. News at deadline. Hospitals 63(5):14, 1989.

35. Hummelstein DU, Woolhandler S: A national health program for the United States: A physician's proposal. N Engl J Med 320(2):102-108, 1989.

36. Iacocca L: Not ready for national health insurance but . . . Houston Chronicle, April 16, 1989, Sec H, p 1.

37. Sick health service. The Economist, July 16, 1988, pp 19-22.

38. Ellwood explains his theory, terminology and outcomes method of managing care. Mod Healthc 19(2):30, 1989.

39. Fuch VR: The ratio of medical care. N Engl J Med 311:1572-1573, 1984.

40. Studnick J: Differences in length of stay of Medicaid and Blue Cross patients and the effect of intensity of services. Public Health Rep 94(5):43845, 1979.

41. Presgrove M: Indigent patients: More nursing or less revenue. Nurs Manage 16(1):47-51, 1985.

42. Peters TJ, Waterman RH: In Search of Excellence. New York, Harper & Row, 1982.

43. Young JL, Mortenson LE, New MS: Hospital reimbursement, charges, and profit and loss for cancer and cancer-related DRGs. Oncol Issues 3(4):9-15, 1988.

44. Mortenson LE, Young JL, Ney MS: Variations in cancer DRG profit and loss by hospital size and region of the nation. Oncol Issues 3(4):16-20, 1988.

45. Katterhagen JG, Clarke RT, Mortenson LE: Understanding the economics of outpatient care. Oncol Issues 4(1):11-14, 1989.

46. Mortenson LE, Winn R: The potential negative impact of prospective reimbursement on cancer treatment and clinical research progress. Cancer Prog Bull 9(3):7-9, 1983.

47. Medicare regulations: final report. Federal Register 49(1):234, January 3, 1989.

48. The Cancer Letter 15(11):1-6, March 17, 1989.

49. Coffey R, Wallen J: Hospital cost and clinical research project. Washington, DC, National Center for Health Services Research, National Cancer Institute, 1985.

50. Reese GJ: Cost-effectiveness in oncology. Lancet 2:1405-1407, 1985.

51. Yasko J: Biological response modifier treatment: Reimbursement—present status and future strategies, Oncol Nurs Forum Suppl 15(6):28-34, 1988.

52. Jensen J: Consumers consider quality in deciding on a hospital, but measurements differ. Mod Healthc 19(10):88, 1989.

53. Report on the responsible conduct of research in the health sciences. Cope Magazine 3(6):12, 13, 1989.

54. Oncology Forum: Is the current system of reimbursement for experimental cancer treatment appropriate for the patient and/or oncologist? Cope Magazine 3(6):17-18, 1989.

55. Mortenson LE: Insurers target chemotherapy payments. Wall Street Journal 83(92):A16, May 11, 1989.

56. Mortenson LE: Audit indicates half of current chemotherapy uses lack of FDA approval. Oncol Issues 3(1):21-25, 1988.

57. FDA review of new indications is lengthy, costly process. Oncol Issues 3(1):19, 1988.

58. HCFA studies outpatient chemotherapy payment levels. Oncol Issues 3:7, 1988.

59. Medicare demands supervision fee refunds in Indiana. Oncol Issues 4:5, 1989.

60. US Department of Health and Human Services: Cancer rates and risks (3rd ed). Washington, DC, National Institutes of Health, 1985, pp 33-35.

61. Baird S: Changing economics of cancer care, challenges, opportunities. Proceedings of the Fifth National Conference on Cancer Nursing. New York, American Cancer Society, 1987, pp 1-16.

62. O'Grady E: Health investment: Firms back worker wellness. Houston Post (Business Section), June 12, 1989, p 1.
63. Kramer M, Schmalenberg C: Magnet hospitals talk about the impact of DRGs on nursing care. Nurs Manage 18(10):33-40, 1987.
64. Mowry, Mychelle, Korpman: Do DRGs reimbursement rates reflect nursing costs? J Nurs Adm 15(7,8):29-35, 1985.
65. American Nurses' Association Center for Research: DRGs and Nursing Care. (HCFA Grant No. 15-C-98421/7-02.) Kansas City, Mo, The Association, 1985.
66. Prospective Payment Commission: Medicare prospective payment and the American health care system. Report to the Congress. Washington, DC, The Commission, 1989.

Chapter 55

Ethics in Cancer Nursing Practice

Constance T. Donovan, RN, MSN, FAAN

INTRODUCTION

The tremendous advances in health-related science and technology of the second half of the twentieth century have resulted in an increased ability to exert control over the lives of human beings. This phenomenon has created an urgent need for a new emphasis on the ethical dimensions of decision making in health-related matters.[1] In fact, an entire field called bioethics (health care ethics, medical ethics, biomedical ethics) has emerged.

Gorovitz,[2] in 1978, defined this field as follows: "Bioethics is the critical examination of the moral dimensions of decision-making in health related contexts and in contexts involving the biological sciences." Questions about what is right or what should be done are raised, and the issues are organized in a way that allows for rational deliberation. Complexities are revealed about such situations as allowing a person with refractory leukemia to die or performing clinical phase I cancer studies. In the process of deliberation, conflict between ethical principles comes to light as alternative choices are considered. While no one "right" ethical answer or set of rules is produced, the potential of wrong action toward persons is minimized. In addition, choices based simply on current practices, universalization of personal convictions (frequently and emotionally expressed as "I feel"), or scientific knowledge can be avoided. In essence, more morally responsible choices in health-related matters can emerge.

Within nursing, considerable attention has been given to the question of whether nursing ethics is a subcategory of or separate from medical ethics. In general, there is a growing concern to develop nursing ethics as a unique field. Scholars in nursing ethics have been engaged in a continuing discourse regarding the moral foundation of nursing[3-6] and the extent to which nursing should borrow from the ethical theory approach or the moral development approach to ethics.[7] Although it is uncertain as to the degree to which the current lack of clarity about nursing ethics has created confusion within the nursing community and impeded integration of ethics into nursing curricula, Thompson and Thompson[8] concluded that formal preparation for ethical decision making lags behind our recognition of the need.

With increasing responsibility and expanding areas of professional decision making, cancer nurses are among those who have become increasingly aware of the importance of being prepared to participate in making ethical choices. They recognize that simple answers based on general statements about patients' rights are inadequate, do not identify the role of nursing in the ethical decision-making process, and certainly do not convince professional colleagues. These colleagues may view a particular situation as requiring only a clinical-scientific decision, rather than a decision that includes an ethical dimension. On the other hand, attempts to resolve ethical dilemmas by focusing strictly on the legal aspects often lead to frustration, because what is legal may not be congruent with what should be done ethically.

This chapter explores the influence of the nurse-patient relationship on bioethical decision making and examines issues that are most relevant to cancer nursing. To provide background for these discussions, the initial section focuses on information about ethical dilemmas and models of ethical reflection.

BACKGROUND INFORMATION

Ethical Dilemmas

Recognition of the fact that every health care decision has a value component is fundamental to the ethical practice of nursing. Although clinical-scientific data contribute to judgments, final decisions involve either the implicit or explicit consideration of values. Alternative actions reflect these values.

Actions are not always preceded by extensive ethical analysis. Veatch[9] notes that numerous health decisions are either so ordinary or have such obvious moral choices that immediate actions are possible. Veatch[9] points out, however, that it is only because some general guidelines have emerged as a result of our previous experiences that we are able to act without being immobilized by ethical considerations. Other situations do present serious dilemmas that require ethical deliberation before action is taken. The alternative choices of action within the situation represent conflicting moral claims for which no best choice is easily identified. Davis and Aroskar[1] define a dilemma as a choice between equally unsatisfactory alternatives and indicate that such questions as the following are asked: What should I do? What is the right thing to do? What harm and benefit result from this decision or action?

An example from the recent past where the alternatives were equally unsatisfactory involved pain management. Before approaches were developed to control the pain of persons with terminal cancer without endangering life, a choice often had to be made between preserving life and relieving suffering. Should a high dose of pain medication be administered or withheld? The best choice was not always easily decided nor mutually agreed on by patient, physician, and nurse.

Ethical problems are not limited, however, to specific patient situations. At times, choices must be defended on the policy-making level, as in the use of human subjects in experimentation and in the allocation of limited health care resources.

Choosing the best or right action requires careful deliberation. The data must be carefully collected. Davis and Aroskar[1] note that "the process of reflective thinking provides data by asking questions related to identifying the actors in the situation, the required action(s), possible and probable consequences of the proposed action(s), the intention or purpose of the action(s), the range of alternatives or choices, and the context of the action(s)." Once the data have been collected, the formulation of the problem is reviewed to be sure that it has been identified accurately and to clarify the values or moral principles that are in conflict.

Models for Ethical Reflection

What is a morally right act? To provide for careful analysis of choices and to move toward deciding the best choice of action, one must have knowledge of the various models of ethical reflection. Veatch[9] describes normative ethics as that area of ethics that determines whether there are general principles or norms related to a situation that make actions right or wrong. Beauchamp[10] describes normative ethics as divided into two fields: applied and general. In applied ethics, general ethical principles such as utility, truth telling, and keeping promises are used to resolve problems. In general ethics, the general ethical principles are organized into a system that is referred to as an ethical theory or position. The two dominant positions in the West are utilitarianism and formalism.

Taylor[11] describes *utilitarianism* as a teleologic ethical system (from the Greek word *telos*, meaning end or purpose) in which an action is morally right if it brings about good consequences. Therefore, in a utilitarian system, it is the goodness or badness of the consequences of actions that make them right or wrong. Taylor[11] describes *formalism* as a deontologic system (from the Greek word *deon*, meaning duty) in which an action is right if it accords with a moral rule and wrong if it violates such a rule, regardless of the end or purpose of the action. In formalism, there exists a set of conditions that are necessary and sufficient for any rule of moral obligation to apply to an action.

In using the utilitarian position to determine which alternative action in a situation of choice will provide the greatest general happiness, one can employ either of two approaches, the act-utilitarian or the rule-utilitarian approach.

The following case study may be used to consider each of these approaches:

Mrs. H. has had a diagnosis of advanced cancer of the esophagus. Her children report that Mrs. H.'s husband has recently died. They insist that they do not wish their mother to be told about her diagnosis because they believe that she will "give up." They request that she be told that she has a narrowing in her esophagus. One day Mrs. H. says to her primary nurse, "I know I'm very sick; I can't eat very much." The next day she asks the same nurse to tell her what is wrong. Should Mrs. H. be told her diagnosis?

According to the act-utilitarian approach, an attempt would be made to predict the possible consequences for the alternative choices of action: (1) withholding information about the diagnosis of esophageal cancer and (2) explaining to Mrs. H. that she has cancer of the esophagus. The consequences would be listed as empiric statements based on experience or knowledge. Some argue that a possible consequence for the first action is that Mrs. H. will maintain hope and for the second action is that Mrs. H. will become anxious and depressed. After all the possible consequences for each action are outlined, each con-

sequence would be assigned a happiness value, and the alternative with the greatest general happiness value for the greatest number involved would be selected.

In the rule-utilitarian approach, the alternative actions would be compared with an established rule that would have predetermined, by a listing of consequences, the actions that would produce the greatest general happiness for the greatest number of persons involved. An example of such a rule might be that depression and fear should be prevented. The alternative that is consistent with the rule would then be considered the right choice.

Finally, according to the deontologic approach, the method would be simply to compare alternative actions with rules or ethical principles such as keeping promises and telling the truth. These principles are seen as independent of consequences or of the good to be achieved. The alternative that is consistent with all appropriate principles would be viewed as the right action. For example, in the case study, telling the patient about her diagnosis might be seen as the right action because it is consistent with the principles of telling the truth and allowing self-determination.

Each of these approaches seems to have practical limitations. For example, in the utilitarian approach, consequences may be hard to predict or validate, and estimates of happiness values may be difficult to determine. In the deontologic approach, if both alternatives are consistent with some principles and conflict with others, choosing the right action might be difficult.

The adequacy of each theory can also be questioned. For the utilitarian approach, achieving the greatest happiness for the greatest number of persons could mean infringing on the rights of some. As an example, consider a clinical study in which cancer cells are to be injected into persons who do not have cancer and who have not consented to the procedure. It could be argued that the happiness of the majority resulting from the knowledge obtained would definitely outweigh the unhappiness of the research subjects. Therefore it could be decided that undertaking such a study is a right act. Some argue, however, that respect for the rights of individuals is of more fundamental moral value than the greatest happiness for the greatest number.[12] Thus, at times, using the concept of greatest happiness as a central focus for ethical decisions may be inappropriate.

For the deontologist, a difficulty unfolds when duties and obligations conflict. Davis and Aroskar[1] explain: "It does not resolve the dilemma for the nurse who decides to follow the rule that one should always tell the truth but realizes that the truth will undoubtedly hurt a particular patient in a given situation where the principle of telling the truth conflicts with the principle of doing no harm."

To avoid the limitations of each of these models, some authors[13,14] have arrived at a pluralistic model in which consideration is given to both consequences and inherent characteristics. Thus, in the situation of telling the truth, one relevant factor considered would be the duty to tell the truth, but the significance of consequences also would be recognized.

Although these and other models do not provide answers and, indeed, should not be used as "recipes," disciplined ethical reasoning is used to try to arrive at decisions about morally right actions.

NURSE-PATIENT RELATIONSHIPS IN CANCER CARE

It can be argued that attention to what constitutes an ethical dilemma, patterns of ethical reasoning, and analysis of ethical issues, although essential to ethical deliberation, is not sufficient; that is, the relational aspect inherent in the clinical situation must also be taken into consideration. In fact, several authors[15-17] have suggested that the key to creating an ethical climate lies in the relationship between the health professional and the patient; they note that the type of relationship will affect directly who makes the decision and how and what kinds of decisions are made.

Several models of the nurse-patient relationship were identified by Gadow[18] in 1977: nurse as healer, parent surrogate, physician surrogate, health educator, patient advocate, and contracted clinician. Gadow[18] noted, however, that each type of relationship raised some ethical questions, such as the following:

Does the nurse, if acting as parent surrogate, have the right to act paternalistically when the patient does not make "health" decisions? Does the nurse, if acting in contractual partnership with the patient, have the right to withdraw care when the patient refuses to assume responsibility for his or her health? Does the nurse, if acting as healer, analogous to the physician, have the right to cultivate the placebo effect that is thought to accompany all the actions of a healer, even to the point of patient deception? Or does the nurse, if acting as patient advocate, have an obligation to protect the patient from every erosion of human dignity and value, including deceptions in the name of health?

Faced with these alternative conceptions and their related ethical difficulties, what has been nursing's choice? American nursing, in general, seems to have rejected most of these models, including the "nurse as parent surrogate" conception, in which the nurse decides what is best for the patient. Rather, the numerous articles and books that have been written promoting the role of the nurse as patient advocate[19-25] suggest that nursing has adopted the "nurse as patient advocate" conception of the nurse-patient relationship.

However, there is a need to clarify the meaning of advocacy in nursing.[26,27] For example, advocacy at times seems to mean assuring the quality of care for groups of patients, whereas at other times, it seems to mean being a spokesperson for the patient or information provider and "watchdog" as the patient representative model and the patient's rights model, respectively, suggest. In addition, there are those times when advocacy seems to mean promoting and enhancing patient autonomy (self-determination).

Ultimately, it may be decided that the concept of advocacy in nursing should encompass a variety of meanings.

However, careful analysis would be required for clarification of each meaning and to avoid including morally incompatible meanings. Consider, as an example, the various meanings identified above in which the nurse's involvement could range from political action or negotiation for change, to protection of particular patients' human rights or best interests, to interactions with patients that promote their autonomy. It is not entirely clear whether all these meanings represent a commitment to the same moral position. For example, if protection of a patient's best interests could be interpreted to mean that, in general, the nurse could act without the competent patient's permission or could decide what was in the competent patient's best interest, then such a paternalistic position clearly would be incompatible with the moral position of the promotion of patient autonomy.

Gadow[28-31] offers one of the most instructive analyses of the meaning of advocacy in the patient-nurse relationship. She characterizes advocacy as based on the primacy of the human right of freedom of self-determination,[28] and describes it as

the effort to help persons become clear about what they want to do, by helping them discern and clarify their values in the situation, and on the basis of that self-determination, to reach decisions which express their reaffirmed, perhaps recreated, complex of values. Only in this way, when the valuing self is engaged and expressed in its entirety, can a person's decision be actually self-determined instead of being a decision which is not determined by others.[29]

Thus, in Gadow's view, advocacy involves "nurse-patient interactions that enhance the patient's autonomy."[31] In some instances, this may mean that the nurse must respect a patient's truly autonomous choice not to know particular information. Gadow contrasts this view of advocacy with both paternalism, in which decisions are made by the nurse without ascertaining or respecting the patient's wishes, and consumerism, in which the patient is supplied with the facts and then left unassisted to reach a decision.[31]

It could easily be argued that patients with cancer are in particular need of the type of advocacy that enhances autonomy. Not only is their autonomy diminished by disease, treatment, and, all too frequently, the health care system, but they are also confronted with many difficult choices.

Clinical observation suggests that cancer care nurses are very much aware of the vulnerability of the patients they care for. Accordingly, they inform patients about decisions that they need to make and assist them in their understanding of treatment options. To the extent that they also assist patients to identify and clarify their beliefs, values, and goals in relation to the available options, they would, in Gadow's view of advocacy,[31] be truly involved in a patient-nurse relationship that enhances patient autonomy.

Cancer care nurses are also concerned about those patients who are unable to communicate their values. (Gadow uses the term silent patients "because all that can be known with certainty about them is that communication—not necessarily competence—is lacking."[32]) Gadow notes that although the values of some silent patients can be known through advance directives or proxy instructions from someone who knows the patient's values well enough to decide as he or she would, access to the values of other silent patients has not seemed possible.[32] For these other silent patients, it is tempting for nurses to abandon the moral position of advocacy for self-determination and to adopt another moral approach, such as utilitarianism or beneficence (promoting the individual patient's best interest as defined by the professional).[32]

Gadow notes the moral chaos for the nurse that results from changing moral positions from patient to patient. She proposes that if the nurse considers himself or herself to be a full-fledged advocate for patient self-determination, the nurse must set aside the notion that the only access to patients' values is through standard communication and consider ways of illuminating the subjective world of silent patients.[32]

MAJOR BIOETHICAL ISSUES

Telling the Truth

Cancer care nurses' commitment to patient self-determination is implicit in a document entitled *Standards of Oncology Nursing Practice*, which was developed jointly by members of the American Nurses' Association (ANA) Council on Medical-Surgical Nursing Practice and the Oncology Nursing Society (ONS).[33] Of particular interest is the section on planning care, in which the outcome criteria for Information reads as follows:

> The client—1) Describes the state of the disease and therapy at a level consistent with his or her educational and emotional status. 2) Participates in the decision-making process pertaining to the plan of care and life activities. 3) Identifies appropriate community and personal resources that provide information and services. 4) Describes appropriate actions for highly predictable problems, oncological emergencies, and major side effect of the disease or therapy.[33]

This content, as well as some content in other sections, suggests that two major assumptions underlie this document: individuals generally desire to exercise their moral right to obtain information; and cancer care nurses should have the competence, collaboration with colleagues, and rapport with patients necessary to fulfill their moral obligation (duty, responsibility) to provide the information or to see that it is provided.

The implementation of the ANA/ONS standards in relation to information giving remains a challenge. Two central questions emerge: (1) Exactly what information should individuals with a diagnosis of cancer be given concerning such matters as the seriousness of their illness or the specifics of various treatment options? (2) Should the nurse be the one to tell the patient?

Traditional and recent views of truth telling

The issue of truth telling historically has received little attention in the medical profession's codes and oaths.[34] This avoidance of the issue of veracity, which Beauchamp and Childress[35] describe as including the obligations to disclose information, not to lie, and not to deceive, seems to have been related to the desire to be free to choose, in each particular situation, the types of information that would result in the greatest good for the particular person and prevent harm, including suffering, fear, and anxiety. Veatch[36] refers to this approach to moral reasoning as individualistic, situational, and a special sort of utilitarianism. From this position, each individual situation is viewed as unique, the greatest good is considered only in relation to potential benefit or harm, with a special emphasis on eliminating harm. Because truthful information was often viewed as harmful (as an example, the effect of telling the patient of a terminal diagnosis), one can see why concealment, evasion, and withholding of information were not prohibited and, in fact, were often justified.

In recent years, professional views regarding truth-telling have undergone a gradual shift.[36] In a 1953 study about disclosure of a cancer diagnosis, Fitts and Ravdin[37] found that 3% of physicians who responded always told their patients and 28% usually did, but 57% usually did not tell and 12% never told. By the early 1970s, studies about physicians' stated policies of disclosure revealed the following information: 25% always told their patients of any diagnosis of a malignancy and only 9% never told[38]; 13% always and 80% usually told the patient with a critical illness the nature of his disease[39]; and 53% always or frequently told terminal patients of their prognosis.[40] However, by 1979, Novack and colleagues,[41] who asked questions almost identical to those asked by Oken in 1961,[42] found that 98% of physicians reported that their usual policy was to tell patients their cancer diagnosis; in contrast, Oken[42] had found that only 12% of physicians usually told their patients.

The reason for this shift in physicians' stated policies of disclosure is not entirely clear. (The issue of actual practices of disclosure will be considered in the section on the Realities of Daily Practice.) Gadow[43] notes that professionals' empirical beliefs regarding truth telling have changed; in the past, professionals emphasized the potential dangers of truth telling, whereas now, other beliefs regarding the potential therapeutic value of truth telling and the potential negative consequences of not telling the truth seem to prevail. Thus, in the weighing of benefit versus harm, it becomes clear why it is more likely that the contemporary professional will decide to tell the truth in the majority of cases. However, such an approach to decision making is paternalistic; that is, the criterion of benefit versus harm is used and the professional decides. In essence, the professional is deciding whether and how much truth will benefit the patient. And, as Gadow notes: "Candor is no less paternalistic a response than deception."[43]

Novack and colleagues[41] offer several other possible reasons for the shift in disclosure practices. One reason is the availability of more treatment options for cancer, including research therapies. Such availability of options clearly has influenced the information given to individuals with cancer, because professionals are now required to disclose information necessary for consent to, or refusal of, further medical treatment. This necessary information includes two major types: information about diagnosis and prognosis and information about diagnostic and therapeutic procedures and alternatives, including their risks and benefits.[44]

Disclosure of information

In general, there are two major contexts in which the disclosure question arises: that in which consent to, or refusal of, treatment is not at issue and that involving consent to, or refusal of, standard or research therapies or procedures.

For patients with a diagnosis of terminal cancer, when no cancer treatment options are available, there is an ethical obligation of veracity that requires disclosure of information regarding diagnosis and prognosis and any other information that affects the patient's understanding and decision making. However, it is important to note that, first, there is no legal obligation of veracity in these situations that do not involve consent; that is, the law requires only disclosure of information about procedures to which patients consent.[35] Second, some argue that limited disclosure and deception can sometimes be justified even though violations of the rules of veracity are viewed as prima facie wrong.

Bok[34] states that the three major arguments for not being truthful with patients are (1) that truthfulness is impossible, (2) that patients do not want bad news, and (3) that truthful information harms them. After careful analysis of each argument, Bok concludes that the three arguments that defend lies to patients do not serve as a counterweight to the right to be informed.

Beauchamp and Childress,[35] in an analysis of the same three arguments, came to a similar conclusion. They point out that some health professionals justify not telling the truth on the basis of their assessment that some patients, particularly the very sick and dying, indicate by various signals that they do not want to know the truth about their condition, despite the conclusions of opinion surveys that they do want to know.[35] Beauchamp and Childress[35] caution that such claims set dangerous precedents for paternalistic actions under the guise of respect for autonomy. They and other authors[44,45] suggest that the best policy is to ask the patient at various points during the illness about the extent to which he or she wants information or autonomy in decision making.

When standard or experimental treatment or procedures are proposed for patients with cancer, professionals have both an ethical and a legal obligation to disclose information necessary for consent or refusal. This information is of two major types: information about diagnosis and prognosis and information about diagnostic and therapeutic procedures and alternatives, including their risks and benefits.[44]

For situations involving research treatments or procedures, the US Department of Health and Human Services (DHHS)[46] presents the kind of information that must be included to constitute "informed consent." These basic elements of informed consent are listed below:

1. A statement that the study involves research, an explanation of the purposes of the research and of the expected duration of the subject's participation, a description of the procedures to be followed, and identification of any procedures that are experimental

2. A description of any reasonably forseeable risks or discomforts to the subject

3. A description of any benefit to the subject or to others that may reasonably be expected from the research

4. A disclosure of appropriate alternative procedures or courses of treatment, if any, that might be advantageous to the subject

5. A statement describing the extent, if any, to which confidentiality of records identifying the subject will be maintained

6. For research involving more than minimal risk, an explanation as to whether any compensation and medical treatments are available if injury occurs and, if so, what they consist of or where further information may be obtained

7. An explanation of who to contact for answers to pertinent questions about the research and about the research subject's rights, and who to contact in the event of research-related injury to the subject

8. A statement that participation is voluntary, refusal to participate will involve no penalty or loss of benefits to which the subject is otherwise entitled, and the subject may discontinue participation at any time without penalty or loss of benefits to which the subject is otherwise entitled.

The following additional elements should be included when appropriate:

1. A statement that the particular treatment or procedure may involve risks to the subject (or to the embryo or fetus, if the subject is or may become pregnant) that currently are unforeseeable

2. Anticipated circumstances under which the subject's participation may be terminated by the investigator without regard to the subject's consent

3. Any additional costs to the subject that may result from participation in the research

4. The consequences of a subject's decision to withdraw from the research and the procedures for orderly termination of participation by the subject

5. A statement that significant new findings developed during the course of the research that may relate to the subject's willingness to continue participation will be provided to the subject

6. The approximate number of subjects involved in the study

Although some of the elements listed apply only to research consent, many are appropriate for consent to standard therapy. However, since these elements identify only the kind of information that must be disclosed, it is still necessary to make judgments about exactly what information to disclose to the patient in each of these categories. Clearly, some standard for making judgments is necessary. From court cases, two standards of disclosure have emerged: the professional practice standard and the reasonable person standard. In addition, some have proposed a third: the subjective standard.

In the professional practice standard, adequate disclosure is determined by inquiring into the customs of the other practitioners in the community.[35] Thus the customary practices of physicians establish the amount and kind of information that patients should be told. A major objection to this standard, therefore, is that it can affect the patient's right of autonomous choice[35] in that some patients may want more information than is uniformly disclosed.

In the reasonable person standard, the information that must be disclosed is that which a reasonable person, in the patient's position, would want to know to decide whether to undergo the treatment or procedure. From court cases, this has come to mean that physicians must include in their disclosure the diagnosis, the nature and purpose of the proposed treatment, the risks and consequences of the proposed treatment, the probability that the proposed treatment will be successful, feasible treatment alternatives, and the prognosis if the proposed treatment is not given.[47]

A major difficulty with this standard is that the informational needs of an "objective, reasonable person" may not be the same as the informational needs of an individual patient. Thus some have proposed a third standard: the subjective standard. According to this standard, professionals must disclose what a reasonable person would want to know, modified by what the practitioner knows or ought to know about the unique needs and desires of the patient.[48]

In addition to a consideration of disclosure standards that address adequacy of information, problems that involve the question of when less than complete disclosure is justified must also be considered.

Legally, exceptions to the disclosure necessary for consent have been allowed in emergency situations and in situations involving competency, waiver, and the like. Exceptions also have been permitted when, in the judgment of the physician, the information would potentially be harmful to an emotionally unstable individual.[35] This latter exception, termed the therapeutic privilege, is not only controversial but is also not uniformly defined across legal jurisdictions. After careful analysis, Beauchamp and Childress[35] conclude that there are difficult and rare nonresearch situations in which a physician's judgment of the patient's welfare takes precedence over the patient's right to information.

Other questions regarding less than complete disclosure have arisen in the context of randomized clinical trials. Included is the question of whether patients should be told about the fact that therapy will be selected by chance and not by clinical judgment. It has been concluded that, in general, there is no ethical justification for not providing complete disclosure in randomized clinical trials, including information about the method of assignment.[35]

In summary, although withholding of information may be justified in a few situations, in general, competent patients, unless they specifically ask not to be informed, should be given complete information. It appears that the subjective standard is most in concert with advocacy for patient autonomy.

Realities of daily practice

A great deal of intellectual and emotional turmoil is involved in deciding exactly what information to give to patients with a diagnosis of cancer. Despite the fact that physician self-reports indicate that they usually favor disclosure, the majority of physicians, according to the study by Novack et al,[41] also report making exceptions to their usual policy of disclosing information, which are manifested in the timing, pattern, and completeness of disclosures. Blumenfield and colleagues[49] found that, although 90% of medical residents held that patients have a right to be told, only 47% thought that the patient should be informed as soon as possible. Other researchers have found evidence that physicians are distinguishing between telling the truth and telling the "complete truth" and between the right to know for patients who ask and for those who do not ask.[50]

Clinical observations seem to agree with these findings. For example, information about the extent of the disease may be withheld; some medically acceptable alternative treatments or the availability of clinical trials may not be discussed; and information about a plan to reduce drug doses to decrease toxic effects and about the disease implications of such a plan may be withheld. Thus, despite a tendency toward more full disclosure, the information necessary for patients to reach a truly autonomous choice may not, in some instances, be provided.

The following case study is an example of the complexity of the current intellectual and emotional pressures. It combines the issues of providing adequate disclosure about the nature, benefits, and risks of treatment and of the withholding of information about the extent of disease.

A 72-year-old competent woman with a left mastectomy was hospitalized for symptoms resembling a stroke. She was aware that she had breast cancer and that she was receiving chemotherapy for metastatic disease. During this hospital admission, she was informed by her physician that she had a brain lesion that was a metastasis from the breast cancer. After receiving information about the nature, benefits, and risks of the proposed treatment and the effects of no treatment, she consented to treatment. The physician and family decided, however, to withhold information that she had multiple brain lesions. This decision was based on the fact that her brother had died of a primary brain tumor, and it was predicted that disclosure of information about the multiple lesions would be too upsetting for her. The woman did not request any further information about the brain metastasis. However, she did ask the nurse, one day, whether her liver scan was positive or negative. At that point, the physician entered the room and asked the nurse to step outside. He informed her that he, with the concurrence of the family, had decided not to tell the woman that her liver scan was positive. They believed that if the woman knew about the liver involvement, she would not only recognize that her time was limited and consequently become very depressed but also refuse current treatment for her brain metastasis as well as any future cancer therapy.

This situation raises at least two major concerns. First, should family members be given information about a competent patient without the competent patient's consent? (This question will be considered in the section on Confidentiality.) Second, does the nurse have any responsibility in this situation of limited disclosure and apparent invalid consent? (The patient's consent to the current therapy for brain metastasis and to any future cancer therapy is not valid because the patient was not fully informed about the extent of disease and thus about the degree of potential benefit.)

The almost total focus in the literature on the physician's role and responsibility in informed consent suggests that it is totally the prerogative of the physician to decide whether information should be given to a particular patient and to disclose such information. Furthermore, feedback to nurses in many instances in daily practice seems to support this traditional position. However, careful reflection leads to the suggestion that nurses do have a moral responsibility in matters of disclosure.

Role of the nurse

In a consideration of the role of the nurse in disclosure of information, the key issue seems to be as follows: Is the question of whether information should be given to a particular patient with a diagnosis of cancer essentially a medical-scientific one or a moral one? Yarling,[51] in his discussion about whether persons with terminal cancer should be informed about their condition, clearly argues that such questions are essentially moral ones. He notes that although telling the patient requires medical-scientific knowledge, the decision to inform is a moral decision because it recognizes the patient's moral right to such information. Accordingly, Yarling[51] concludes that no one professional group has a special position in making judgments about whether to inform persons with terminal cancer of their condition. Medical expertise cannot be generalized to other areas; therefore nurses and physicians stand as moral equals.

It follows, therefore, that questions regarding disclosure of information in the context of consent to medical treatment or procedures are also essentially moral ones that require morally responsible judgments on the part of nurses as well as physicians. In fact, Pellegrino[52] argues that, although physicians are legally responsible for obtaining a valid consent, all team members are morally responsible for the quality of the consent. Clearly, disclosure of information, an element of informed consent, is an important factor influencing the quality of the consent.

Given that nurses have moral responsibility in disclosure matters and that physicians and nurses may disagree as to the kind and amount of information to provide, it is important that nurses be prepared to articulate their ethical position clearly. Ordinarily, these disagreements involve a physician's decision to limit disclosure rather than to provide complete and full information. The physician may justify, on the basis of acting in the patient's best interests, plans to withhold such information as the extent of disease, a terminal diagnosis, a medically acceptable alternative treatment, or the amount of expected benefit from treatment. Furthermore, the physician may "order" the nurse to avoid disclosing such information. If, however, the nurse, after careful thought, thinks that plans to interfere with the person's right to self-determination are not justified, what course of action should the nurse take?

Initially, the nurse makes an effort to engage the physician in a thoughtful and respectful dialogue. Concurrently, the nurse could also, if the patient wishes, assist the patient to identify the information that he or she might want to know to reach a decision about treatment or care. Through such efforts, the disagreement might be resolved. For example, the nurse might be persuaded by either the physician's arguments or the patient's explicit requests not to be told certain information to change her or his position, or the physician might be persuaded by either the nurse's arguments or the patient's specific requests for information to change her or his position, or the physician and nurse might agree to a mutually acceptable compromise position, such as a plan to assist the patient to ask questions regarding diagnosis, care, and treatment and to provide the information (which was previously to be withheld) within the context of these specific questions.

If, however, the disagreement is not resolved, the nurse will consider the following question: Does the nurse's moral obligation regarding disclosure extend to informing the patient about such matters as diagnosis and medical treatment? There are two distinct contexts in which this question can be asked: (1) the patient is not asking the nurse for information or has directly and specifically requested not to be told, and (2) the patient directly and clearly asks the nurse for information.

In the first context, which through therapeutic interaction is always subject to change, the patient is not exercising his or her moral right to information, and therefore the corresponding moral responsibility for the nurse to disclose the information does not exist.[51] The patient does not have a moral obligation to know. However, it is important to note that if procedures or treatments are being proposed, any consent would be without legal effect.

The second context, however, is more common. Yarling[51] argues as follows regarding disclosure of a terminal diagnosis: Given that the nurse has the medical knowledge and psychosocial skills necessary to make a competent disclosure, collaborates and communicates with the physician before responding to facilitate quality care, and has the requisite rapport with the patient, as evidenced by the patient's asking the nurse, the nurse can be seen as having the moral obligation to disclose the information. The same argument could be applied to situations involving procedures and treatments.

Legally, the situation of the nurse who discloses information that the physician has withheld and perhaps has "ordered" the nurse not to disclose is ambiguous. Would the nurse be seen as interfering with the patient-physician relationship? There seems to be room for precedent-setting action by nurses. Besch[53] takes the following position:

> If one profession has not adequately met the patient's needs or has neglected to tell the patient facts he might consider relevant in making a decision, it is the responsibility of another profession to meet these needs. One does not need permission to foster patient autonomy. The only permission necessary is the patient's. If there is some question that a doctor-patient relationship has been interfered with, it seems reasonable that the patient is capable of deciding this for himself.

This position seems to suggest that prior communication with the physician about plans for disclosure is not necessary. However, communicating with the physician differs from requesting the physician's permission, and communication with the physician before responding to the patient is desirable because it provides the possibility of facilitating quality care. Furthermore, such communication offers the opportunity for further ethical deliberation, which could help to prevent such situations from arising in the future.

Informed Consent

A review of the history of informed consent in the twentieth century reveals that it emerged from two different ethical concerns.[54] In the early years, the primary concern was the protection of the patient from harm and the promotion of the patient's welfare, which, in the research situation meant reduction of risk and avoidance of unfairness and exploitation. During the last two decades, the protection of autonomy has emerged as the primary concern and, indeed, the primary justification for the requirements of informed consent. Thus the primary goal of informed consent in medical care and in research is now considered to be that of enabling individuals to make autonomous decisions about whether to authorize medical and research interventions.[35] This more recent ethical perspective is consistent with twentieth-century American case law, which typically appeals to the right of self-determination as the justifying principle for the requirement of informed consent.[54]

Not surprisingly, the focus of the professional's obligation in informed consent has been influenced by this more recent ethical perspective and case law. In the past, the emphasis was on disclosure of information; now, the focus increasingly is on the *quality* of a patient's or subject's understanding and consent.[35] This shift in emphasis suggests that informed consent increasingly is being viewed as an active ongoing process rather than an isolated event.

The standard elements of informed consent, which can be viewed as imposing conditions for valid consent, have been listed as follows by Beauchamp and Childress[35]: I. Threshold Element: Competence; II. Information Elements: Disclosure of information, Understanding of in-

formation; III. Consent Elements: Voluntariness, Authorization. The following is a discussion, based on the work of Beauchamp and Childress,[35] of each of these conditions.

Competence

To determine whether one ought to solicit a decision from a particular patient, one must determine whether the individual is capable of adequate decision making. Incompetent patients would be unable to give a valid consent or valid refusal of consent to medical procedures. In the following considerations, the term "competence" will not be used in the legal sense but rather will refer to decision-making capacity.

Unfortunately, there is no established standard of competence. Thus determining whether a person is capable of adequate decision making requires judgments about (1) what capacities are needed (capacities range from ability to evidence a choice to ability to reach a reasoned decision), (2) the threshold required for each of the selected capacities, and (3) how these thresholds will be determined.[35]

Decisions by professionals will vary in relation to how the professional balances concerns about benefit and harm with concerns about autonomy; that is, if the professional's primary concern is protection of autonomy, then a less stringent level of capacity and testing will be decided on, but if the primary concern is that patients receive the best medical care, then a more stringent level of capacity and testing will be required.[35] (The reader is referred to Drane's model[55] of competency as an instructive example of how concerns about benefit and harm might be balanced with the importance of autonomy.

Another instructive example of the process of determining competence is offered by Brody,[56] who suggests that there are five capacities that constitute the patient's competency to participate in health care decision making: (1) the ability to receive information, (2) the capacity to remember the information received, (3) the ability to make a decision and give a reason for it, (4) the ability to use the relevant information in making the decision, and (5) the ability to assess the relevant information appropriately.

Brody[56] notes, in his discussion, that it is relatively easy to test, through mental-status examinations, the first two components—that is, to test whether a patient can receive information and the status of the patient's short-term memory—whereas the latter three components are more difficult to define and assess. For example, is the patient not coming to a decision because he is being careful or because, continually vacillating, he cannot make a decision? Is the patient not using the relevant information because he cannot understand it or is denying it or because he finds the information not relevant from the perspective of his values? Does the patient come to a decision that differs from the professional's because the patient is more or less optimistic than the professional or because he truly cannot appropriately estimate outcomes?

The process of determining competence is complex, and the judgments involved are often difficult. However, the importance to patients of a careful evaluation is enormous in that it protects competent patients from being declared incompetent simply because they refuse treatment that professionals judge to be essential to health and protects incompetent patients from being considered competent simply because they agree with the professionals' treatment plan.

Finally, even if a patient is determined, by careful evaluation, to have adequate decision-making capacity, professionals must take the law into account. In general, persons less than 18 years of age are not seen as legally competent to consent, although exceptions may apply, depending on the nature of the decision. However, whether young persons have legal authority to consent should not influence their involvement in the decision-making process. Their role in this process should be consistent with their decisional capacity.

Disclosure of information

The reader is referred to the previous discussion in the section on Telling the Truth.

Understanding of information

Studies suggest that attaining the comprehension necessary for valid consent may be difficult. On the day after signing consent forms for cancer treatment, only 60% of the 200 patients studied by Cassileth et al[57] understood the purpose and nature of the treatment, and only 55% were able to identify one major risk. Similarly, Muss et al[58] found that only 29% of the patients they studied could recognize the purpose of their treatment even though they had signed the consent form. Parenthetically, even if patients in these studies were able to recall the material, this would not necessarily be evidence of comprehension and certainly would not indicate whether patients believed what was disclosed.

Many of the environmental, patient, and communication barriers to achieving comprehension are well known. Thus the focus here will be on those that are less frequently discussed: the framing of information about risk and acceptance of information.

A recent study by McNeil and colleagues[59] reveals that presenting risk information as a gain or a loss influences choices. Three groups of people—outpatients with chronic medical problems, radiologists, and graduate students in business—were asked to make a hypothetical choice between two alternatives for lung cancer: radiation therapy and surgery. In all three groups, preferences were affected by how the information was framed. When the information about surgery was framed in terms of probability of dying, 42% preferred radiation. However, when the information about surgery was framed in terms of probability of survival, only 25% chose radiation over surgery.[59] The implication of this important study is clear: patient comprehension is affected by how risk information is framed.

Distinguishing between patient comprehension of information and patient acceptance of information is important. Some patients may understand the information disclosed and yet may not believe it. For example, a patient may be given all appropriate information about the diagnosis and the proposed radiation therapy treatment and may demonstrate an understanding of the material, and yet he may refuse treatment because he does not believe that he has cancer. As another example, a patient may demonstrate full understanding about a phase 1 clinical trial, but his agreement to participate is based on the false belief that he will be cured; that is, he does not believe the information about the purpose of the study.

Some might argue that false beliefs are evidence of lack of understanding and that it is not possible to judge a patient as comprehending if he evidences false beliefs. There seems to be a difference, however, between objective understanding of disclosed information and subjective integration of that information. If so, then it is possible to judge a patient who has false beliefs as having comprehension of the disclosed information. Interventions to assist these individuals include more than providing information or simply correcting a false belief that is based on misinformation. Thus the reason for suggesting that comprehension and acceptance not be conflated becomes clearer.

Voluntariness

The key question in determining whether the patient is free to act is as follows: Is the patient free from controlling influences? In general, influences can be divided into three major categories: coercion, manipulation, and persuasion.[35]

Beauchamp and Childress[35] view coercion as the intentional use of "a credible and severe threat of harm or force to control another." An example of coercion is a threat by a professional to abandon a patient unless the patient complies with treatment. In contrast, persuasion occurs when a person is convinced by logical reasoning to believe in something. Manipulation consists of getting people to do what the manipulator wants by means other than coercion or persuasion, such as lying, withholding of information, or distortion of the facts.

Influences that are coercive or manipulative are controlling influences; influences that are persuasive are not controlling in that they appeal to reason. However, professionals must be aware that some attempts to persuade may bypass reasoning or irrationally influence the patient and thus become controlling; for example, distressing information may overwhelm a patient with fear and panic and thus bypass reasoning; patients who are weak and dependent may not be able to resist influences that they ordinarily would and thus even attempts at rational persuasion may irrationally influence them.[35]

Authorization

Simply electing a medical intervention is not sufficient. The patient must give approval or consent.

Summary

For the consent of a patient or subject to be considered valid, the consent must be competent (legally), voluntary, informed, and comprehending. *Since all members of the health care team are morally responsible for the quality of the consent,[52] nurses should be prepared to participate in disclosure of information, evaluation of decision-making capacity, facilitation of understanding, and mitigation of patients' vulnerabilities. In addition, they should ensure that consent has actually been given before proceeding with treatment.*

Research Involving Human Subjects

Cancer care nurses continually are involved in research involving human subjects. This involvement may be as investigator, member of a research team or institutional review board, clinician, or user of results. Therefore an understanding of the ethical considerations of the conduct of clinical research is essential.

Six general ethical norms emerge from the various codes and regulations on research involving human subjects.[60] There should be (1) good research design, (2) competent investigators, (3) a favorable balance of harm and benefit, (4) informed consent, (5) equitable selection of subjects, and (6) compensation for research-related injury.

The reader is referred to the American Nurses' Association's *Human Rights Guidelines for Nurses in Clinical and Other Research.*[61] The following discussion will address some of the ethical concerns in clinical research from two broad perspectives: the design of the research and the involvement of human subjects.

Research design

Good research design is one of the conditions necessary for justifying research on human subjects. Evidence of this requirement can be found in the Nuremberg Code[62] and the Declaration of Helsinki[63]:

> The experiment should be so designed and based on the results of animal experimentation and a knowledge of the natural history of the disease or other problems under study that the anticipated results will justify the performance of the experiment. [Nuremberg Code 3]
> Biomedical research involving human subjects must conform to generally accepted scientific principles and should be based on adequately performed laboratory and animal experimentation and on a thorough knowledge of the scientific literature. [Helsinki 1.1]

In addition, the US Department of Health and Human Services (DHHS) regulations[46] (Section 26.111a) charge the institutional review board (IRB) to make a determination of the "importance of the knowledge that may reasonably be expected to result." Levine[60] suggests that this statement may be construed as a charge to the IRB to make determinations as to the adequacy of research design.

Generally, a review of research design involves attention to scientific validity, benefit-risk ratio for the human subject, investigator bias, and methods of analysis. Consider the situation of the controlled clinical trial with a randomization procedure. Such a design could certainly minimize investigator bias, but the benefit-risk ratio for the human subjects also must be explored. Rutstein's commentary[64] on a proposal to perform internal mammary artery operations for angina pectoris (which uncontrolled evidence had suggested might be helpful) on one group of patients and sham operations on the control group is instructive for two reasons: It demonstrates the ethical importance of benefit-risk ratio considerations, and it serves to highlight the tremendous need for stronger research guidelines. Rutstein[64] states:

> Although scientifically sound, I do not believe that it is ethical to perform sham operations on human subjects because of the operative risk and the lack of potential benefit to the patient. Instead, controlled studies could have been performed with randomly allocated control patients being given the best medical treatment of the time together with a period of bed rest similar to that of the surgical convalescent.

Current DHHS regulations clearly mandate a favorable balance between the projected benefits and the projected harms[46]: "Risks to the subjects (must be) reasonable in relation to anticipated benefits, if any, to subjects, and the importance of the knowledge that may reasonably be expected to result" (DHHS, Section 46.111a).

Identifying a design that is both scientifically valid and meets the benefit-risk requirements calls for careful deliberation. Sutnick and colleagues[65] demonstrate such deliberations in their discussion regarding studies to test the effectiveness of screening methods. First, a controlled clinical trial could be designed in which an identified population at high risk for cancer could be randomly divided into two subgroups, one receiving the screening techniques and the other serving as the control subjects; no change in care would be offered to the control group. Sutnick and colleagues[65] point out that such a design raises serious ethical questions. For example, the control group, known to be at high risk for cancer, will most likely not receive any benefits and might indeed be harmed. This potential harm could arise from the possibility that the control group "for whom more extensive screening procedures are not recommended will have the false security of feeling that they are not required."[65]

The authors[65] therefore consider the possibility of telling the control group about their increased risk and advising them to have periodic examinations. They decide, however, that such an action would probably minimize the difference between the subgroups and render the information obtained from the study less conclusive. Finally, they conclude that an alternative design is needed. They suggest an adaptive design in which the study group is selected from a large population that is already under medical surveillance for other reasons: "In this way, a representative sample could be selected for the institution of screening procedures and appropriate follow-up, while prospective or even retrospective examination of the records of the remainder of the population, or of a similarly selected or evenly matched sample population, could serve as the control observations."[65]

Decisions about benefits and risks are not limited, however, to the preimplementation period:

> During the course of the experiment the scientist in charge must be prepared to terminate the experiment at any stage, if he has probable cause to believe . . . that a continuation . . . is likely to result in injury, disability or death to the experimental subject. [Nuremberg Code 10[62]]
>
> The investigator . . . should discontinue the research if in his/her . . . judgment it may, if continued, be harmful to the individual. [Declaration of Helsinki 111.3[63]]
>
> Where appropriate, the research plan makes adequate provision for monitoring the data collected to insure safety of the subjects. [DHHS, Section 46.111a[46]]
>
> An IRB shall have authority to suspend or terminate approval of research . . . that has been associated with unexpected serious harm to subjects. [DHHS, Section 46.113[46]]

Clearly, to make such decisions in situations involving controlled clinical trials with randomization procedures, the method of data analysis must be valid.

Research subjects

Usually, concerns regarding the ethical involvement of human subjects focus on such considerations as whether there is good and ethical research design, including a favorable balancing of harms and benefits along with measures to maximize benefits and reduce harms; adequate provisions for the protection of privacy and maintenance of confidentiality of data; and valid consent. Although these considerations are both essential and important, explicit attention must also be given to the equitable distribution of the harms and benefits of research. This concern raises questions regarding subject selection. The following discussion highlights considerations and recommendations on subject selection by Levine.[60]

Selection of subjects based exclusively on informed consent may result in inequitable distribution of the harms and benefits of research. Although truly autonomous persons are capable of adequately negotiating informed consent, those with diminished autonomy may not be able to look after their own best interests; that is, they may accept an unfair share of the burdens of research participation. Levine[60] defines those persons who are incapable of protecting their own interests as vulnerable and includes uneducated subjects; seriously ill persons who are desperate and willing to take any risk for a possibility of relief; those with dependent relationships who fear that they will place their relationships in jeopardy if they refuse to cooperate with the investigator; members of minority groups who are impoverished, seriously ill, or dependent; and elderly persons with reduced capacities.

Involving vulnerable persons in research is not forbidden by codes and regulations, but it must be justified. Justification becomes more difficult, however, as the degree of risk and the degree of vulnerability increase. Therefore, efforts must be made to reduce the ethical problems associated with selecting vulnerable persons as

research subjects. In general, these efforts are directed toward improving the quality of the consent. This may include clarifying the fact that individuals have a right to refuse to participate in research or to withdraw at any time without prejudicing their care or relationships. If, however, patients' capacity for consent cannot adequately be increased, then they should be excluded from the study and less vulnerable persons from the populations being studied should be selected.[60]

In the field of cancer medical research, one area of intense concern regarding patient vulnerability is the situation of phase 1 clinical studies.[66] In these studies, patients with advanced cancer whose disease is not amenable to known effective treatment constitute the population from which subjects are selected. In addition, these studies ordinarily offer only a remote possibility of any medical therapeutic benefit for enrolled patients[67]; the potential benefit is for future patients with cancer.

Some might suggest that members of this population be considered as a vulnerable group. This does not seem appropriate, because they are not homogeneous in regard to such factors as degree of desperateness or willingness to take any risk, perceptions of imminent death, and concerns about prejudicing their relationships with professionals. To consider these persons as vulnerable would suggest, among other things, that all patients with advanced cancer whose disease is not amenable to therapy are incapable of looking after their own best interests.

However, the capacity of some does not mean that many other individuals within this population are not vulnerable. Thus it is appropriate to consider each patient as potentially vulnerable and to take measures to improve the quality of consent in the event that it is needed. Such measures may include defining more clearly the fact that the expected benefits are for future patients; assuring patients that their relationships and care will not be prejudiced if they refuse to participate; and outlining the kind of care (eg, support, symptom control, and monitoring for unexpected events) that can be provided if the patient does not participate. In some instances, it may be necessary for the investigator to decide or for other health professionals to recommend that a patient not be selected for study.

Confidentiality

Basic to an understanding of the issues of confidentiality is an appreciation of the fact that privacy and confidentiality are two distinct concepts even though the concepts partially overlap and the terms are often used interchangeably. Privacy can be defined as "the freedom of the individual to pick and choose for himself the time and circumstances under which, and most importantly, the extent to which, his attitudes, beliefs, behavior and opinions are to be shared with or withheld from others."[68] Respect for privacy requires that professionals not invade patients' privacy (through such activities as taking a personal history; touching, listening to, or observing the body; or conducting tests) without their permission.

In the situation of a patient's voluntary admission to a

hospital, there is both explicit and implicit consent to limited losses of privacy. However, the patient's voluntary admission to the hospital does not grant unlimited access.[35] The right to restrict some access is reflected in the American Hospital Association's *Statement on a Patient's Bill of Rights*,[69] which states that persons not directly involved in a patient's care must have the permission of the patient to be present.

In contemporary society, the most poignant example of a privacy issue is the screening and testing of individuals to determine whether they have antibodies to the human immunodeficiency virus (HIV). Some proposed policies would infringe on privacy in that they would not involve permission or consent; that is, screening or testing would be mandatory. Whether such infringements are justified and, if so, under what conditions remain matters of continuing debate. The point is that this particular aspect of the acquired immunodeficiency syndrome (AIDS) debate is about whether intrusions into individuals' privacy are justified, not about what to do with the private information (that persons have detectable antibodies or AIDS) once it is generated; the question of what to do with, or how to manage, private information is a confidentiality issue.

In general, respect for confidentiality requires that private information that is shared by a patient, whether through words or an examination, not be disclosed to others without the patient's authorization. Although most professionals accept this ideal, there are informational needs in the contemporary health care setting that have altered the meaning of confidentiality.[35] The large and diversified health care team needs relevant information to provide care for the patient; therefore, in most cancer care settings today, information shared by the patient with one health professional is usually disclosed to other health professionals involved in the patient's care, except for information that is judged to be "confidential." In addition there are numerous other persons with legitimate needs and responsibilities to examine the patient's chart.

The difficulty is that many patients do not know about these practices. In addition, judgments about what information is too "confidential" to disclose, either verbally with other members of the health care team or in the chart, are made by the health professional. Patients should be informed about these contemporary practices so that they, not the health care professional, can decide what is too "confidential" to be disclosed.

Bok[70] points out, however, that there are justifiable limits to the obligation of confidentiality. Walters,[71] in an earlier work, identified three possible grounds for violating the principle of confidentiality. First, the principle may come into conflict with the rights of the patient himself. As an example, a temporarily but seriously depressed patient with cancer may tell the nurse "in confidence" that he plans to commit suicide. In such a life-threatening situation, the nurse's duty to act in the patient's best interest might require temporarily interfering with the patient's self-determination by disclosing, without the patient's consent but with the patient's knowledge, the information to a third party.

Second, the principle of confidentiality may be violated

when it conflicts with the rights of an innocent third party.[71] As a contemporary example, a patient, on being told that HIV antibodies have been detected in his serum, not only refuses to tell his wife but insists that the health care professional maintain absolute confidentiality. If the professional is unable to persuade the patient either to disclose the information or to give permission for the disclosure, then a strong ethical argument can be made that the professional should disclose the portion of the information that is necessary to protect the wife from harm.[35] (The reader is referred to a report by the American Medical Association's Council on Ethical and Judicial Affairs[72] for the medical profession's position on and procedures for warning third parties.)

Finally, the principle of confidentiality may be violated when there exists a serious conflict between the principle and the rights or interests of society in general.[71] One type of situation involves persons with communicable diseases. For many years, it was agreed that the mandatory reporting of persons with communicable diseases by health care professionals to public health officials was justified; that is, the public health objectives underlying the reporting requirements were substantial enough to justify the violation of confidentiality. However, in the specific situation of a new disease, AIDS, new and complex questions have been raised. Currently the focus is not, for the most part, on mandatory reporting of AIDS. (All states require the reporting of AIDS, as defined by the Centers for Disease Control, to public health officials.[73]) Rather, the focus is on proposals that would require the mandatory reporting of HIV-positive test results with identifiers. Some would argue that the public health objectives are not substantial enough at this time to justify either a violation of confidentiality or the possibility of serious harm from wrongful and damaging public disclosure of the information.

With the three broad categories of justified exceptions to the obligation for confidentiality in mind, it seems that disclosures of information to family members without the competent patient's consent cannot, in general, be ethically justified. One approach to this not uncommon problem would be to assist patients to clarify and explicitly to communicate what information they want shared and with whom. In this way, disclosures to family members without patient consent would require strong explicit justification by any health team member proposing such action.

CONCLUSION

This chapter focuses on bioethical decision making in the context of cancer nursing practice. Special emphasis is placed on relationships in cancer care and the challenge of protecting and promoting patient self-determination. The issues of telling the truth, informed consent, research on human subjects, and confidentiality are used to illustrate ethical deliberation and explore advocacy nursing.

FUTURE TRENDS

To promote continued growth and development in ethical decision making, cancer nurses may wish to develop a forum for deliberation within their practice settings.[74] These discussions initially could be among nurse colleagues and then expand to include other health care professionals. The outcome of such discussions could be the prevention of some recurring ethical dilemmas; the clarification of professional responsibilities, particularly in relation to persons who have detectable HIV antibodies; the development of research studies; and the identification of areas for action on the public policy level.

One of the most urgent issues in the latter category is the "fair" allocation of limited health care resources; that is, who should receive what kind of care. Cancer nurses must become active in considering these and other questions involving distributive justice.

REFERENCES

1. Davis AJ, Aroskar MA: Ethical Dilemmas and Nursing Practice (ed 2). Norwalk, Conn, Appleton-Century-Crofts, 1983.
2. Gorovitz S: Bioethics and social responsibility, in Beauchamp TL, Walters L (eds): Contemporary Issues in Bioethics. Encino, Calif, Dickenson, 1978, pp 52-60.
3. Yarling RR, McElmurry BJ: The moral foundation of nursing. Adv Nurs Sci 8:63-73, 1986.
4. Bishop AH, Scudder JR: Nursing ethics in an age of controversy. Adv Nurs Sci 9:34-43, 1987.
5. Cooper MC: Covenantal relationships: grounding for the nursing ethic. Adv Nurs Sci 10:48-59, 1988.
6. Packard JS, Ferrara M: In search of the moral foundation of nursing. Adv Nurs Sci 10:60-71, 1988.
7. Yeo M: Integration of nursing theory and nursing ethics. Adv Nurs Sci 11:33-42, 1989.
8. Thompson JE, Thompson HO: Teaching ethics to nursing students. Nurs Outlook 37:84-88, 1989.
9. Veatch RM: Case Studies in Medical Ethics. Cambridge, Mass, Harvard University Press, 1977.
10. Beauchamp TI: Ethical theory, in Beauchamp TL, Walters L (eds): Contemporary Issues in Bioethics. Encino, Calif, Dickenson, 1978, pp 1-5.
11. Taylor P: Utilitarianism, in Beauchamp TL, Walters L (eds): Contemporary Issues in Bioethics. Encino, Calif, Dickenson, 1978, pp 12-22.
12. Campbell AV: Moral Dilemmas in Medicine. New York, Churchill Livingstone, 1975.
13. Veatch RM: Death, Dying, and the Biological Revolution: Our Last Quest for Responsibility (ed 1). New Haven, Conn, Yale University Press, 1976.
14. Childress J: Ethical issues in the experimentation with human subjects. Conn Med 43:26-31, 1979.
15. Pellegrino ED: Protection of patients' rights and the doctor-patient relationship. Prev Med 4:398-403, 1975.
16. Curtin LL: The nurse as advocate: A philosophical foundation for nursing. Adv Nurs Sci 3:1-10, 1979.
17. Bandman EL: The rights of nurses and patients: A case for advocacy, in Bandman EL, Bandman B (eds): Bioethics and Human Rights. Boston, Little, Brown, 1978, pp 332-338.
18. Gadow S: Humanistic issues at the interface of nursing and the community. Conn Med 41:357-361, 1977.
19. Donahue MP: The nurse: A patient advocate? Nurs Forum 17:143-151, 1978.
20. Kohnke M: The nurse as advocate. Am J Nurs 80:2038-2040, 1980.
21. Laszewski M: Patient advocacy in primary nursing. Nurs Adm Q 5:28-30, 1981.
22. Brower HT: Advocacy: what it is. J Gerontol Nurs 8:141-143, 1982.
23. Fay P: In support of patient advocacy as a nursing role. Nurs Outlook 26:252-353, 1978 (editorial).
24. Namerow MJ: Integrating advocacy into the gerontological nursing major. J Gerontol Nurs 8:149-151, 1982.
25. Ash CR: Are you an advocate? Cancer Nursing: An International Journal for Cancer Care 7:447, 1984 (editorial).
26. Winslow GR: From loyalty to advocacy: a new metaphor for nursing. Hastings Cent Rep 14:32-40, 1984.
27. Nelson ML: Advocacy in nursing. Nurs Outlook 36:136-141, 1988.
28. Gadow S: Advocacy nursing and new meanings of aging. Nurs Clin North Am 14:81-91, 1979.
29. Gadow S: Existential advocacy, in Spicker SF, Gadow S (eds): Nursing: Images and Ideals. New York, Springer, 1980, pp 79-101.
30. Gadow S: A model for ethical decision-making. Oncol Nurs Forum 7:44-47, 1980.
31. Gadow S: An ethical case for patient self-determination. Semin Oncol Nurs 5:99-101, 1989.
32. Gadow S: Clinical subjectivity: advocacy with silent patients. Nurs Clin North Am 24:535-541, 1989.
33. American Nurses' Association, Oncology Nursing Society: Standards of Oncology Nursing Practice. Kansas City, Mo, American Nurses' Association, 1987.
34. Bok S: Lying: Moral Choices in Public and Private Life. New York, Pantheon Books, 1978.
35. Beauchamp TL, Childress JF: Principles of Biomedical Ethics (ed 3). New York, Oxford University Press, 1989.
36. Veatch RM: Death, Dying, and the Biologic Revolution: Our Last Quest for Responsibility (ed 2). New Haven, Conn, Yale University Press, 1989.
37. Fitts WL Jr, Ravdin IS: What Philadelphia physicians tell patients. JAMA 153:901-904, 1953.
38. Friedman HJ: Physician management of dying patients. Psychiatry Med 1:295-305, 1970.
39. Mount BM, Jones A, Patterson A: Death and dying: Attitudes in a teaching hospital. Urology 4:741-747, 1974.
40. Travis TA, Noyes R Jr, Brightwell DR: The attitude of physicians toward prolonging life. Int J Psychiatry Med 5:17-26, 1974.
41. Novack DH, Plumer R, Smith RI, et al: Changes in physicians' attitudes toward telling the cancer patient. JAMA 241:897-900, 1979.
42. Oken D: What to tell cancer patients: A study of medical attitudes. JAMA 173:1120-1128, 1961.
43. Gadow S: Advocacy and paternalism in cancer nursing, in McCorkle R, Hongladarom G (eds): Issues and Topics in Cancer Nursing. Norwalk, Conn, Appleton-Century-Crofts, 1986, pp 19-28.
44. Schoene-Seifert B, Childress JF: How much should the cancer patient know and decide? CA 36:85-94, 1986.
45. Angell M: Respecting the autonomy of competent patients. N Engl J Med 310:1115-1116, 1984.
46. US Department of Health and Human Services: Final reg-

ulations amending basic HHS policy for the protection of human research subjects: final rules: 45 CFR 46. Federal Register: Rules and Regulations 46:8366-8392, 1981.

47. Rosoff AJ: Informed Consent. Rockville, Md, Aspen, 1981.
48. Veatch RM, Fry ST: Case Studies in Nursing Ethics. Philadelphia, JB Lippincott, 1987.
49. Blumenfield M, Levy N, Kaufman D: The wish to be informed of a fatal illness. Omega 9:323-326, 1978–1979.
50. Hatfield CB, Hatfield RE, Geggie PHS, et al: Attitudes about death, dying, and terminal care: differences among groups at a university teaching hospital. Omega 14:51-63, 1983–1984.
51. Yarling RR: Ethical analysis of a nursing problem: the scope of nursing practice in disclosing the truth to terminal patients—an inquiry directed to the National Joint Practice Commission of the AMA and the ANA. Part I and Part II. Supervisor Nurse 9:28-34, 40-50, 1978.
52. Pellegrino ED: The moral foundations for valid consent. Proceedings of the American Cancer Society Third National Conference on Human Values and Cancer. New York, American Cancer Society, Inc, 1981, pp 171-177.
53. Besch LB: Informed consent: a patient's right. Nurs Outlook 27:32-35, 1979.
54. Faden RR, Beauchamp TL (in collaboration with King NNP): A History and Theory of Informed Consent. New York, Oxford, 1986.
55. Drane JF: The many faces of competency. Hastings Cent Rep 15:17-21, 1985.
56. Brody B: Life and Death Decision Making. New York, Oxford, 1988.
57. Cassileth BR, Zupkis RV, Stuton-Smith K, et al: Informed consent—why are its goals imperfectly realized? N Engl J Med 302:896-900, 1980.
58. Muss HB, White DR, Michielutte R, et al: Written informed consent in patients with breast cancer. Cancer 43:1545-1550, 1979.
59. McNeil BJ, Pauker SG, Sox HC, et al: On the elicitation of preferences for alternative therapies. N Engl J Med 306:1259-1262, 1982.

60. Levine RJ: Ethics and Regulation of Clinical Research (ed 2). New Haven, Conn, Yale University Press, 1988.
61. American Nurses' Association: Human Rights Guidelines for Nurses in Clinical and Other Research. Kansas City, Mo, American Nurses' Association, 1985.
62. Nuremberg Code, 1964, in Reich WT (ed): Encyclopedia of Bioethics, vol 4. New York, The Free Press, 1978, pp 1764-1765.
63. World Medical Association Declaration of Helsinki as Revised by the 29th World Medical Assembly, October, 1975, in Beauchamp TL, Walters L (eds): Contemporary Issues in Bioethics. Encino, Calif, Dickenson, 1975, pp 405-407.
64. Rutstein D: The ethical design of human experiments, in Beauchamp TL, Walters L (eds): Contemporary Issues in Bioethics. Encino, Calif, Dickenson, 1975, pp 421-426.
65. Sutnick A, et al: Ethical issues in investigation of screening strategies. Med Pediatr Oncol 3:133-136, 1977.
66. Lipsett MB: On the nature and ethics of phase 1 clinical trials of cancer chemotherapies. JAMA 248:941-942, 1982.
67. Lipsett MB: Ethics of phase 1 clinical trials. JAMA 249:883, 1983.
68. Kelman HC: Privacy and research with human beings. J Soc Issues 33:169-195, 1977.
69. American Hospital Association. Statement on a patient's bill of rights. Hospitals 4:41, 1973.
70. Bok S: The limits of confidentiality. Hastings Cent Rep 13:24-31, 1983.
71. Walters L: Ethical aspects of medical confidentiality, in Beauchamp TL, Walters L (eds): Contemporary Issues in Bioethics. Encino, Calif, Dickenson, 1975, pp 169-175.
72. Council on Ethical and Judicial Affairs. Ethical issues involved in the growing AIDS crisis. JAMA 259:1360-1361, 1988.
73. Gostin LO: Public health strategies for confronting AIDS: legislative and regulatory policy in the United States. JAMA 261:1621-1630, 1989.
74. Donovan CT: Toward a nursing ethics program in an acute care setting. Top Clin Nurs 5:55-62, 1983.

Chapter 56

Unproven Methods of Cancer Treatment

Connie Henke Yarbro, RN, BSN

INTRODUCTION

Defined as "methods that have not been shown to be active in tumor animal models or in acceptable clinical trials and yet are promoted as effective methods for the cure, palliation, and control of cancer," unproven methods are a major concern for health care professionals in the United States.[1] Unproven, unorthodox, and alternative treatments have existed for decades and continue to be a problem today, with the public spending four billion dollars a year on unproven cancer cures.[2,3] Questionable nutritional supplements alone are a two-billion-dollar-a-year business in the United States.[4] According to Cassileth and colleagues,[5-8] more than half of all cancer patients eventually try an unproven method either in conjunction with conventional treatment or as a substitute for treatment.

In a discussion of unproven methods, it is important to remember that for thousands of years, individuals in need of medical care have turned to those who were offering what they felt or hoped would meet their needs. Only in relatively recent times has the scientific method, in conjunction with organized medicine and government, been able to provide a measure of confidence in a given treatment's safety and efficacy.

HISTORICAL PERSPECTIVES

Before the Food and Drug Act of 1906, thousands of unproven treatments were promoted to the American public. Often the treatments were not harmful in themselves, but as an anonymous physician of the era noted in a letter to the *National Quarterly Review,* "Quackery kills a larger number annually than the disease it pretends to cure."[9]

Advertisements frequently guaranteed the effectiveness of a particular treatment. For example, promotions for "Dr. Chamlee's Cancer Specific," which appeared in the 1930s, informed readers that "any lump in [a] woman's breast is cancer" and "any tumor, lump, or sore on the lip, face, or anywhere six months is, nearly always, cancer."[9] Dr. Chamlee's treatment involved "no knife or pain, no x-ray or other swindle." The promoter of this treatment was so confident that he required no payment until the person was cured. He further promised to pay $1000 to any individual he failed to cure of cancer. With sufficient information to evaluate these treatments, fewer qualified medical experts to consult with, and human nature being what it is, it is not difficult to understand how such a promoter could make a fortune.

Even well-intentioned and educated individuals were duped. In 1748 the Virginia General Assembly, whose members included George Washington and James Madison, appointed a committee to investigate the efficacy of Mary Johnson's recipe for curing cancer. The cure included sorrel, bark celandine, and springwater. Witnesses' statements that they had been cured of various cancers were read into the Assembly's record, and in good time the legislators voted that Mrs. Johnson's recipe was indeed effective in treating cancer and consequently awarded her 100 pounds for her achievement.[10]

The promotion of unproven methods was not significantly affected even by the passage of the Food and Drug Act in 1906. Janssen[11] reported that in 1910 a crucial test of the new law found the US Supreme Court ruling that the law involved only the truthful labeling of ingredients used in drugs, not the false therapeutic claims on the drug label. Justice Oliver Wendell Holmes, Jr, concluded that individuals could not be prosecuted for what he termed "mistaken praise" of their treatments even though the claims were false.

Noting the dangers of permitting unsafe and ineffective drugs on the market, President Taft exhorted the Congress, in 1911, to pass tougher legislation:

> There are none so credulous as sufferers from disease. The need is urgent for legislation which will prevent the raising of false hopes of speedy cures of serious ailment by misstatements of facts as to the worthless mixtures on which the sick will rely while their disease progresses unchecked.[12]

In 1912 Congress passed the Sherley Amendment, which stated that it was a crime to make false or fraudulent claims regarding the therapeutic efficacy of a drug. The problem encountered with this legislation was that it was necessary to prove that the promoter intended to defraud the public. Mistaken claims could still be made, and patients could continue to be defrauded. In 1938 Congress eliminated this difficulty by passing legislation that required scientific proof of safety before a drug could be marketed. This law was the direct result of a disaster in which over 200 individuals lost their lives. A drug promoter had marketed a sulfanilamide with a diluting agent consisting of automobile antifreeze.

In 1962 Congress clarified some of the language of the previous legislation and further added that drugs must demonstrate efficacy in addition to safety before they can be marketed. Thus a process was created by which a substance can become approved for prescription use. First, a sponsoring group submits data, generally first from animal studies that demonstrate some measure of safety and probable efficacy. The sponsor then files an Investigational New Drug (IND) application with the Food and Drug Administration (FDA). If approved, clinical testing with human volunteers is permitted. Following the completion of clinical testing, the company may make the drug available if it can be determined reliably that the drug is indeed safe and effective.

The Food and Drug Commissioner[13] noted that the Food and Drug Act of 1962 means that the "the absolute freedom to choose an ineffective drug was properly surrendered in exchange for the freedom from danger to each person's health and well-being from the sale and use of worthless drugs." This is, in fact, the same decision made by those in government who have decided over the years that only persons certified by experts may practice medicine and are qualified to help the patients who would choose to seek their assistance.[13] Although the Food and Drug Act of 1962 frequently has been challenged over the years by those who promote unproven methods, the act was upheld by a decision of the US Supreme Court in 1973.

MOTIVATIONS FOR THE USE OF UNPROVEN METHODS

People in the twentieth century seek unproven methods in conjunction with or in lieu of standard medical procedures for many of the same reasons their ancestors did. Following are some of the more common reasons:

- "I have nothing to lose."

- "If it won't hurt me, why not?"

- "I want to feel that I tried everything."

- "They wouldn't put that in the papers if it wasn't true."

- "The doctor told me there is nothing more that can be done."

- "I heard of a person who was terminal, took it, and was cured."

Cancer creates many fears, such as fear of death, an uncertain future, pain, mutilation, loss of family, dependency, alienation, and costly medical care. Given these fears, it is not difficult to understand that many individuals with cancer are in great need of hope and are likely to seek out those individuals who seem most capable of providing this desired commodity. Unfettered by standard methods, ethics, and regulations, a purveyor of unproven methods has a distinct advantage over individuals within the established medical system. The current norm is for a person to be informed of treatment alternatives, all of which necessarily have risks that are inextricably linked with a potentially positive outcome. Emotionally, an individual may regret having ever gone to the physician who diagnosed cancer. Cancer patients want a treatment without risks and pain and with a good probability of cure. Yet they are confused and frustrated by some reports claiming that cancer is a curable disease with a cure rate approaching 50% and others claiming that no major advances have been made in treatment of the major types of cancer.[7,8] Turning to some dietary or enzyme therapy that promises no side effects or uses "the body's natural defenses" may coincide with patients' fantasies about being cured. That is, by utilizing unconventional therapy, the patient hopes for an unconventional cure.[14]

The use of an unproven method may provide an individual with a greater sense of control. This desire for control may partially be a response to fear but may also be a reaction to the feeling of being merely a passive recipient of treatments designated by the health care team rather than being a partner in the fight against the disease.

Better educated and highly motivated patients fighting their disease are more likely to turn to unproven methods because the promoters of such methods falsely promise that "you can control your disease."[5,15,16] The age-old cry of the quack, placing the blame of failure on the patient, remains: "It is the patient's fault if it fails. You came to us too late."[17] Inasmuch as the provider of unproven methods is often supplying an illegal or unapproved therapy requested by the patient with cancer, a bond may easily be formed between them. This relationship may assist the person with cancer in rebelling against his or her fate and the medical system that provided the fearful diagnosis of cancer. The promoter of unproven methods often appears to be an underdog battling the medical system to make some new risk-free treatment available to neglected people with cancer. Those individuals within the conventional medical system may be seen as profiting from the plight of the poor and sick. The purveyors of unproven methods frequently suggest that the government and organized medicine are in a conspiracy against curing cancer. It is easy for the cancer patient to identify with the isolation projected by the marketer of unproven methods. Patients with cancer frequently resent those who do not have it. It is perfectly acceptable for an individual to feel this way, but it is also important for the health care professional to ensure that this anger does not interfere with communication. The patient with cancer who is made to feel persecuted might seek out someone who "understands," even if—or especially if—the new care provider is also at odds with established medicine.

Other influences for using unproven methods can come from pressures exerted by family or friends.[18] The family often plays the most important role in providing emotional support. Family members, who have many of the same fears as the patient with cancer, are susceptible to the same influences. They often share responsibility for deciding the patient's treatment, and this responsibility itself can be overwhelming and frightening. "We want to feel that we tried everything" is commonly heard from concerned family members. The health care provider also may hear an unspoken wish to avoid guilt if the patient with cancer does not recover. Not being in a position to understand completely what treatments can and cannot do, the family may feel that the best course is to try everything with the hope that something will work. In turn, the patient with cancer may feel obligated to meet the family's expectation to submit to these treatments or may be afraid of alienating his or her support system at this crucial time by doing otherwise. In contrast, others might want to try everything. In such instances the family might feel pressured to unearth "cancer cures," and friends may bring in newspaper articles or stories that tell of someone who was cured by some method or another. Although the friend's intentions are admirable, such information might foster feelings of guilt in the patient with cancer or in the family members if these avenues are not explored.

Even with the best intentions of all parties concerned, the course of the disease can be torturous for everyone. How difficult this time will be greatly depends on the types of personalities and relationships that existed before the cancer was diagnosed, the quality of communication that takes place, the availability of accurate information on treatment options and outcomes, and the effects of disease and therapy.

UNPROVEN METHODS: 1940s TO 1970s

Unproven approaches to cancer treatment have existed for centuries, and a specific alternative seems to develop and thrive during each decade. Examples of unorthodox approaches, listed according to their eras of popularity, are identified in Table 56-1. We have gone from the nineteenth-century "holistic," or "natural," movement to the so-called-drug approach of the early and mid 1900s, and back to the holistic, natural, or diet-oriented regimens of today.[7] According to Cassileth et al,[5-8] among all unproven therapies today, the most commonly used are, in order of frequency, metabolic therapy, diet therapy, megavitamin therapy, mental imagery, faith or spiritual healing, and "immune" therapy. The following discussion will review the alternative approaches from the era of the 1940s through the 1980s.

Koch Antitoxin Therapy: 1940s to 1950s

First mentioned in 1919,[19] the Koch antitoxin therapy was a popular unproven cancer treatment during the 1940s and 1950s. The treatment consisted of extremely pure distilled water mixed with one part per trillion of a chemical called glyoxylide. Glyoxylide is merely glyoxylic acid with water removed. Glyoxylic acid is a normal body constituent, but it would take nearly a trillion of the 2 mL ampules that Koch distributed to equal the quantity the body produces normally in a single day.[13] Koch proposed that cancer was caused by a microorganism that was susceptible to the differential poison in his antitoxins. Associated therapies included enemas and a special diet. Over 3000 health practitioners in the United States employed this regimen, paying $25 per ampule for it and charging patients as much as $300 for a single injection.[11] The Koch Cancer Foundation promoted the treatment through lectures, pamphlets, and magazines. In 1942 the Food and Drug Administration held hearings across the United States in an effort to gather information regarding the promotion and use of the Koch antitoxins. In 1943, Dr. Koch was indicted. Although 43 expert witnesses testified that the Koch method was a worthless cancer therapy, the defense produced 104 witnesses who alleged that the treatment was useful in the management of some 69 diseases, including herpes zoster, appendicitis, allergies, and cancer. A mistrial was declared after the jury could not come to a unanimous decision.

TABLE 56-1 EXAMPLES OF MAJOR UNORTHODOX APPROACHES 1800—PRESENT

Era Popular In US	Unorthodox Approach
1800–1850	Thompsonianism Belief: All disease results from one general cause (cold), and can be cured by one general remedy (heat). Opposed "mineral" drugs and the "tyranny" of doctors. Remedy: Emetics and hot baths.
1850–1900	Homeopathy Belief: Like cures like ("Law of Similia"); disease results from suppressed itch ("psora"). Remedy: More than 3000 different drugs, each a highly distilled organic or inorganic substance.
1890–	Naturopathy Belief: Disease results not from external bacteria but from violation of natural laws of living; drugs are harmful; "natural" products and activities cure. Remedy: Diets, massages, colonic irrigation.
1890–	Early Osteopathy and Chiropractic Belief: Mechanistic view of the body; disease caused by dislocation of bones in spine. Rejected drugs and germ theory. Remedy: Spinal manipulation.
1900s	Tablet and Ointment Cancer Cures Bye, Buchanan, Chamlee, Curry, Leach (Cancerol), Mixer, Griffith (Radio-sulpho), Warner, Wells (Radol).
1920s	"Energy" Cancer Cures Abrams (Radio Wave cure}, Brown (Radio Therapy), Kay (cosmic energy "vrilium"), Ghadiali (Spectro-Chrome Light Therapy); Cayce's psychic diagnoses and treatments
1940s	Koch's Glyoxylide
1950s	Hoxsey's Cancer Treatment
1960s	Ivy's Krebiozen
1970s	Laetrile
1980s	Metabolic Therapies Diet, High Colonics, Vitamins, and Minerals

Source: Reprinted with permission from Cassileth B: Unorthodox cancer medicine. Cancer Invest 4:591-598, 1988. By courtesy of Marcel Dekker, Inc.

In 1943 the Canadian Cancer Foundation issued a report on a clinical trial using the Koch method. None of the patients in the study benefited from the treatment.[20] In 1948 Koch closed his laboratory and moved to Brazil. Three years later the Federal Trade Commission issued a court order forbidding the promotion of Koch antitoxins because of their lack of therapeutic value. Although Koch's antitoxins are illegal in the United States, they can be obtained through the underground medical community or in Mexico.

Hoxsey Method: 1950s

Promoted since the early 1920s, the Hoxsey method aimed to restore the body to physiologic "normalcy."[21] Hoxsey maintained that cancer was a result of a chemical imbalance that caused the body's healthy cells to mutate and become cancerous. The aim of the therapy was to restore the chemical environment and kill the cancerous cells. Hoxsey's Herbal Tonic consisted of several different formulas: the "black medicine" was composed of cascara (a laxative) in an extract of licorice root, alfalfa, burdock root, red clover blossoms, buckthorn bark, barberry root, pokeweed, and prickly ash bark; the "pink medicine" contained potassium iodide and lactated pepsin.[21] Hoxsey claimed that a horse his grandfather owned had been cured of a leg cancer after eating a mixture of these plants, and this chance event led to his using this form of therapy for cancer in humans. Except for potassium iodide and the laxative, which are effective drugs but have no value in treating cancer, all the other ingredients have been discarded as medically ineffective.[11]

Hoxsey began promoting his treatment in the early 1920s, at which time it was called "Hoxide." After having been convicted of practicing medicine without a license in Illinois and Iowa, Hoxsey opened a small clinic in Dallas, Texas, and a second clinic in Portage, Pennsylvania, where Hoxsey's medicines were given in tablet form. The Hoxsey therapy was available at the clinic until 1960, when a federal court injunction, after 10 years of litigation, declared the sales of the treatment illegal.[11]

During the 10 years of litigation, a University of British Columbia panel investigated the Hoxsey method and found "that the methods of diagnosis are inadequate, that the treatments for internal cancer do not affect the progress of the disease, that no serious attempt is made to follow up treated cases in order to evaluate results, and that no significant research has been done."[22]

The Food and Drug Administration (FDA) investigated nearly 400 cases of persons who claimed to be cured of cancer through the use of the Hoxsey method. No case of a bona fide cure was discovered. Janssen[11] notes that one group of persons had never been diagnosed as having cancer, a second had received conventional therapy in addition to the Hoxsey treatment, and the final group still had cancer or had died from it. At the time the Hoxsey Clinic was closed, more than 10,000 individuals were enrolled as current patients. The FDA estimated that more than $50 million had been spent for the Hoxsey drugs.[23]

As of 1985, Hoxsey's medicines were thriving at the Bio-Medical Center in Tijuana, Mexico. The cost of therapy ranged from $150 to $450 for the blood test and examination to $2000 for the herbal remedies and physician consultation. A down payment of 30% was required.[24]

Krebiozen: 1960s

Krebiozen was allegedly first produced by a Yugoslavian physician named Steven Durovic. Durovic claimed that the first 200,000 doses (2 g in all) were obtained from blood extracted from some 2000 Argentinian horses. The horses were said to have been previously inoculated with a special mold before the blood sample was obtained.

Dr. Andrew C. Ivy, professor emeritus of the University of Illinois, endorsed the substance as an effective cancer therapy in the mid-1950s. Thousands of physicians across the country used Krebiozen as an investigational drug and charged nine dollars per ampul.[11] In 1961 the National Cancer Institute (NCI) obtained a sample of Krebiozen, and the substance was identified as creatine monohydrate, an amino acid found in all animal tissue.[25] Subsequent investigation of samples of Krebiozen actually distributed to physicians found that pre-1960 samples contained mineral oil and a small amount of amyl alcohol and methylhydantoin.[26]

The Krebiozen Research Foundation submitted 504 case records to the NCI in an effort to demonstrate therapeutic efficacy and help justify a clinical trial. A team of 24 scientists reviewed these records and unanimously concluded that Krebiozen is an ineffective drug.[27] Although no clear scientific evidence of efficacy has been brought forward, the treatment was available until 1977.[11]

Laetrile: 1970s

Laetrile is a term applied to various cyanogenic glucosides, derived from a variety of food products (eg, apricot pits, peaches, cherries, and almonds). It is also known as amygdalin and "vitamin B_{17}." It has been known as a killer of people since the Pharoahs' priests in ancient Egypt used it in the form of a water extract of peach kernels as the official means of execution of their enemies. Laetrile has been a quack remedy since 1840, 10 years after its isolation in pure form by two French chemists.[28] Ernst T. Krebs, Sr, a physician, claimed to be the first individual to use a cyanogenic glucoside as an anticancer agent. In the 1940s, Dr. Krebs used amygdalin, derived from apricot kernels, and found it to be too toxic for use in humans despite what he claimed were encouraging results. In 1952 his son, Ernst Krebs, Jr, reported that he had made an empiric apricot formula that was safe for parenteral administration.

Kreb's patent on laetrile was for a chemical different from amygdalin, and yet amygdalin is what is typically distributed as laetrile.[13] Laetrile's purported mechanism of action has changed over the years. Perhaps the most common hypothesis is that an enzyme called β-glucosidase is present in cancer cells in larger quantities than in healthy tissue. In turn, normal tissue is alleged to have greater quantities of the enzyme rhodanese, which supposedly is not present in cancerous tissue. The theory notes that the β-glucosidase in the cancerous tissues causes the laetrile to be broken down into glucose and mandelonitrile, which breaks down further into hydrogen cyanide (a toxic substance) and benzaldehyde (a mild anesthetic). The cyanide kills the cancer cells while the healthy tissue is protected by rhodanese, which converts cyanide into nontoxic sodium thiocynate. Manner et al[29] expand this theory and suggest, for example, that benzaldehyde may interfere with respiration in cancer cells. They also claim to have demonstrated a differentiation in quantities of rhodanese and β-glucosidase in the directions predicted by theory. However, this result is inconsistent with the findings of other investigators.[30-32] Greenberg[32] theorized that the majority of the parenterally injected laetrile is probably excreted intact in the urine.

Claims have been made that laetrile is a nontoxic form of "vitamin B$_{17}$," and that taking this vitamin can prevent cancer. Because no disease state exists in the absence of laetrile, however, it does not fulfill the requirements of a vitamin.[33] Evidence suggests that laetrile has toxic effects. The gastric lumen is thought to have enzymes capable of breaking laetrile down into hydrogen cyanide and mandelonitrile.[34] Numerous reports have associated cyanide toxicity with the ingestion of fruits or seeds containing cyanogenic glucosides, including amygdalin.[35-39] Ingestion of laetrile with certain other foods, such as sweet almonds, lettuce, certain fresh fruits, or mushrooms, can potentiate the toxic reaction. In addition, a number of deaths attributed to cyanide poisoning from oral laetrile have been reported,[28,40,41] and laetrile by enema is so poisonous.[42,43]

Another area of potential risk for the laetrile user is that the FDA has no control over the manufacture, importation, and distribution of laetrile. Laetrile that is used in the United States is either imported illegally or brought in under court order (exempting the substance from FDA supervision). There have been reports of fungal contamination of parenterally formulated laetrile, variations in dosage, and mislabeling of contents of laetrile imported from Mexican manufacturers.[44] For the cancer patient, whose immune system may already be compromised, an infection resulting from contamination could be fatal.

With regard to tests of efficacy, it is worth noting that laetrile has been the most extensively tested unproven method of all time. Numerous animal studies[45-49] and two retrospective studies have showed no therapeutic benefit.[50,51] Throughout the 1970s the FDA took legal action against many of the proponents of laetrile, there was a movement to legalize laetrile in many states, and approximately 75,000 US cancer patients were seeking laetrile therapy; many of these patients were discontinuing effective conventional therapy.[52] Laetrile was a billion-dollar-a-year industry in 1979.[28] Thus, in 1980, the FDA gave approval to the NCI for the first prospective clinical trial of laetrile and once again demonstrated laetrile to be ineffective against cancer.[53]

Today, many of the proponents of laetrile have changed their strategy of using it as a single agent and are combining it with vitamins, enzymes, or so-called metabolic therapy. For example, the Centro Medico Del Mar, in Tijuana, which is known for its laetrile treatments, has provided a therapy program consisting of laetrile, enzymes, diet, detoxification with enemas, "vaccines," vitamin A, and extracts of thymus tissue. The treatments last approximately 3 weeks and cost about $4000.[24]

MOST POPULAR UNPROVEN METHODS OF TODAY

Metabolic Therapy

Developed by German physician Dr. Max Gerson in the 1920s, metabolic cancer therapy proposes that constipation, or inadequate elimination of wastes from the body, interferes with metabolism and healing. Cure can be achieved through manipulation of diet and "detoxification," or purging the body of so-called toxins. There are many adaptations of Dr. Gerson's original program, but all have a consistent approach, which includes (1) avoidance of exposure to carcinogens, (2) positive mental outlook, and (3) eliminating wastes from the body. The diet is high in potassium, low in sodium, low in fats and oils, and includes reduced amounts of animal proteins. Individuals are encouraged to drink raw vegetable and fruit juices, take coffee enemas, and ingest supplemental vitamins, minerals, and enzymes.[54]

Cassileth et al[5] reported that 45% of the patients in their study used metabolic therapy with or without conventional therapy. Metabolic therapies are available from individual practitioners and clinics in the United States, Europe, and Canada, with the majority of such therapy given at the Gerson Therapy Hospital, in Tijuana, Mexico.[7,16,24] Treatment in the Mexican clinic costs approximately $3000 to $4000 and lasts from 3 to 6 weeks.[55] There is a long waiting list of US patients to receive a 1-week treatment, for $1700, of 13 glasses of carrot juice per day and coffee enemas.[24] Repeated enemas and purgatives are more likely to lead to metabolic imbalance than to correct it, and coffee enemas have killed people.[56,57] There are no objective data showing that the Gerson method has any benefit in the treatment of cancer.[58]

Harold Manner, PhD, is another proponent of metabolic cancer therapy. He is founder and president of the Metabolic Research Foundation, in Glenview, Illinois. He supervises his Tijuana Clinic, in Mexico, and has 168 Manner Metabolic Clinics in the United States, Canada, Japan, and Scotland. He claims that "metabolic therapy" enhances the body's immune system, causing tumors to disappear. The "Manner cocktail" consists of an intravenous solution of 10mL dimethyl sulfoxide, 25 g vitamin C, 9 g laetrile, and 5% dextrose given over a 2-week period at a cost of approximately $6000.[24] There are various protocols for this metabolic therapy, which may also include coffee enemas, megavitamins, and enzymes.[59] More important, there is no objective evidence that Harold Manner's metabolic therapy has any benefit in the treatment of cancer.[59]

Macrobiotic Diets

Over the years, a variety of diet therapies have been purported to be useful in the treatment of cancer. The macrobiotic diet is probably the most common today and is promoted both as a cure for cancer and a preventive measure. This diet has its origin in Zen mysticism, which proposes two antagonistic and complementary forces, yin and yang, governing everything in the universe. Each food can be classified as yin or yang, whereas each tumor can be classified as being caused by an imbalance of either yin or yang. The diet is matched to the tumor to restore the balance between yin and yang, resulting in a cure or prevention, as the case may be.[16] In addition to diet, balance is also achieved through cooking techniques and a correct attitude toward life.[60]

The original version of the diet, developed by George Ohsawa (1893–1966), involved 10 macrobiotic diets ranging from diet −3 to diet 7. As an individual progresses from diet −3 toward diet 7, more and more foods are forfeited, until in diet 7 the diet exclusively consists of cereal grains. In the 1970s, Michio Kushi,[61] recommended a more "standard macrobiotic diet" that was less restrictive than diet 7. This standard approach consists of 50% to 60% whole cereal grains, 20% to 25% vegetables, 5% to 10% soups, 5% to 10% beans and sea vegetables, occasional fish and fruits, and liquids used sparingly. The foods that are not allowed because they are excessively "yin" or "yang" include meat, animal fat, poultry, eggs, dairy products, bananas, citrus fruits, potatoes, tomatoes, spinach, coffee, sugar, and vitamin supplements.[61] Thus the macrobiotic diet uses only plant proteins and is high in bulk and low in fat. It is necessary to consume a large quantity of macrobiotic foods to meet the daily recommended energy allowance. For example, a healthy man who requires 2700 kilocalories would need 17 cups of food in volume.[62] Kushi[61] also recommends that modern medicine be avoided except for emergency lifesaving treatment.

Macrobiotic therapy may result in malnutrition and may cause a variety of serious health problems.[63] With adequate planning, vegetarian diets may be nutritionally sound, but the diet recommended by Kushi is unsound. The American Cancer Society[64] (ACS) recently reviewed the literature and available information and found no objective evidence that macrobiotic diets are of benefit in the treatment of cancer. There are also no valid data on the efficacy of the macrobiotic diet in the prevention of cancer.[63]

Megavitamins

The use of supplemental vitamins is another approach that has been exploited and promoted as an unproven method for the treatment of cancer. Megadoses of vitamin C, vitamin A, and pangamic acid ("vitamin B₁₅") have been alleged to have antitumor properties. However, excessive vitamin intake can be useless and, more important, very toxic.

Vitamin C

Vitamin C, consumed in megadoses, is probably the most popular self-administered vitamin supplement. Vitamin C has been promoted as a remedy for conditions ranging from the common cold to arthritis. It gained popularity as a therapy for cancer when Cameron and Pauling[65] published a study claiming that patients with terminal cancer who received massive doses of vitamin C survived much longer. However, their study was not valid because they selected the patients who received vitamin C and the control subjects were selected from files; thus the groups were not comparable.[66] Objective studies have shown such therapy to be worthless.[28,67,68] In fact, megadoses of vitamin C may cause severe kidney damage,[69] release cyanide from laetrile,[70] and cause death if administered intravenously.[67,71,72]

Vitamin A

Megadoses of vitamin A have also become popular, used either alone or in combination with other agents, for the treatment of cancer. Doses of vitamin A supplements as low as five times the recommended dietary allowance (RDA) may be toxic; moreover, vitamin A has no clear value in the treatment of cancer.[73]

Pangamic acid (vitamin B₁₅)

Pangamic acid is a vitamin in name only, has no standard identity, and does not exist except as a label.[16] In the United States, it is illegal to sell this agent as either a drug or a food supplement.[74-76] There is evidence that the two most widely used chemicals in products labeled "B₁₅" or "pangamate" are diisopropylamine dichloroacetate (DIPA-DCA) and dimethylglycine hydrochloride (DMG), which actually may promote the development of cancer.[77,78]

Mental Imagery: Simonton Method

The Cancer Counseling and Research Center (CCRC), in Fort Worth, Texas, was established by O. Carl Simonton, a board-certified radiologist, and Stephanie Matthews-Simonton, a motivational counselor. The Simontons hypothesized that attitude and stress could be crucial factors in both causation and potential cure of cancer. It is their belief that a positive mental attitude can improve an individual's physiologic responses, resulting in improved response to standard therapies. Patients with cancer and their partners are taught to use mental imagery and relaxation techniques to visualize cancer cells as weak and sick and to imagine body defenses as a strong army that attacks and eliminates cancer cells.[79] The Simontons strongly advocate that individuals who participate in their counseling sessions continue to receive conventional medical treatment.

Although the scientific and medical communities support the notion that a positive mental attitude may increase patient comfort and promote a sense of control and well-being, the following problems remain concerning the Simonton method:

1. There are no carefully controlled clinical studies that show an objective benefit of the Simonton method for the treatment of cancer.

2. Patients may be made to feel guilty by leading them to believe that they are responsible for the development of cancer because they have a particular personality type.
3. If individuals become overly reliant on the Simonton method, they may be encouraged to abandon standard medical therapy.

Until such time as the efficacy of the Simonton method is documented by carefully controlled clinical studies, the American Cancer Society has determined that the Simonton method should be listed as an unproven method.[80]

The CCRC enrolls many patients and families in each session, and many people derive benefit from the sessions (ie, improved confidence, sense of well-being, and improved quality of life). In counseling patients about available options, nurses can point out potential benefits of the Simonton program while stressing that the method has no scientific documentation of effectiveness.

Spiritual, Faith, or Mind Healing

Many people find empowerment and comfort through various aspects of spiritual or faith healing. Cassileth and Brown[7] noted that in their study of 378 patients, 71 were attracted to this method of therapy, which involved use of prayer, "laying on of hands," incantation, or other ways of obtaining divine intervention to rid themselves of the disease. Many patients resort to commercialized faith healers who defraud people of their money by claiming that they can cure cancer. Other healers, such as Louise Hay, espouse self-love as a way to improve health and a possible cure.[81] Holland[18] notes that some methods that require patients to accept the idea that emotions contributed to their cancer may render patients even more vulnerable to guilt and depression. More important, these methods may be more hazardous to the patients' well-being than is usually recognized.

Immunoaugmentive Therapy

Dr. Lawrence Burton (doctor of zoology) is the originator of immunoaugmentive therapy (IAT) for cancer; treatment is given at his Immunology Research Center, located in the Bahamas. IAT is based on the theory that stimulation of the immune system will enable the body's normal defenses to destroy tumor cells. Although the therapeutic approach is based on reasonable scientific theory, scientific documentation of results of this therapy is lacking.[82] Evidence reported in 1985 suggested that his therapy not only is worthless but in fact may spread hepatitis and acquired immunodeficiency syndrome (AIDS).[83]

The ACS maintains a file of unproven methods and is therefore a good resource for information concerning them. Table 56-2 lists a variety of unproven methods that have been used for cancer diagnosis, prevention, or treatment.[84]

PROMOTERS OF UNPROVEN METHODS

Promoters of unproven cancer treatment methods survive, thrive, and grow rich. They invest time, effort, and money in public relations and media presentations that use legitimate scientific words or phrases in a misleading and deceptive manner while retaining their emotional impact. The promoters and purveyors omit the facts that their remedies have never been objectively tested and found valid. They omit citing the lack of benefit resulting from their regimen. Instead, they rely on testimonials and anecdotes that do not separate fact from fiction or from coincidence resulting from the natural history of the disease.[16]

In the last decade, the strategies used by the promoters of unproven treatment methods have become more sophisticated. Several points should be made about these new strategies: (1) the public's reasonable interest in nutrition, good mental attitude, and physical fitness is being exploited for personal profit; (2) the prevention of cancer is represented by purveyors of unproven methods as achievable with their remedies at a time when health professionals and the government also are emphasizing prevention; (3) there has been a movement to combine many questionable methods to make objective evaluation difficult; and (4) a rising distrust of health professionals is being exploited.[16,17] Highly motivated and better-educated individuals are more likely to turn to unquestionable methods because of the promise that "you can control your disease."[5,15]

The Subcommittee on Unorthodox Therapies of the American Society of Clinical Oncology[85] lists 10 questions to ask in making a decision as to whether a treatment should be suspected of being questionable (Table 56-3). Although these questions were developed as a guide for the layperson, they are also an excellent resource for the health professional.

INTERVENTIONS

The health care professional who discusses unproven methods of treating cancer with a patient or a family member must first assess the underlying motivations of the individual's desire to use these therapies. What information has the patient heard regarding the method in question? Where was the information obtained? What does the individual perceive as the benefits of pursuing this therapy? If a family member is asking about such a method, has the individual discussed this therapy with the patient?

Individuals who raise questions regarding unproven methods are usually aware that such techniques are not likely to be approved by the health care professional. For the professional, these questions provide an opportunity to discover unmet needs of the patient and family and to assess their understanding of the therapies that have been

TABLE 56-2 Unproven Methods for Diagnosis or Treatment of Cancer

Alkylating punch	Compound X	Helt "cancer serum" and	Nichols escharotic method
Almonds	Contreras methods	Gruner blood smear test	Nieper
Aloe vera plant	Cresson method	Hoxsey method or Hoxsey	
American International	Crofton immunization	chemotherapy	Olive oil
Hospital's program	method	Hubbard E. Meter	OM-12
Anti-cancer factor in clams	Cytec system	Hypnosis	Oncone juice
Anticacergen Z-50 and			Orgone energy devices
Zuccala lytic test	Diamond carbon compound	Immuno-augmentation	Oscilloclast
Antineol	DMSO	cancer therapy program	
Arthur morphologic	Dotto electronic reactor	Iscador	Pap-Chek, Female
immunostatus differentials	Drown radio-therapeutic	Issels combination therapy	laboratory testing
Asparagus oil	instrument		Polonine
		Kallzyne	Psychic methods
Bacteria enema	Esterlit	Kanfer neuromuscular or	
Bamfolin	Ferguson plant products	handwriting test	Rand coupled fortified
H. H. Beard methods	Fonti methods	KC-555	antigen (RCFA) and
Bio-medical detoxification	Francis diet	Kelley malignancy index	Delayed double diffusion
therapy	Fresh cell therapy	and ecology therapy	(3-D) test
Bonifacio anticancer goat	Frost method	Koch antitoxins	Revici cancer control
serum			
	Ganner petroleum or	Laetrile	Samuels causal or
Cancer lipid concentrate	"Petroleum pal"	Lewis method	"endogenous
and the malignancy index	Germanium	Livingston vaccine	endocrinotherapy"
Carcin and neo-carcin	Gerson method		Sander's treatment
Carrot/celery juice	Gibson method	M-P virus	Simonton method
Carzodelan	Glover method	Makari intradermal cancer	Snake meat
Cath$_2$O$_2$LIC therapy	Goat's milk	test	Snake oil capsules
Cedar cones	Grape cure	Manner's metabolic cancer	Spears hygienic system
CH-23	Greek cure	prevention program	Staphylococcus phage
Chamonils		Marijuana	lysate or Lincoln
Chaparral tea	H. 11	Megadose vitamin therapy	bacteriophage lysate
Chase dietary method	Hadley vaccine and blood	Mexican clinics and hospitals	Sunflower seeds
Chelation	and skin test	Millet bread	
Cinical El Buen Samaritano	Haematoxylon dissolved in	Millrue	Ultraviolet blood irradiation
C.N.T.	DMSO	Miniburg system	intravenous treatment
Coffee enemas	Heat therapy or	Mucorhicin	
Coley's mixed toxins or	hyperthermia	Multiple enzyme therapy	Wigmore program
mixed bacterial toxins	Hemacytology index (HCI)		
(MBT)	Hendricks natural immunity	Naessens serum or anablast	Zen macrobiotic diet
Collodaurum and	therapy		
bichloracetic acid			
Kahlenbury			

Source: Reprinted with permission from Miller NJ, Howard-Ruben J. Unproven methods of cancer management: Part I. Background and historical perspective. Oncol Nurs Forum 10(4):46, 1983.

administered. If the patient receives a strong negative response concerning the unproven method, the communication channel between the health care professional and the patient will likely be impaired. A nonjudgmental attitude facilitates the caregiver's assessment of the patient's and family's motivations for wanting to try an unproven method. In turn, the patient and family will likely be more receptive to the information provided by a nonjudgmental health care professional.

Anything that can be done to make the patient feel a part of the therapeutic effort may help prevent the use of unproven methods by the patient. Information on exercise or nutrition provided in a positive context will help

the patient feel less isolated. Keeping the patient and family well informed by answering questions concerning the type of therapy being received will also combat feelings of isolation. Pamphlets available from the ACS or NCI may increase communication because they provide background material that can put the health care team's information into perspective. The goal of communication is to have the patient feel that he or she is being treated humanely. The person who feels like an adversary of the health care team is not likely to see the hospital staff as human beings. Many individuals will say that health care professionals could cure cancer if they wanted to but that there is no profit in doing so. Those who make such statements forget

TABLE 56-3 Ten Questions to Ask in Deciding Whether a Treatment is Questionable

1. Is the treatment based on an unproven theory?

2. Is there a purported need for special nutritional support?

3. Is there a claim for painless, nontoxic treatment?

4. Are claims published only in the mass media and not in reputable peer-reviewed scientific journals?

5. Are claims for benefit merely compatible with a placebo effect?

6. Are the major proponents recognized experts in cancer treatment?

7. Do proponents claim benefit for use with proven methods of treatment? For prolongation of life? For use as a cancer preventive?

8. Is there a claim that only specially trained physicians can produce results with the drug, or is the preparation secret?

9. Is there an attack on the medical and scientific establishment?

10. Is there a demand by promoters for "freedom of choice" regarding drugs?

Source: Subcommittee on Unorthodox Therapies, American Society of Clinical Oncology: Ineffective cancer therapy: A guide for the layperson. J Clin Oncol 1:154-163, 1983.

that health care professionals are human and that their loved ones also die of cancer.

In evaluating communication patterns, the health care professional also needs to examine communications between the patient and family. The family may become preoccupied with seeking various therapies as a means of coping with stress. Such a situation may be sufficiently intense to cause the family to engage in a conspiracy to exclude the patient from the decision-making process. The patient then becomes alienated from the family's communication system and from the psychologic and physical support that is so important. The family must be made aware of the impact of their actions on the patient. A social worker, chaplain, or patient-family support group might facilitate more effective intrafamily communication.

Frequently, discussion will focus on the use of unproven methods for individuals who are terminally ill. For many such patients, standard therapy will be able to extend life. Should "terminal" be used to describe a state in which no therapeutic modalities can be effective? Palliative care may still be able to extend the person's life, whereas an unproven method may shorten it. When a patient is interested in experimental research, the options should be explored by the physician. In all instances the issue of quality of life versus quantity of life should be discussed. The advantages and disadvantages for each individual

should be examined. For many, a second opinion concerning therapeutic options may prove helpful. Second opinions can provide two positive outcomes:

1. They can make the patient aware of additional therapeutic alternatives.
2. They reassure both patient and family that the therapeutic assessment that has been made is likely a sound one.

The health care professional must be informed both regarding technical information on the most frequently encountered unproven methods and regarding the particular aims of a given individual's therapy. The health care professional should be able to explain the risks of unproven methods, such as toxic effects and, in instances where the unproven method is being used as the sole form of therapy, the risk of further progression of disease. For individuals who are using an unproven method in combination with standard therapy, it is still important to be aware of possible side effects. A drug analysis may prove valuable for any substances that the patient has been given from an unproven methods clinic. For example, one Mexican clinic provided a "vitamin" that was actually a potent chemotherapeutic agent. The patient was at the same time taking standard chemotherapy at a university medical center. Fortunately, the physicians discovered the true identity of the "vitamin" after noting an unusually low white blood cell count.[14] The risks of adverse effects can be increased when drugs are mixed with unorthodox substances, and the patient must be informed that all risks may not even be known.

Finally, health care professionals who are caring for patients with cancer must be kept informed regarding hospital, state, and federal policies regarding any drug—experimental, standard, or unproven. The term "unproven," as originally noted, suggests that the substance is being promoted even though it has not been proven effective. However, the fact that a promoted therapy has not been proven effective does not necessarily mean that it has no therapeutic value. It must be tested to determine its safety and efficacy. The present system permits the scientific method to play a strong role in determining what therapies will be on the market, and improvements are continually being made in methods of evaluation. In this way the health care consumer is protected from unsafe and fraudulent therapies.

REFERENCES

1. Olson KB: Drugs, cancer and charlatans, in Horton J, Hill GJ (eds). Clinical Oncology. Philadelphia, WB Saunders, 1977, pp 182-191.
2. House Subcommittee on Aging: Quackery: A 10-Billion-Dollar Scandal—Report. Committee publication No. 98-435. Washington, DC, Government Printing Office, 1984, pp 1-250.

3. House Subcommittee on Aging: Quackery: A 10-Billion-Dollar Scandal—Hearing. Committee publication No. 98-463. Washington, DC, Government Printing Office, 1984.

4. Herbert V, Barnett S: Vitamins and "Health" Foods: The Great American Hustle. Philadelphia, George F Stickley, 1981.

5. Cassileth B, Lusk E, Strouse T, et al: Contemporary unorthodox treatments in cancer medicine. Ann Intern Med 101:105-112, 1984.

6. Cassileth B: Unorthodox cancer medicine. Cancer Invest 4:591-598, 1986.

7. Cassileth B, Brown H: Unorthodox cancer medicine. CA 38:176-186, 1988.

8. Cassileth BR, Berlyne B: Counseling the cancer patient who wants to try unorthodox or questionable therapies. Oncology 3:29-33, 1989.

9. Janssen WF: The cancer "cures": A challenge to rational therapeutics. Anal Chem 50:197A-202A, 1978.

10. Grant RN, Bartlett I: Unproven cancer remedies: A primer, in Unproven Methods of Cancer Management. New York, American Cancer Society, 1971.

11. Janssen WF: Cancer quackery: the past in the present. Semin Oncol 6:526-536, 1979.

12. Message from President Taft. Congressional Record 62 Cong., 1 Sess. 2380 (June 21, 1911).

13. Kennedy D: Commissioner decision on status. Federal Register 42:39806-39967, 1977.

14. Luurs KJ: Unproven methods of treatment, in Groenwald SL (ed): Cancer Nursing Principles and Practice. Boston, Jones & Bartlett, 1987, pp 405-413.

15. Hiratzka S: Knowledge and attitudes of persons with cancer toward use of unproven treatment methods. Oncol Nurs Forum 12:36-41, 1985.

16. Herbert V, Yarbro CH: Nutrition quackery. Semin Oncol Nurs 2:63-69, 1986.

17. King M: Falling victim twice. Cancer News 39:8-11, 1985.

18. Holland JC: Why patients seek unproven cancer remedies: A psychological perspective. CA 32:10-14, 1982.

19. Koch WF: A new and successful treatment and diagnosis of cancer. Detroit Med J, 1919.

20. Letter to the Editor: Senator Langer abuses franking privilege by circulation of propaganda for Koch's cancer quackery. JAMA 137:1333, 1948.

21. Hoxsey HM: You Don't Have to Die: The Amazing Story of the Hoxsey Cancer Treatment. New York, Milestone Books, 1956.

22. Mather JM: Report of a committee of faculty members of the University of British Columbia concerning the Hoxsey treatment for cancer. Unpublished report, December 19, 1957.

23. Press Release HEW-020: US Department Health, Education, and Welfare, Food and Drug Administration. Washington, DC, Stepember 21, 1960.

24. Kreiger L: Unorthodox clinics flourishing in Tijuana. Am Med News 3:25-27, 1985.

25. Holland JF: The Krebiozen story: Is cancer quackery dead? JAMA 200:213-218, 1967.

26. American Cancer Society: Unproven methods of cancer management. New York, American Cancer Society, 1971.

27. Report of Director, National Cancer Institute, to Secretary of Department of Health, Education, and Welfare concerning decision of the Institute not to undertake clinical testing of Krebiozen. Washington, DC, FDA Records 539.1.PX, October 16, 1963.

28. Herbert V: Nutrition Cultism: Facts and Fictions (ed 3). Philadelphia, George F. Stickley, 1981.

29. Manner HW, DiSanti SJ, Michalsen TL: The Death of Cancer. Evanston, Ill, Advanced Century Publishing, 1978.

30. Conchie J, Findlay L, Levvy GA: Mammalian glycosidases: Distribution in the body. Biochem J 71:318-325, 1959.

31. Gal EM, Fung FH, Greenberg DM: Studies on the biological action of malonitriles. II. Distribution of rhodanese (transulfurase) in the tissues of normal and tumor-bearing animals and the effect of malononitrile thereon. Cancer Res 169:449-450, 1952.

32. Greenberg DM: The vitamin fraud in cancer quackery. West J Med 122:345-348, 1975.

33. Greenstein JP: Quantitative nutritional studies with water-soluble chemically defined diets. I. Growth, reproduction and lactation in rats. Arch Biochem Biophys 72:396-416, 1957.

34. Everly RC: Laetrile: Focus on the facts. CA 26:50-54, 1976.

35. Grabois B: Exposure to hydrogen cyanide in processing of apricot kernels. Monthly Review: New York Department of Labor 33:33-36, 1954.

36. Sayre JW, Kaymakcalan S: Cyanide poisoning from apricot seeds among children in central Turkey. N Engl J Med 270:1113-1115, 1964.

37. Gunders AE, Abrahamov A, Weisenberg E: Cyanide poisoning following the ingestion of apricot (Prunus armeniaca) kernel. J Israel Med Assoc 76:536-538, 1969.

38. Humbert JR, Tress JH, Braico KT: Fatal cyanide poisoning: Accidental ingestion of amygdalin. JAMA 238:482, 1977 (letter).

39. Sadoff L, Fuchs K, Hollander J: Rapid death associated with laetrile ingestion. JAMA 239:1532, 1978.

40. Herbert V: Laetrile: The cult of cyanide—Promoting poison for profit. Am J Clin Nutr 32:1121-1158, 1979.

41. Vogel SN, Sultan TR: Cyanide poisoning. Clin Toxicol Exp Ther 18:367-383, 1981.

42. Ortega JA, Creek J: Acute cyanide poisoning following administration of laetrile enemas. J Pediatr 93:1059, 1978.

43. Eisele JW, Reay DT: Deaths related to coffee enemas. JAMA 244:1608-1609, 1980.

44. Food and Drug Administration: Toxicity of laetrile. FDA Drug Bull 7:25-32, 1977.

45. Wodinsky I, Swiniarsky JK: Antitumor activity of amygdalin as a single agent and with beta-glucosidase on a spectrum of transplantable rodent tumors. Cancer Chem Rep 59:939-950, 1975.

46. Hill GJ, Shine TE, Hill HZ, et al: Failure of amygdalin to arrest B16 melanoma and BW5147 AKR leukemia. Cancer Res 36:2102-2107, 1976.

47. Stock CC, Tarnowski GS, Schmid FA, et al: Antitumor tests of amygdalin in transplantable animal tumor systems. J Surg Oncol 10:81-88, 1978.

48. Stock CC, Martin DS, Suguira K, et al: Antitumor tests of amygdalin in spontaneous animal tumor systems. J Surg Oncol 10:89-123, 1978.

49. Ovejira AA, Houchens DP, Barker AD, et al: Inactivity of DL-amygdalin against human breast and colon tumor xenografts in athymic (nude) mice. Cancer Treat Rep 62:576-578, 1978.

50. California Medical Association, Cancer Commission: The treatment of cancer with "Laetriles." Calif Med 78:320-326, 1953.

51. Ellison NM, Byar DP, Newell GR: Special report on laetrile: the NCI laetrile review. N Engl J Med 299:549-552, 1978.

52. Henney JE: Unproven methods of cancer treatment, in DeVita VT, Hellman S, Rosenberg SA (eds): Cancer Principles and Practice of Oncology (ed 2). Philadelphia, JB Lippincott, 1985, pp 2333-2342.

53. Moertel CG, Fleming TR, Tubin J, et al: A clinical trial of

amygdalin (laetrile) in the treatment of human cancer. N Engl J Med 306:201-207, 1982.

54. Gerson M: The cure of advanced cancer by diet therapy: A summary of 30 years of clinical experimentation. Physiol Chem Phys 10:449-464, 1978.

55. Donsbach KW, Walker M: Metabolic Cancer Therapies. Huntington Beach, Calif International Institute of National Health Sciences, 1981.

56. Istre GR, Kreiss K, Hopkins RS, et al: An outbreak of amebiasis spread by colonic irrigation at a chiropractic clinic. N Engl J Med 307:339-342, 1982.

57. Markman M: Medical complications of "alternative" cancer therapy (letter). N Engl J Med 312:1640-1641, 1985.

58. American Cancer Society: Unproven methods of cancer management: Gerson method of treatment for cancer. CA 23:314-317, 1973.

59. American Cancer Society: Unproven methods of cancer management: The metabolic cancer therapy of Harold W. Manner, Ph.D. CA 36:185-189, 1986.

60. Ohsawa G: Cancer and the Philosophy of the Far East. Binghamton, NY, Swan House Publishing, 1971.

61. Kushi M: Macrobiotic Approach to Cancer. Wayne, NJ, Avery Publishing Group, 1982.

62. Arnold C: The macrobiotic diet: A question of nutrition. Oncol Nurs Forum 11:50-53, 1984.

63. Bowman BB, Kushner RF, Dawson SC, et al: Macrobiotic diets for cancer treatment and prevention. J Clin Oncol 2:702-711, 1984.

64. American Cancer Society: Unproven methods of cancer management: Macrobiotic diets for the treatment of cancer. CA 39:248-251, 1989.

65. Cameron E, Pauling L: Supplemental ascorbate in the supportive treatment of cancer, prolongation of survival time in terminal human cancer. Proc Natl Acad Sci USA 73:3685-3689, 1976.

66. Sampson WI: When the big C is a vitamin. Coping 2:35, 1988.

67. Marshall CW: Vitamins and Minerals: Help or Harm? Philadelphia, George F Stickley, 1983.

68. Creagan ET, Moertel CG, O'Fallon JR, et al: Failure of high-dose vitamin C to benefit patients with advanced cancer. N Engl J Med 301:687-690, 1979.

69. Swartz RD, Wesley JR, Somermeyer MG, et al: Hyperoxaluria and renal insufficiency due to ascorbic acid administration during total parental nutrition. Ann Intern Med 100:530-531, 1984.

70. Backer RC, Herbert V: Cyanide production from laetrile in the presence of megadoses of ascorbic acid. JAMA 241:1891-1892, 1979.

71. Herbert V: The rationale of massive-dose vitamin therapy: Megavitamin therapy—hot fiction vs cold facts, in Whilte PL, Selvey N (eds): Proceedings of the Fourth Western Hemisphere Nutrition Congress. Acton, Mass, Publishing Sciences Group, 1975, pp 84-91.

72. Hodges RE: Nutrition in Medical Practice. Philadelphia, WB Saunders, 1980.

73. Herbert V: Toxicity of 25,000 IU vitamin A supplements in "health" food users. Am J Clin Nutr 36:185-186, 1982.

74. Herbert V: Pangamic acid (vitamin B_{15}). Am J Clin Nutr 32:1534-1540, 1979.

75. Herbert V, Herbert R: Pangamate (vitamin B_{15}) in Ellenbogen L (ed): Controversies in Nutrition. New York, Churchill Livingstone, 1981, pp 159-170.

76. McPherrin EW, Herbert V, Herbert R: "Vitamin B_{15}": Anatomy of a Health Fraud. New York, American Council on Science and Health, 1981.

77. Colman N, Herbert V, Gardner A, et al: Mutagenicity of dimethylglycine when mixed with nitrite: Possible significance in human use of pangamates. Proc Soc Exp Biol Med 164:9-12, 1980.

78. Gelernt MD, Herbert V: Mutagenicity of diisopropylamine dichloroacetate, the "active constituent" of vitamin B_{15} (pangamic acid). Nutr Cancer 3:129-133, 1982.

79. Simonton OC, Matthews-Simonton S, Creighton J: Getting Well Again: A Step-by-Step, Self-Help Guide to Overcoming Cancer for Patients and Their Families. Los Angeles, Jeremy P. Tarcher, 1978.

80. American Cancer Society: Unproven methods of cancer management: O. Carl Simonton, MD. CA 32:58-61, 1982.

81. Irish AC: Maintaining health in persons with HIV infection. Semin Oncol Nurs 5:302-307, 1989.

82. Easy cures for cancer still find support. JAMA 246:714-716, 1981.

83. OT briefs. Oncol Times 7:26, 1985.

84. Miller NJ, Howard-Ruben J: Unproven methods of cancer management. Background and historical perspectives. Oncol Nurs Forum 10:46-52, 1983.

85. Subcommittee on Unorthodox Therapies, American Society of Clinical Oncology: Ineffective cancer therapy: A guide for the layperson. J Clin Oncol 1:154-163, 1983.

Chapter 57

Teaching Strategies: The Public

Marion E. Morra, MA

INTRODUCTION

Communicating to and educating the public in the area of health has been a responsibility of nurses for many years. Health care professionals in the cancer field view themselves as role models, not only to the patients they serve but also to the public at large.

DEFINITION OF TERMS

There are many definitions of health education. Some relate to the field of education as a whole; others are based in the areas of communications, behavior, and marketing.

The President's Committee on Health Education views health education as a process that bridges the gap between health information and health practices. Health education motivates the person to take information and do something with it—to keep healthier by avoiding actions that are harmful and by forming habits that are beneficial.[1] The World Health Organization (WHO) defines health education as any combination of planned activities leading to a situation where people want to be healthy, know how to obtain health, do what they can individually and collectively, and seek help when needed.[2] Green et al[3] have a broader definition: Health education is any combination of learning experience designed to facilitate voluntary adoption of behavior conducive to health. This increases the scope as well as the purpose of health education, allowing for a wide variety of programs, activities, and methods to enrich the field.

THEORIES AND MODELS

Health education embodies theories in the fields of education, psychology, and communications. Following are several theories relating to health education.

The Health Belief Model

The Health Belief Model, often considered the basis for health behavioral research, was developed in the 1950s[4] and established a framework for explaining and predicting why people engage in specific preventive behaviors. The Health Belief Model provides insight into how an individual makes such a decision. Based on the tenet that the beliefs and values acquired over a lifetime affect a person's decisions, it combines variables such as the person's perception of being susceptible to that condition, the perceived seriousness of the problem, and the availability of specific actions that prevent or treat the condition. This model is discussed in detail in Chapter 6.

PRECEDE

The PRECEDE model of health education[3] provides an organizing framework within which more detailed theories might be integrated. The PRECEDE (an acronym for predisposing, reinforcing, and enabling causes in educational diagnosis and evaluation) framework is highly focused on intervention, be it with people whose health is in question or with those who control resources or rewards, such as community leaders, parents, peers, teachers, or health care professionals. PRECEDE has seven phases: (1) assessment of social problems of concern, (2) identification of specific health-related problems, (3) identification of specific health-related behaviors linked to the health problems, (4) categorization of factors that have direct impact on these behaviors (predisposing, enabling, or reinforcing factors), (5) assessment of relative importance of factors and resources available to influence them, (6) development and implementation of programs, and (7) evaluation.

PAR

The PAR (population attributable risk) theory[1] is based on the incidence of a disease with a fraction of a population due to exposure to a specific risk factor. It then focuses on those priority health behaviors that must influence the health of the target communities.

Communications Theory

In communication theory,[5] six basic elements are described as essential to any process of communications: (1) a source (that constructs a message), (2) an encoder (that produces it), (3) the message itself, (4) a channel (that carries it), (5) a decoder (that translates it), and (6) a receiver (that gets the message). Within the source and the receiver, four factors impinge on the success of communications: communications skills, attitudes, knowledge level, and social or cultural systems.

Social Marketing Theory

Social marketing is a theory that introduces the principles and practices of marketing to social issues, causes, and ideas.[6] It takes the attitudes and needs of the target audience into account in planning programs and campaigns. A social marketer uses research as a basis for segmenting audiences, positioning the offering, and identifying audience needs, wants, expectations, satisfactions, and dissatisfactions. In addition to the offering, social marketing contains other essential elements, such as price strategies, channel strategies, and communications. It embraces classic health promotion models and other behavioral theories and disciplines. Social marketers believe in designing related products and services, making them available when and where consumers are, and using effective channels to promote the wares.

Since health behavior is caused and determined by

many factors, education must incorporate different methods and channels to effect changes in behaviors.

BARRIERS TO EDUCATING THE PUBLIC

The National Cancer Institute (NCI) has defined several barriers to the publics' acceptance of health messages[7]:

1. Health risk is an intangible concept. Many people underestimate their risk of common health problems, such as cancer, stroke, and diabetes. People believe a serious illness will not happen to them, regardless of their actual risk.
2. The public responds to easy solutions. People are more likely to respond to simple actions (such as getting a blood test for cholesterol checking) than to a more complicated one (such as quitting smoking).
3. People want absolute answers. In the cancer field, there are not many firm answers from scientists.
4. The public may react unfavorably to fear. Frightening information may result in denial, hysteria, anxiety, and helplessness, which may be compounded if there are not immediate actions to take.
5. The public doubts the verity of science. People may not believe a scientist's prediction.
6. The public has other priorities. Many times daily problems are more important than intangible health information.
7. The public holds contradictory beliefs. Even though an individual believes "it can't happen to me", he or she can still believe "everything causes cancer" and can find no need to alter behavior. Only 38% of the population believes that life-style is related to cancer.[8]
8. The public lacks a future orientation. Many Americans, especially lower socioeconomic groups, have trouble relating to the concept of changing their behaviors for something that may not happen to them.

It is important to take such barriers into consideration during the various phases of program development. It may be possible to turn barriers into opportunities, thus creating better programs.

DEVELOPMENT OF PROGRAMS

The extent of the planning process for a health education program will depend on many factors. For example, a nationwide program will entail a more extensive planning process than will a program carried out in one community. However, several planning steps should be considered for every program and a decision made on their applicability to each situation.

The Office of Cancer Communications of the NCI outlines six stages in developing health communications programs[7]:

Stage 1: Planning and Strategy Selection

Careful assessment is made of the problem to determine whether it can be addressed by communication strategies. During this phase, information is gathered and available data are reviewed to identify existing activities and any gaps that must be addressed. Goals and objectives are written to establish what the program will accomplish. Target audiences are defined and described. The direction the program will take and the strategy for reaching the target audiences are planned. Major obstacles and barriers are identified. Resources needed to carry out the strategies are identified. Finally, a program plan and timetable are produced.

Stage 2: Selecting Channels and Materials

In this stage, the decisions made in the planning process are used to select the kinds of materials needed to reach the target audience. An assessment is made on whether existing materials can be used or adapted or whether new materials must be produced. Decisions about how the target audience will be reached (channel to be used) are also made during this stage—whether it will be a face-to-face campaign, one delivered in a classroom or a worksite, one using mass media or community groups, or a combination of more than one channel.

Stage 3: Developing Materials and Pretesting

If new materials are to be developed, this state is essential. Pretesting is used to determine whether materials produced by you or by someone else will be suitable for use with a specific target audience. This phase assures that all messages in the materials reinforce each other, are based on the strategies determined in Stage 2, and are presented in a way that is understandable to the target audience. Both the written material and the illustrations are pretested to be sure they convey the proper response. For example, when the NCI tested the phrase "cancer prevention" with an apple substituted for the "o" in prevention, it found respondents failed to link apples to either good health or prevention and thus did not use it.[7]

Stage 4: Implementing the Program

During this stage, the program is introduced to the target audience. The promotion and distribution of the materials is begun. Before starting this stage, it is essential to assure that all materials are ready in sufficient quantities, that promotion plans are in place, and that methods of tracking progress (process evaluation) have been developed. The written program plan for this phase will also contain a strategy for informing and working with other organizations involved, information on when resources are needed, when specific events are planned, and ways to identify potential problems. Specific periodic assessments are planned to determine whether the target audiences and time schedule are being reached, whether some strategies are more successful than others, how the program is operating, whether the target audience is responding, and whether the resources are being used as planned. Written progress reports and modification of program components are important aspects of this phase.

Stage 5: Assessing Effectiveness

Assessment of the effectiveness of the program is based on the goals and objectives planned in Stage 1 and used throughout the life of the program. This stage determines the outcome or results of the program, that is, whether the target audience learned, acted, or made a change. Outcome evaluation usually consists of a comparison of target audience awareness, attitudes, or behavior before and after the program.

Stage 6: Feedback

Using the information gathered at each stage—about the audience, the messages, the channels of communication, and the program's intended effect—this phase prepares to improve an ongoing program, revise it, or plan a new cycle of program development. It is also a time for sharing what has been learned about others, such as writing an article, sending materials to a related clearinghouse or agency, or presenting a poster or an abstract at a professional meeting.

OPPORTUNITIES AND CHALLENGES

The NCI, in establishing its Year 2000 goal to achieve a 50% reduction in the 1985 cancer death rate, has set a challenge for concentrated efforts by health organizations, voluntary and professional associations, government agencies, industry, and the media. The Year 2000 goal offers a framework for action and has been further enhanced by the setting of cancer-control objectives[9] based on the goal (Table 57-1). The prevention objectives center on the reduction of smoking—responsible for some 30% of all cancer deaths—and on diet, which is associated with several cancers, including colorectal cancer, the leading cause of cancer deaths after lung cancer.[9] The screening objective relate to detecting cervical and breast cancers in asymptomatic women. There are effective screening tech-

TABLE 57-1   Cancer Control Objectives to Meet Year 2000 Goal

Action	Target	Rationale	Year 2000 Objectives
Prevention	Smoking	The causal relationship between smoking and cancer has been scientifically established.	Reduce the percentage of adults who smoke from 34% to 15% or less.
			Reduce the percentage of youths who smoke by age 20 from 36% to 15% or less.
	Diet	Research indicates that high-fat and low-fiber consumption may increase the risk for various cancers.	Reduce average consumption of fat from 37% or 38% to 30% or less of total calories.
			Increase average consumption of fiber from 8 to 12 g to 20 to 30 g per day.
Screening	Breast	The effectiveness of breast screening in reducing mortality has been scientifically established.	Increase the percentage of women ages 50 to 70 who have an annual physical breast examination coupled with mammography from 45% for physical examination alone and 15% for mammography to 80%.
	Cervix	The effectiveness of cervical screening in reducing mortality has been scientifically established.	Increase the percentage of women who have a Pap smear every 3 years from 79% (ages 20 to 39) to 90% and from 57% (ages 40 to 70) to 80%.
Treatment	Transfer of research results to practice	Review by NCI of clinical trial and NCI's SEER Program data indicates that, for certain cancer sites, mortality as shown by SEER data is greater than that experienced in clinical trials.	Increase adoption of state-of-the-art treatment.

Source: National Cancer Institute: Cancer Control Objectives for the Nation: 1985-2000. NCI monograph no. 2, Appendix B. Bethesda, Md, Division of Cancer Prevention and Control, The Institute, October 1986.

niques available for both types of cancers, and women who are diagnosed early have excellent prognoses. These objectives form a strong basis for program planning and offer widespread opportunities. These opportunities also offer many challenges to health education. A few will be discussed further: segmenting audiences, reaching the disadvantaged, and using the media as a gatekeeper.

Segmenting Target Audiences

A major challenge in public education is to identify the main audience for the program. The most basic way to segment audiences is by age into adult and child learners. Factors other than age, however, must be taken into account, including sex, education, income levels, race and ethnic origin, attitudes, and beliefs. Audience segmentation has become so complex that it encompasses an entire new field of study called psychographics.

Psychographics

Psychographics, sometimes referred to as attitudinal or life-style research, segments the country into neighborhood types, personality types, media users, product and brand buyers, and benefit seekers. Its roots come from sociology, political science, and developmental psychology. Psychographics goes beyond demographics in identifying smaller, more targeted clusters in the population. One branch of psychographics is called *geodemographics*. Based on the theory that people in similar neighborhoods have similar life-styles, geodemographics divides the country into neighborhoods with specific characteristics. Using these techniques in the cancer field can give direction into who is the targeted learner—who is at highest risk and who is most needy of learning about the particular issue—as well as what kind of message to deliver.

The NCI reinforces the need for segmenting audiences to increase the likelihood that the targeted learner is reached by the educational program. Several studies on the national level have detailed cancer prevention opportunities as well as the knowledge, attitude, and behavior of specific target groups. The NCI outlines several opportunities for health education in cancer prevention[8]:

1. The lung cancer rate for women is rising much faster than that for men and has surpassed the death rate for breast cancer. The American Cancer Society (ACS) has found that 20% more women are heavy smokers (a pack or more a day) than in the 1960s.[10]
2. Cigarette smoking among adolescent girls (ages 17 to 19) is now greater than among boys in the same age group. Young women are starting to smoke at an earlier age (50% before 10th grade). The ACS estimates that female smokers are starting to smoke an average of 9 years earlier than they did in the 1960s.[10]
3. Women older than 50 who have annual physical breast examinations and mammograms can reduce their risk of breast cancer death by as much as 30%, but only 15% of women age 50 and over have an annual mam-

mogram and only 45% have a physical breast examination.
4. Since many cancers (breast, prostate, colorectal) occur more often in people age 50 or over, this age group is a prime target for early detection tests.[11]

Primary and secondary targets

In segmenting audiences, it may be useful to identify both primary and secondary audiences. A "primary" target audience is one that will be affected in some way by the messages given. A "secondary" target audience is one that has some influence on the primary audience or who must do something to help cause the change in the primary target audience. For instance, women over age 50 may be the primary audience for a mammography education program. Physicians serving this population can be a secondary target audience to be reminded to refer these women for the screening test.

One of the steps to developing a successful education program is to get to know as much as possible about the target audience and to write as detailed a description as can be defined. Items that should be delineated include[7]:

- Age, sex, ethnic background, area of residence or work
- Knowledge, attitudes, and behavior as related to the patterns to be changed
- Available health-related services and patterns of use
- Media preference and habits
- Information sources considered credible by the potential target group.

Obtaining information about audiences

There are many ways to obtain information about potential target audiences. Census data, reports from Chambers of Commerce, health departments, economic development agencies, and local hospitals can all offer demographic information. Advertising agencies, television and radio stations, newspapers, and media guides can provide data on the use of the media and the composition of the media's audiences. Knowledge and attitudes of various groups are available from polling companies, voluntary health agencies, health professional organizations, and universities. Library searches may yield useful data for audience segmentation.

New data may be needed to pinpoint specific information about the target audience. Focus group interviews is one method often used to provide insight into the beliefs, perceptions, and feelings about topics among a particular group of people. Usually consisting of 12 to 14 persons, a focus group is good for stimulating discussion of issues and for gathering opinions in a short time. However, it is not a representative sample of target populations, usually has too few participants for concensus or decision making, and depends greatly on a skilled moderator. Focus groups can be especially useful for testing materials before production in the areas of appropriate language, the appeal of a message, or the appeal of a particular spokesman to a specified target population. For instance, the NCI, in planning a major national survey on public knowledge attitudes of breast cancer, conducted separate focus groups with white, black, and Hispanic men and women to help develop the wording for specific questions. Focus groups can also be used to (1) clarify the results of survey research (especially if the results are different from those expected), (2) to generate hypotheses, or (3) to give depth to feelings about health-related issues.

Personal interviews, either by mail, telephone, or at home, are another method to gather vital data but are more expensive to conduct. If the questions that need answering are few, it may be possible to add them to an ongoing survey (such as polls that are conducted by newspapers or other enterprises to determine consumer attitudes). Mailed questionnaires are a relatively inexpensive way to reach large numbers of people. However, response rates may be low, respondents may not be representative of the whole sample, and minimum information may result. Telephone interviews generally give a higher response rate but may limit the questionnaire length. Interviews in the home, although they may give the most information, also cost the most.

Whatever the method used, it is worth the time to identify the people who are most important to reach so that pertinent messages can be developed and communication channels established. In this process, decisions can be made about audiences that will not be targeted, assuring that the available resources will be used in the most cost-effective manner.

Reaching the Disadvantaged

In 1987 and 1988, the NCI's National Advisory Board sponsored public hearings in Los Angeles, Atlanta, Miami, Dallas and Philadelphia. As a result of these hearings, the Board recommended intensified efforts to provide cancer information, prevention, and early detection programs to special population groups for whom a combination of economic disadvantage and indigenous cultural factors impede access to the health care system.[12] Groups to be included are the poor, older Americans, blacks, Hispanics, Asian-Americans, and native Americans.

Several studies[13-17] have defined serious cancer problems in the disadvantaged populations. For instance, from 1978 to 1981, blacks experienced annual cancer mortality substantially higher than did whites for several cancer sites (cervix, uterus, esophagus, larynx, lung, pancreas, prostate, and stomach).[13] Blacks delay for 3 to 12 months before seeking diagnosis and treatment for cancer.[8] There is also evidence of a relationship between low socioeconomic levels and cancer incidence. Several racial and ethnic groups have severe problems in this area (Table 57-2). For example, women of lower socioeconomic status are less likely to have regular examinations, such as Papanicolaou (Pap) tests for cervical cancer.[17] Hispanic

TABLE 57-2 Sociodemographic Characteristics of United States Population Subgroups

Characteristics	Ethnic/Racial Background				
	White	Black	Hispanic	Asian Pacific	Native American
Percentage of total US population	79.6	11.5	6.4	1.6	0.9
Median age	31.6	24.9	23.2	28.7	22.4
Percentage high school graduates	88	79	58	75	31
Median annual income in dollars	23,270 ±	13,270 ±	16,228 ±	22,713*	15,900*
Percentage below poverty level	11‡	34‡	30§	13.1*	29*
Percentage unemployed	8.6§	18.9§	13.8§	4.7*	13§
Average fertility rate per family	1.7†	2.3†	2.3†	—	4.0†
Percentage of households headed by women	10.9	37.7	23	11	24

*1979
†1980
‡1981
§1982

Source: Reprinted with permission from Ramirez AG, MacKellar DA, Gallion K: Reaching minority audiences: A major challenge in cancer reduction. Cancer Bull 40:334-343, 1988. Copyright Medical Arts Publishing Foundation, Houston, Texas.

women have twice the incidence of cervical cancer as do non-Hispanic white women.[14]

Other issues related to ethnic minorities create special requirements for cancer prevention information. On the average, blacks are less aware of cancer signs, available treatment options, and early detection techniques and their importance.[13] Both blacks and Hispanics underestimate the prevalence of cancer and have a fatalistic attitude about the disease.[17] There are also voids in almost every area of research in the minority population. For instance, the literature on the black population and cancer prevention research, cancer intervention studies, and clinical trials studies is particularly scant,[18] signalling a major opportunity for nurses.

There are several strategies for implementing health education programs in communities where the socioeconomically disadvantaged live and work. It is useful, especially in the early planning stages, to make a list of leaders who can provide information and access into the community. The list includes those persons who are respected and have personal contacts with the specific audience to be reached. The influentials can include any of the following categories[8]: church leaders, leaders in the school system, merchants and other members of the business community, members of the media, health care providers, government and civic leaders, officers of fraternal orders, and leaders in teenage communities. The influential leaders can help identify the needs of the community and assist with education programs where people live, work, and play.

Social service and health organizations are an important point of entry into these communities. A program's success can be increased by coordinating with these trusted and respected organizations and working through their existing programs. Creating special health events that address the concerns of the audience and adding them to established neighborhood-based efforts can also help ensure success.

Health education programs must take into consideration the many socioeconomic and cultural characteristics among minorities. The following considerations must be addressed during the development stage to assure successful programs for reaching the socioeconomically disadvantaged audiences.

1. *The family.* The family is a dominant influence on many minority populations and can be a credible source of health-related information. On the other hand, depending on factors, such as the disease being discussed or the type of program being planned, the family can also be a major barrier. For instance, in the Native American population, tribal elders may need to be used as role models to assure the program's success.

2. *The community.* Many minority groups, especially those who have recently come to this country, strongly identify with neighborhood and community groups. In rural areas and in some neighborhoods, the community may act as an extension of the family and become the focus of social interaction. There may be a distinct microculture, such as a religious society, within a community. Knowing the community structure is essential. It can open up different lo-

cations for presenting health education messages—such as in churches and barber shops, libraries and malls, and gyms and bodegas (stores in Hispanic neighborhoods).

3. *The language.* Language can be a significant barrier, especially in those areas where new settlers to the country are located. It is crucial, when producing materials in different languages, to involve persons who understand the nuances of the language. In some communities, language can be a major obstacle to conducting successful health education programming, and extra time and planning will be needed to ensure success.

4. *Folk beliefs and traditions.* Some minorities have strong beliefs and traditions in folk medicines, depending on cultural mores. Programming may need to incorporate these beliefs and traditions to enhance messages or at least to determine their potential impact.

5. *The influence of poverty.* Some people who live in poverty develop a sense of powerlessness, a loss of control over the outcomes of day-to-day living. Self-esteem may be lost, along with the hope for a better life. In addition, some may have a short-term perspective in living. The day-to-day stresses of crime and drugs, of foraging for meals and an existence, make issues like cancer risk seem unimportant. These influences create serious obstacles to programming for health education on issues such as cancer prevention and behavioral changes.

Reaching the Elderly

As people grow older, there seems to be a greater need to reach them, especially with messages concerning cancer screening. Approximately 50% of all cancers occur in persons over 65, with certain ones (stomach, prostate, colon and rectum in men, breast in women) accounting for over 50% of invasive cancers in persons over 60.[10] Stromborg-Frank[11] notes that the elderly are being divided into three categories: young-old (65 to 74 years), older-old (75 to 85 years) and old-old (85 years and over), a practice that helps in delivering public education messages, since cancer incidence of specific sites varies significantly with age.

The elderly population provides different challenges and obstacles to anyone presenting health education messages. These individuals have beliefs and attitudes acquired over a lifetime that may significantly influence their health practices.

A study conducted at Fox Chase Cancer Center[17] showed that most older people did not realize they are at increased risk for cancer. In addition, more than 50% of the older people surveyed believed cancer treatments are worse than the disease and had negative attitudes about physicians (80% thought that physicians cause patients to worry because they do not explain everything). In general, older persons are usually not as aware of their risk of developing cancer, are less likely to participate in screening programs, and are less likely to practice self-examination. The elderly also are more apt to underreport significant symptoms and thus present to the health care system with more advanced disease. This may be due to the fact that aches and pains are seen as more normal occurrences among the elderly and taken for granted rather than viewed as a potential symptom of disease.[19]

Dellefield[19] defines several topics that must be addressed in educating older persons: (1) the increased risk of developing cancer with advancing age, (2) the seven warning signals of cancer, (3) normal vs abnormal changes of aging, (4) the health maintenance practices recommended by the ACS, (5) the benefits of early detection in relation to reduced morbidity and mortality, (6) the acceptability and management of cancer treatments, (7) the skills and coping strategies needed to make the elderly more successful as patients in the contemporary health care system, and (8) the community resources available to provide early detection services and assistance in developing better self-care skills.

On average, the elderly do not learn as quickly and as easily as do younger persons. They may not see and hear as well. They may have had many negative lifetime experiences with cancer and cancer treatment. In preparing materials and in presenting programs to this target group, special attention must be paid to specific strategies to overcome these barriers.

Socializing and social atmospheres are attractive to this target population. Taking advantage of already existing meetings, such as senior citizens groups, may add to a program's success. Using positive, wellness-related tactics is another strategy. A gastroenterologist in Connecticut found that entitling his program "The Care and Feeding of Your Digestive Tract" rather than "Cancer of the Colon" increased his audiences twofold. Older Americans are an important group to target. They present special problems and have distinct barriers that must be overcome if programming is to be successful. Table 57-3 summarizes the strategies for reaching special audiences.

TABLE 57-3 Reaching Special Audiences

Production of Materials	Strategies for Older Learners	Strategies for Lower Socioeconomic Groups
Use language appropriate to different cultural groups (one word may have different meanings to different groups).	Keep learning sessions brief (10 to 15 minutes) and pace instruction.	Work through existing programs and agencies.
Understand values and customs for each cultural group.	Avoid rushing the learner.	Work through people already trusted in the community.
Identify channels that will be credible and most capable of reaching minority audiences.	Proceed from the simple to the complex.	Try to create programs incorporating your needs into already ongoing programs.
Use current information to choose the best channels and message strategies.	Focus and maintain attention on a single well-defined piece of information.	
Develop separate message appeals for each minority group, since perceived needs, values, and beliefs may differ.	Use concrete examples, short sentences, slow speech, and much repetition.	Use concern for family as a motivator.
	Use redundant or multiple cuing; say it, draw it, write it.	Stress payoffs for changing attitudes or beliefs.
Use simply written print materials, reinforced with graphics and pretested.	Allow the initial learning tasks to proceed slowly.	Create simple, concrete messages.
Pretest both print and graphics. People perceive graphics and illustrations in different ways, just as words have different meanings.	Do not present new information until earlier concepts have been mastered.	Use visual materials—people learn more by seeing than by any other method.
	Allow ample time for learning tasks involving psychomotor skills.	
Use bilingual materials to ensure that intermediaries and family members who are most comfortable with English can help readers understand content.	Deemphasize tasks involving abstract reasoning.	Use both visual and written materials to reinforce messages.
	Minimize the number of alternative responses available.	
Do not simply translate print materials from the English; rewrite the material, since concepts and appeals may differ by culture just as the words do.	Compensate for sensory changes by using non-glare lighting, large print, mid- to low-pitched speaking voice, and a quiet environment.	Repeat the same message and same themes.
	Use social support to reinforce learning.	Use television as a primary channel.
Consider audiovisual materials or interpersonal communication that may be more successful for some messages and audiences.	Provide positive feedback to make learner aware of progress.	Use personalized, direct mail messages.
	Express warmth and respect.	

Source: Adapted from National Cancer Institute: Making Health Communications Programs Work: A Planner's Guide. Bethesda, MD, Office of Cancer Communications, The Institute, NIH pub. no. 89-1493, 1989; and Dellefield ME: Informational needs and approaches for early cancer detection in the elderly. Semin Oncol Nurs 7:156-168, 1988.

Making Written Materials Easier to Read

One of the major problems facing those producing printed health communications materials is how to make them easy to read. About 20% of the adult American population reads at or below the fifth-grade level. An additional 35% reads at the fifth- to tenth-grade level.[20] Yet cancer materials being used for general information and education are written at higher levels. For instance, the NCI pamphlet "Goods News for Blacks About Cancer" is written at a seventh-grade level. The ACS pamphlet "Fry Now, Pay Later," about skin cancer, is written at an 11th-grade level. A Readers Digest article, "Why Can't We Get the Medicine We Need," tests at a 14th-grade level.

In the area of patient information, there is also a wide gap between the readability level of commonly used health-teaching materials and patients' reading comprehensive skills. Much of the material is written at a 10th-grade level, although the average patients have word-recognition skills at about the seventh-grade level; they state, however, that they are high school graduates.[20]

Both the NCI and the ACS are working to produce more materials in easy-to-read language and format. A series of simple, one-page cards on each of the major cancer sites has been produced by the ACS (Figure 57-1) with the message in English on one side and Spanish on the other. These have a fifth-grade readability level.

Performing readability tests

Readability testing measures the approximate level of education needed to understand printed materials. Most of the formulas used to test how readable an item is take into account the difficulty of the words being used and length of sentences. Short sentences and words of two syllables or less make materials easier to read. The Office of Cancer Communications of the NCI reviewed twelve readability formulas and chose the SMOG grading system for testing its own materials because it is easy to use and accurate.[7]

A basic description of how the SMOG system is used follows:

1. Pick 10 consecutive sentences near the beginning, in the middle, and at the end of the material (30 sentences total).
2. Count the words that have three or more syllables, including repeats of those words.
3. Using the conversion numbers listed below, find the approximate grade level that a person must have reached to understand fully the text being examined (the grade will be plus or minus 1.5 grades).

Word count	Grade level
0-2	4
3-6	5
7-12	6
13-20	7
21-30	8
31-42	9
43-56	10
57-72	11
73-90	12
91-110	13
111-132	14
133-156	15
157-182	16
183-210	17
211-240	18

Guidelines for producing simpler material

To produce materials that will be understandable to the general audience, use the following guidelines:

- Pick short words—two syllables or less.
- Create short sentences. It makes you write more simply.
- Use short paragraphs—limit each one to one idea.
- Pick simple language.
- Write to one person, using action verbs and a conversational style.
- Use the same words to describe an item. Do not say "cancer" one time and "tumor" the next.
- Use examples to illustrate important points.
- Do not use abbreviations.
- Repeat the same information in several ways. Write it. Show a picture or sketch of it. Make a chart out of it.
- Use subheads to tell the reader what is coming.
- Break up the text with graphics at key points, using bold face type, bullets, underlining, or boxed text.
- Summarize at the end of major points.
- Do a readability test; if the level is too high, go back and try again.

THE MEDIA AS GATEKEEPER

The media is an essential part of many programs for communicating with and educating the public. The mass media, which includes radio, television, wire service, newspapers, and magazines, can also involve other channels such as direct mail, billboards, and transit cards. Mass media transmits information quickly to a broad audience and is probably the public's main source of information. The media plays an important role for some target au-

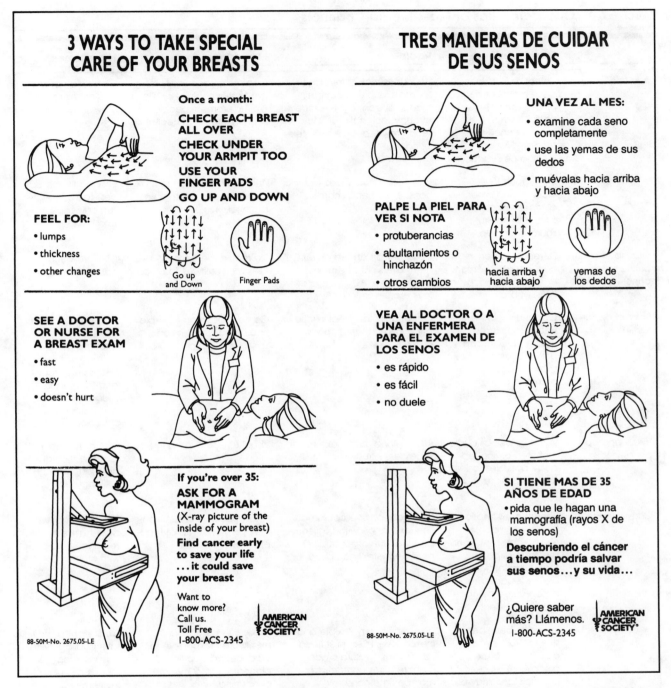

FIGURE 57-1 The American Cancer Society has published a series of educational cards, with English on one side and Spanish on the other, written at a fifth-grade level. (Source: American Cancer Society: Three Ways to Take Special Care of Your Breasts. Atlanta, Ga, The Society, pub no. 88-2675.05-LE, 1988.)

diences, since the average American has a television set turned on for almost 7 hours a day and individual family members watch television approximately 3 hours each. In addition, most Americans read a newspaper daily.

Drawbacks of Mass Media

Mass media has several drawbacks when used for public education about cancer: (1) its main purpose is to inform and entertain rather than to educate, (2) it is difficult to use for transmitting complex messages, (3) it has major constraints on space and time, and (4) it carries a high risk of miscommunication, particularly if the material is controversial (Table 57-4).

Public service announcements (PSAs), which the mass media will carry for free for nonprofit organizations, are often thought of as the major use of the mass media for public education purposes. Since deregulation, however, television and radio stations are no longer required to

TABLE 57-4 Characteristics of Mass Media Channels

	Television	Radio	Magazines	Newspapers
Audiences	Potentially largest/wide range of audiences, but not always at times when public service announcements (PSAs) are most likely to be broadcast.	Various formats offer potential for more audience targeting than television (eg, teenagers through rock stations). May reach fewer people than television.	Can more specifically target to segments of public (young women, people with an interest in health)	Can reach broad audiences rapidly.
	Can reach low-income and other audiences not as likely to turn to health sources for help.	Can reach audiences who do not use the health care system.	Audience has chance to clip, reread, contemplate material.	Easy audience access to in-depth issue coverage is possible.
Availability of public service announcements	Deregulation ended government oversight of station broadcast of PSAs, public affairs	Deregulation ended government oversight of stations' broadcast of PSAs, public affairs programming.	No requirement for PSA use; PSAs more difficult to place.	PSAs are virtually nonexistent.
Special opportunities	Opportunity to include health messages through broadcasts, public affairs/interview shows, dramatic programming.	Opportunity for direct audience involvement through call-in shows.	Can explain more complex health issues, behaviors.	Can convey health news/breakthroughs more thoroughly than television or radio and faster than magazines. Feature placement possible.
Visual and audio appeals	Visual as well as audio make emotional appeals possible. Easier to demonstrate a behavior.	Audio alone may make messages less intrusive.	Visual effects can be intensified	Print may lend itself to more factual, detailed, rational message delivery.
Convenience	Passive consumption by viewer; viewers must be present when message aired; less than full attention likely. Message may be obscured by commercial "clutter."	Generally passive consumption; exchange with audience possible, but target audience must be there when aired.	Permits active consultation; may pass on; read at reader's convenience.	Short life of newspaper limits rereading, sharing with others.
Flexibility	PSAs can be expensive to produce and distribute. Feature placement requires contacts and may be time-consuming.	Live copy is very flexible and inexpensive; PSAs must fit station format. Feature placement requires contacts and may be time-consuming.	Public service advertisements are inexpensive to produce; ad or article placement may be time-consuming.	Small papers may take public service ads; coverage demands a newsworthy item.

Source: National Cancer Institute: Making Health Communications Programs Work: A Planner's Guide. Bethesda, Md, Office of Cancer Communications, National Cancer Institute, NIH pub no. 89-1493, 1989.

donate a specific amount of time to public service programming, and the number of PSAs being carried has diminished. Although well-planned and well-produced PSAs can be effective, many other opportunities exist in the mass media, such as news programs, public affairs programs, interview and talk shows, local television panel discussions, call-in programs, editorials, letters to the editors, and health and political columns.

There are professionals ("media gatekeepers") in the media who decide what material will be used and when it will be used. It is their responsibility to understand what the public wants. If the health information messages or programming do not fit into the gatekeepers' needs, they will not be used or they will be used at odd hours or, in the case of print media, will be placed in nonprominent positions. It is a challenge to produce materials that are appealing to media formats and relevant to media needs as well as to target audiences.

Beliefs Among Gatekeepers

Stuyck and Chilton [21] conducted a study to examine the role of mass media gatekeepers in disseminating cancer information. The study gathered information on the beliefs among gatekeepers of the major health problems, the perception of their roles, and their opinions on materials they received for cancer information. The following are observations and recommendations based on the information gained from the study:

1. Disease mortality and morbidity in themselves do not guarantee media interest. Cancer and acquired immune deficiency syndrome (AIDS) ranked highest as important health care issues. Cardiovascular disease was ranked by less than half to be among the three major health concerns (although heart disease annually kills more than twice as many Americans as does cancer). There was little correlation between the prevalence or impact of disease and related problems and their relative rank among health issues.

2. Health professionals should be armed with information before approaching the media. Most gatekeepers feel a responsibility to educate the public but consider themselves trained to report and write, and they expect health educators to be informed about the issues and about the needs of the media.

3. Health communicators should be aggressive if they wish to achieve results. In the Stuyck and Chilton survey,[21] there was a correlation between how often the gatekeepers were contacted by persons in the cancer field and how often they covered cancer news. Since the gatekeepers did not consider reporting cancer news as a top priority for their media, health communicators must be knowledgeable and active advocates for their causes.

4. The media are more likely to pay attention to information from sources they perceive to be credible. Among seven factors with the potential for influencing news coverage, the credibility of the news source was ranked highest, significantly above others such as management interests and audience or readership surveys. Gatekeepers also said they were most likely to cover a news story from an institution with a reputation in cancer.

5. Media gatekeepers want information they consider useful to their audiences. Gatekeepers showed great interest in helping their audiences become informed consumers in the area of cancer, especially in advances in cancer treatment and risk reduction (tobacco and nutrition).

6. Media gatekeepers want information that is clearly written and is brief. The main reason for not using materials sent to them by health professionals were inappropriate format (43%), lack of space or time (28%), and uninteresting material (18%). Complicated terminology and inability of physicians and scientists to discuss findings in simple language were also cited. Ways in which the information could be improved include tailoring the information to local audiences (29%), making information more concise (18%) or simple and clear (13%), and sending information on a regular basis (8%). Gatekeepers from all types of media were interested in receiving materials they perceived as relevant to their audiences and of help in doing their jobs.

This study emphasizes the importance of looking at material being produced and disseminated through the eyes of the people who control its use, be they news directors or public service directors at radio and television stations or medical reporters, science writers, life-style editors, or journalists in the print media.

EXAMPLES OF PUBLIC EDUCATION ACTIVITIES

If one were to consider all the activities that educate and inform the public about health in the media and in community sites of various descriptions, around the country, they would number in the thousands per month. In the government arena alone, some 20 agencies directly offer information related to cancer prevention and detection (Table 57-5). The activities range from a simple talk before a woman's group to complex curricula proposed for school systems in entire states, from an 8-second mention on a local television news program to the organization of a national 1-day event such as the Great American Smokeout. The evaluation of these programs also varies widely—from none at all to highly sophisticated. Two major activities have been selected and will be considered in this section—smoking-related programs and the Cancer Information Service.

Helping People to Stop Smoking

There have been programs in the United States to help people to stop smoking since the 1950s. Although more than 40 million Americans have stopped smoking since the first Surgeon General's report on smoking and health in 1964, over 50 million Americans continue to smoke.[10] There are more heavy smokers today than ever before.[10] To help these people quit and to make the Surgeon General's goal of a smoke-free society by the year 2000 will require a major effort by all the health groups in this country. It will also require knowledge of the most effective intervention strategies and widespread implementation of these strategies.

The NCI commissioned a comprehensive review and evaluation of smoking cessation methods in the United States and Canada for the years 1978 to 1985, as an update to a review carried out under the auspices of the Centers for Disease Control (CDC) for the years 1969 to 1977 (an earlier review of smoking control methods was supported by the National Clearinghouse for Smoking and Health

TABLE 57-5 Government Agencies as Resources for Cancer Education

Agency	Major Programs	Special Features
CENTER FOR HEALTH PROMOTION AND EDUCATION CENTERS FOR DISEASE CONTROL Building 1 South, Room SSB249 1600 Clifton Road, NE Atlanta, GA 30333 (404) 329-3492	Provides technical assistance to state and local health departments Coordinates Behavior Risk Factor Surveillance System (BRFS). Implements School Health Education Program (SHED). Maintains Health Education Database (HED).	Tracks risk factors in population with BRSF-telephone survey on smoking, alcohol, nutrition. SHFD evaluates impact of program on students' health related behaviors. HED gives on line, computer summary of health education efforts.
CLEARINGHOUSE FOR OCCUPATIONAL SAFETY AND HEALTH INFORMATION NATIONAL INSTITUTE FOR OCCUPATIONAL SAFETY AND HEALTH Technical Information Branch 4676 Columbia Parkway Cincinnati, OH 45226 (513) 684-8326	Provides technical information to Institute's research programs. Gives information to others on request.	
CLEARINGHOUSE ON HEALTH INDEXES NATIONAL CENTER FOR HEALTH STATISTICS Division of Epidemiology and Health Promotion 3700 East-West Highway, Room 2-27 Hyattsville, MD 20782	Provides informational assistance in development of health measures for researchers, administrators and planners.	
CONSUMER INFORMATION CENTER GENERAL SERVICES ADMINISTRATION Pueblo, CO 81009 (303) 948-3334	Distributes consumer publications on many topics, such as food and nutrition, health, and exercise.	Provides *Consumer Information Catalog* from which to order publications.
CONSUMER PRODUCT SAFETY COMMISSION Washington, DC 20207 (301) 492-6800 (800) 638-2772 (Hotline)	Sets standards and conducts information programs on potentially hazardous products, such as carcinogens.	Independent Federal regulatory agency. Has jurisdiction over consumer products in and around home.
FOOD AND NUTRITION INFORMATION CENTER U.S. DEPARTMENT OF AGRICULTURE National Agricultural Library Building-Room 304 Beltsville, MD 20705 (301) 344-3719	Serves information needs of professionals interested in nutrition education, food services and food technology.	Acquires and lends books, journal articles and audiovisual materials.
NATIONAL AUDIOVISUAL CENTER NATIONAL ARCHIVES 8700 Edgeworth Drive Capitol Heights, MD 20743-3701 (301) 763-1896 (301) 763-4385 (TDD)	Distributes more than 8000 programs on over 600 topics, including cancer and environment, cancer detection, smoking, specific cancer sites.	Central source for federally sponsored audiovisuals. Charges for audiovisuals and accompanying materials.
DIVISION OF CANCER PREVENTION AND CONTROL NATIONAL CANCER INSTITUTE National Institutes of Health Bethesda, MD 20892-4200 (301) 496-6616	Plans and conducts basic and applied research programs aimed at reducing cancer incidence, morbidity and mortality. Plans, directs and coordinates the support of basic and applied research on cancer prevention and control at cancer centers and community hospitals. Coordinates programs activities with Federal and state agencies. Establishes liaison with professional and voluntary health agencies, labor organizations, cancer organizations and trade associations.	Activities carried out across five phases of research: hypothesis development, methods testing, controlled intervention, trials, defined population studies and demonstrations relevant to the prevention and management of cancer.

TABLE 57-5 Government Agencies as Resources for Cancer Education (continued)

Agency	Major Programs	Special Features
OFFICE OF CANCER COMMUNICATIONS NATIONAL CANCER INSTITUTE National Institute of Health Bethesda, MD 20892 (301) 496-6631	Provides information on all aspects of the cancer problem to physicians, scientists, educators, Congress, the Executive Branch, the media and the public. Fosters and coordinates a national cancer communications programs designed to provide the public and health professionals with information they need to take more responsible health actions.	The Cancer Information Service (1-800-4-CANCER) is located with this office, with a network of locations across the country.
OFFICE OF PREVENTION, EDUCATION, AND CONTROL NATIONAL HEART, LUNG, AND BLOOD INSTITUTE (NHLBI) National Institute of Health 9000 Rockville Pike Bethesda, MD 20892 (301) 496-5437	Initiates educational activities for NHLBI which fosters informational and educational activities designed to reduce preventable heart, lung, and blood disease morbidity and mortality.	
NATIONAL CLEARINGHOUSE FOR ALCOHOL INFORMATION NATIONAL INSTITUTE ON ALCOHOL ABUSE AND ALCOHOLISM P.O. Box 2345 Rockville, MD 20852 (301) 468-2600	Gathers and disseminates current information on alcohol-related subjects. Provides literature searches, referrals, a library and reading room and summaries of current alcohol-related information.	Responds to requests from the public, health professionals, scientists, and other professionals.
NATIONAL LIBRARY OF MEDICINE NATIONAL INSTITUTES OF HEALTH 8600 Rockville Pike Bethesda, MD 20892 (301) 496-6308 Public Information Office (301) 496-6095 Reference Station	Collects, organizes and disseminates both printed and audiovisual materials, technical and scientific in nature, primarily for medical professionals. Offers extensive computerized literature retrieval service.	Listing of bibliographies, catalogs and indexes with specific ordering instructions is available from the Public Information Office.
NATIONAL MATERNAL AND CHILD HEALTH CLEARINGHOUSE 38th and R Street, NW Washington, DC 20057 (202) 625-8410	Provides information and publications on maternal and child health and genetics, including topics such as smoking and pregnancy and nutrition and pregnancy.	Provides materials to consumers and health professionals.
NATIONAL TOXICOLOGY PROGRAM NATIONAL INSTITUTE OF ENVIRONMENTAL HEALTH SCIENCES M.D. B2-04, Box 12233 Research Triangle Park, NC 27709 (919) 541-3991	Develops and disseminates scientific information regarding potentially hazardous chemicals, including those which can cause cancer. Coordinates research conducted by four agencies of the Department of Health and Human Services.	Information in the form of technical reports is available free of charge to scientists and other health professionals.
OFFICE OF CONSUMER AFFAIRS FOOD AND DRUG ADMINISTRATION 5600 Fishers Lane Rockville, MD 20857 (301) 443-3170	Responds to consumer inquiries. Serves as clearinghouse for consumer publications on a variety of topics including pregnancy, food and nutrition, cosmetics, proper use of drugs and health fraud.	Over 250 publications available free of charge.

TABLE 57-5 Government Agencies as Resources for Cancer Education (continued)

Agency	Major Programs	Special Features
NATIONAL HEALTH INFORMATION CLEARINGHOUSE OFFICE OF DISEASE PREVENTION AND HEALTH PROMOTION P.O. Box 1133 Washington, DC 20013-1133 800-336-4797 (202) 429-9091	Central source of information and referral for health questions from the public and health professionals. Maintains computer database of government agencies, support groups, professional societies and other organizations that can answer questions on specific health topics. Offers library containing medical and health reference books, directories, information files and periodicals; database development on organizations that provide health information; and a number of publications including resource guides and bibliographies.	Among publications prepared are *Prevention Abstracts,* which summarizes prevention-oriented findings in the scientific literature; *Prevention Activities Calendar,* which highlights major prevention events for the month; *Healthfinder Series* which provides resource lists on specific health topics such as exercise for older Americans, health risk appraisals, health statistics and many other issues; *Staying Healthy: A Bibliography of Health Promotion Materials,* which serves as a guide to current information on health promotion and disease prevention topics.
OFFICE ON SMOKING AND HEALTH U.S. DEPARTMENT OF HEALTH AND HUMAN SERVICES Technical Information Center Park Building-Room 1-10 5600 Fishers Lane Rockville, MD 20857 (301) 443-1690	Produces and distributes a number of informational and educational materials. Offers bibliographic and reference services to researchers and others. Produces pamphlets, posters and public service announcements which contain various health messages.	Materials and services are available free of charge.
PUBLIC INFORMATION CENTER ENVIRONMENTAL PROTECTION AGENCY 820 Quincy Street, NW Washington, DC 20210 (202) 829-3535	Provides information on programs and activities of the Environmental Protection Agency including topics such as hazardous wastes, the school asbestos project, air and water pollution, pesticides and drinking water.	
PUBLICATION DISTRIBUTION OFFICE OCCUPATIONAL SAFETY AND HEALTH ADMINISTRATION U.S. Department of Labor 200 Constitution Ave., NW—Room s4203 Washington, DC 20210 (202) 523-9667	Responds to inquiries about a limited number of job-related carcinogens and toxic substances.	Single copies of materials available free to general public, health professionals, industry, educational institutions and other sources.
INFORMATION OFFICE NATIONAL INSTITUTE ON AGING Federal Building, 6th Floor 9000 Rockville Pike Bethesda, MD 20892 (301) 496-1752	Distributes information for older Americans on many topics, including cancer and smoking.	
OFFICE OF MINORITY HEALTH RESOURCE CENTER P.O. Box 37337 Washington, DC 20013-7337 1-800-444-MHRC(6472)	Provides minority health information and referrals. Maintains computerized database of materials, organizations and programs. Provides network of professionals active in the field.	Provides bilingually staffed toll-free number.

Source: National Cancer Institute: Cancer Prevention Resource Directory, Bethesda, Md, Office of Cancer Communications, The Institute, NIH pub no. 86-2827, 1986.

and published in 1969). The conclusions of this review are as follows[22]:

1. Smokers prefer to quit on their own with the help of instructions, medicines, and guides. Less complex quit guides achieve higher success rates. Of people who select to quit on their own, 16% to 20% are not smoking 1 year later. These data are supported by national studies that show that of those who try to quit, 20% report that they succeed. Self-quitting seems to involve cumulative learning over repeated efforts.

2. Many people who quit act on the advice or warning of a health professional. Physician advice and counseling encourage many individuals to attempt to break their cigarette habit. Where the physician adds a stronger message, gives tips on how to quit, or provides follow-up support, the results improve.

3. The nurse is an ideal person to counsel smokers, since the nurse is viewed as a credible health worker. The nurse involves the patient's family in the counseling process so that family members can provide support and encouragement.

4. The roles of other health professionals such as dentists, dental hygienists, physician's assistants, nurse practitioners, inhalation therapists, paramedics, pharmacists, and others have not been studied adequately in terms of their effects on influencing patients to quit smoking.

5. Nicotine chewing gum (Nicorette) can be an effective tool for persons who are motivated to quit. Longer use (6 months to 1 year) appears to improve quit rates. Other methods (counseling, support) should be used to supplement the gum.

6. Hypnosis and acupuncture are popular treatments, but evaluation has been inadequate. In general, counseling and support also are needed.

7. The media reaches a wide number of smokers with instructions on how to quit smoking. Long-term quit rates are low, but these programs could be more effective if combined with group or individual instructions. Use of the telephone to promote maintenance support is noteworthy.

8. Community studies have mixed results but suggest that a combination of mass media and intensive instruction is more successful than media alone.

9. Behavioral techniques reveal a wide range of success. Adversive therapy (electric shock, breath holding, unpleasant taste, etc.) showed poor results. Rapid smoking appears to be effective in the short term. Covert sensitization (use of subject's imagination) has failed to produce long-term results but, like rapid smoking, may be useful combined with other procedures.

10. The worksite offers an excellent opportunity for implementing strategies that lead to cessation of smoking. There is a growing movement to restrict smoking in employee work areas. Some companies offer smoking cessation programs, such as educational programs, distribution of self-help kits, and physician advice during physical examinations and groups.

11. Maintenance support is the critical ingredient in the long-term success of smoking cessation. Successful quitters score higher than recidivists in personal security, ease of quitting on last attempt, expectation of success in giving up smoking, and social support. They had smoked fewer cigarettes a day before quitting and had lower levels of anxiety.

12. Leading causes of relapse are anxiety, stress, anger, frustration, social pressures, weight gain, and lack of inner resources. Being around other smokers, eating, and drinking alcohol or coffee also contribute to relapse.

13. The highest median quit rates for trials with 1-year follow-up were scored by physician intervention programs for patients with cardiac disease (these patients are highly motivated due to life-threatening illness). High quit rates were also scored by physician intervention with patients with pulmonary disorders, risk factor studies, and rapid smoking and satiation when each was combined with other procedures. Support groups and nicotine chewing gum, combined with behavioral treatment or therapy, came next.

14. A significant trend is the increased negative attitude toward cigarette smoking, as exemplified by the numerous regulations for nonsmoking sections in schools, restaurants, worksites, military areas, and other public places.

The smoking, tobacco and cancer program In 1982, the NCI launched an intervention research effort, the Smoking, Tobacco and Cancer Program, which is today supporting 60 intervention trials. These trials are evaluating the use of specific channels (schools, health care providers, mass media and self-help strategies) among target populations (youth, women, ethnic minorities, heavy smokers, and smokeless tobacco users). About half these trials have been completed, with the remaining to be completed in 1992.

These target groups were selected based on the latest smoking statistics. In 1987, 33% of men and 28% of women smoked (down from 53% and 34%, respectively, in 1964). However, because of an increase in total population, there are now 1 million more smokers than existed 10 years ago—over 50 million regular smokers.[10]

There are also many signs of problems among population groups. The proportion of teens, ages 12 through 17, who smoke increased from 12% in 1979 to over 15% in 1985. Smoking quit rates among adults have slowed, with more adults hard-core addicted smokers and more heavy smokers (25 or more cigarettes a day). Black men are more likely to smoke, are more likely to use cigarettes with a higher tar and nicotine content, and are 50% more likely to develop lung cancer than are white men. In addition, the use of smokeless tobacco products has increased, particularly among adolescent males and young men. It is estimated that at least 12 million people used smokeless tobacco in 1985.[10]

The ASSIST/2000 program The ASSIST/2000 program, a new initiative launched by the NCI in the early

1990s, supports large-scale demonstrations in states and large metropolitan areas. It includes a broad range of organizations and community groups capable of working together to coordinate the area's tobacco control resources and to implement intervention trials. The program has two phases: an 18- to 24-month planning phase, and a 5-year implementation phase.

Activities include the training of health care professionals to deliver cessation counseling, the provision of targeted cessation interventions in worksites and other locations, the implementation of tobacco-use prevention curricula in schools, and the use of print and electronic media to cover the smoking issue. The target groups are minorities, women, heavy smokers, low-income smokers, and youth. The lead organizations on the local levels are the state (or local) health departments and the ACS. The interventions will be based on the trials presently underway. An independent evaluation will be conducted using baseline and follow-up surveys of smoking and tobacco use in each geographic area funded. It is estimated that some 20 areas will be funded to begin phase II work in 1992.

The investigators involved in the Smoking, Tobacco and Cancer Program are testing the strategies to be used in ASSIST/2000 and by 1988 had already produced 166 articles in journals and scientific reports on these studies.[23] This scientific base will be used to plan the intervention by the organizations involved. ASSIST/2000 is a massive effort that will provide many challenges and opportunities for nurses.

The Cancer Information Service
As public educator

The Cancer Information Service (CIS), a program of the NCI, is a toll-free telephone service that answers questions about cancer prevention and control, diagnosis, treatment, and rehabilitation. Begun in 1976, the CIS has a network of offices throughout the country based in comprehensive cancer centers, community cancer centers, and hospitals. Using a common number (1-800-4-CANCER), calls are routed automatically to CIS offices in local areas. Since 1976, when the CIS received 47,000 calls, the calls have grown steadily to nearly 400,000 a year in the late 1980s.

CIS counselors, after completing a standardized training program, provide accurate, up-to-date information tailored to the needs of individual callers. The NCI's computerized database, PDQ (Physician's Data Query), which contains state-of-the-art treatment information and NCI-aproved clinical trials, is a major resource for treatment information.

Between 1983 and 1986, almost 50% of inquiries to the CIS were from the general public, that is, people without symptoms. The callers are predominantly white (86%), female (70%), over age 30 (74%), and with at least a high school education (89%). A national user survey, carried out in 1983, of a random sample of over 7600 CIS callers, showed that the respondents found the information help-

ful (94%) and clear and easy to understand (96%). The CIS staff was seen as knowledgeable (95%), courteous (97%), and friendly (97%). Nearly 98% said they would call the service again if they had questions, and more than 50% had already recommended the use of CIS to others. About 93% of the callers reported taking some kind of action, with 58% sharing the information with at least one other person (information from 4091 initial inquiries reached 11,386 people). In addition, 91% indicated the CIS was important in their decisions to take action following the call.[24] As one of the oldest continuously funded programs of the NCI and as its major outreach arm, the CIS has grown in size, in quality, and in the services it offers.

As change agent

The CIS, in addition to its roles in public and patient information and in education, is increasingly acting as a change agent in the area of cancer prevention and risk reduction. In CIS offices across the country, telephone counselors have been trained in techniques to help smokers who wish to quit, based on a research project conducted at the Roswell Park CIS[24] and on basic strategies for behavior change (using a protocol concentrating on steps including precomtemplation, contemplation, action, and maintenance). The counselors assess the individual's needs, identify roadblocks and facilitators to altering personal behavior, and give the appropriate advice, referrals, and written materials to help the caller make the change. A similar training program has been conducted to enable counseling about clinical trials.

A study, currently being conducted at the University of California at Los Angeles and the University of Southern California, uses the CIS as an instrument to increase breast screening among female callers. This project attempts to change the CIS from a passive system, which depends on a specific request from the caller, to an active one, which targets particular subgroups of high-risk callers for specific cancer control messages. All female CIS callers 40 years and older who are not currently being treated for cancer will be randomized within these groups: group I (information about mammography will only be given in response to a specific request by the caller); group II (information about breast screening and age-specific behavioral recommendations will be given, following a strict intervention protocol, to all callers regardless of their initial reason for calling the CIS; and group III (will receive the same intervention as group II but will be contacted 2 weeks after the initial call to reinforce adherence to the behavioral recommendations).

The intervention protocol is grounded in communications and persuasion theory. Assessment of the outcome (self-reported adherence to the mammography recommendations made by the CIS) will be by telephone interview 6 months after the initial call, along with measures of attitudes, barriers, beliefs, and intentions related to mammography.[24]

This new thrust of the CIS into the role of change agent has the potential for major impact. It uses an existing system with a proven track record for satisfying the needs of people who wish cancer information in a new and different way. These studies, showing that a telephone system can be used to reinforce positive health messages and stimulate encouraging behavioral change, could provide a new catalyst to altering knowledge and health practices.

CHALLENGES FOR THE FUTURE

There have been many changes in public information and education during the 1980s. The cancer field, led by the NCI and the ACS, has kept pace, using sophisticated marketing techniques. New opportunities will continue, and health professionals must join with colleagues in other areas to meet them.

As health professionals work toward reaching the NCI's Year 2000 goals, a number of challenges present themselves: how to develop interventions most effectively to reduce the cancer risk, how to implement those interventions to reach the greatest number of people at risk, how to plan public education programs that will use resources, both nationally and locally, to their greatest benefits, and how to plan and implement programs that will be sensitive to the needs of minority and other target audiences. These challenges demand new ways of thinking, new interrelationships, and new methods of operation. Nurses can assume a leadership role in providing innovative, research-based educational opportunities that will help meet these challenges.

REFERENCES

1. Gochman DS: Health Behavior: Emerging Research Perspectives. New York, Plenum Press, 1988.
2. Kolbe LJ: The application of health behavior and research: Health education and health information, in Gochman DS (ed): Health Behavior: Emerging Research Perspectives. New York, Plenum Press, 1988, pp 381-396.
3. Green LW, Kreuter MW, Deeds SG, et al: Health Education Planning: A Diagnostic Approach. Palo Alto, Calif, Mayfield Publishing Co, 1980.
4. Rosenstock IM: Historical Origins of the Health Belief Model. Health Ed monographs 2:328-35, 1974.
5. Berlo DK: The Process of Communication: An Introduction to Theory and Practice. New York, Holt, Rinehart & Winston, 1960.
6. Kotler P, Andreasen AR: Strategic Marketing for Nonprofit Organizations (ed 3). Englewood Cliffs, NJ, Prentice-Hall, 1987.
7. National Cancer Institute: Making Health Communications Programs Work: A Planner's Guide. Bethesda, Md, Office of Cancer Communications, The Institute, NIH pub no. 89-1493, 1989.
8. National Cancer Institute: Making The Right Connection. Bethesda, Md, Office of Cancer Communication, The Institute, 1989.
9. National Career Institute: Cancer Control Objectives for the Nation: 1985-2000. NCI monograph no. 2, Appendix B. Bethesda, Md, Division of Cancer Prevention and Control, The Institute, October 1986.
10. American Cancer Society: Cancer Facts and Figures—1989. Atlanta, Ga, The Society, 1989.
11. Stromborg-Frank M: The role of the nurse in early detection of cancer: Population sixty-six years and older. Oncol Nurs Forum 13(3):66-74, 1986.
12. National Cancer Institute: Fighting Cancer in America: Findings and Recommendations of the 1987-88 Public Participation Hearings of the National Cancer Advisory Board on Cancer Prevention and Early Detection. Bethesda, Md, Office of Cancer Communications, The Institute, 1989.
13. US Department of Health and Human Resources: Report of the Secretary's Task Force on Black and Minority Health (Vol III), Cancer, 1986. Washington, DC, US Government Printing Office, 1986.
14. US Department of Health and Human Resources: Report of the Secretary's Task Force on Black and Minority Health (Vol VIII), Hispanic Health Issues. Washington, DC, US Government Printing Office, 1986.
15. Porter/Novelli: Cancer Prevention and Control Needs of Disadvantaged Americans: An Exploratory Study. Atlanta, Ga, The American Cancer Society, 1988.
16. Ramirez AG, MacKellar DA, Gallion K: Reaching minority audiences: A major challenge in cancer reduction. Cancer Bull 40:334-343, 1988.
17. Wilson CM, Rimer BK, Bennett DJ, et al: Educating the older cancer patient: Obstacles and opportunities. Health Ed Q 10:76-87, 1984.
18. National Cancer Institute: Annotated Bibliography of Cancer-Related Literature on Black Populations. Bethesda, Md, The Institute, Division of Cancer Prevention and Control, NIH pub no. 89-3024, 1989.
19. Dellefield ME: Informational needs and approaches for early cancer detection in the elderly. Semin Oncol Nurs 7:156-168, 1988.
20. Doak CC, Doak LG, Root JH: Teaching Patients with Low Literary Skills. Philadelphia, JB Lippincott, 1985.
21. Stuyck SC, Chilton JA: Examining the role of mass media gatekeepers in disseminating cancer information. Cancer Bull 40:334-343, 1988.
22. Schwartz JL: Review and Evaluation of Smoking Cessation Methods: The United States and Canada, 1978-1985. Bethesda, MD, National Cancer Institute, Division of Cancer Prevention and Control, NIH pub no. 87-2940, 1987.
23. National Cancer Institute: Assist/2000: American Stop Smoking Intervention Study. Presentation to Board of Scientific Counselors. Bethesda, Md, The Institute, Division of Cancer Prevention and Control, October, 1988.
24. Ward JD, Duffy K, Sciandra R, et al: What the public wants to know about cancer: The Cancer Information Service. Cancer Bull 40:384-389, 1988.
25. National Cancer Institute: Cancer Prevention Resource Directory. Bethesda, Md, Office of Cancer Communications, The Institute, NIH pub no. 86-2827, 1986.
26. American Cancer Society: Three Ways To Take Special Care of Your Breasts. Atlanta, GA, The Society, pub no. 88-2675.05-LE, 1988.

Chapter 58

Teaching Strategies: The Patient

Barbara D. Blumberg, ScM

Judith (Judi) L. Bond Johnson, RN, PhD

INTRODUCTION

Approximately 75 million, about 30%, of Americans now living are expected to get cancer.[1] Given the complexity of the disease, along with the wide range of physiologic and economic accompaniments, one would expect the education of patients and their family members to be of prime concern. Within the broader context of cancer education itself, the education of those who are ill has been overshadowed by public and preventive efforts.[2]

HISTORICAL PERSPECTIVE

Patient education itself is not a new concept in health care. For years doctors and nurses, in the course of regular contact with patients, have explained illness and its consequences. As a rule, however, these efforts have been sporadic and lacking in consistency.[3]

Literary references to patient education first appeared in the 1950s. A prime factor responsible for increased attention to the field was the development of prepaid health care plans. A basic tenet of these plans was that informed self-care could reduce the costs of long-range patient care.[4] Patient education was viewed by some as a factor that facilitated such self-care.

At a 1964 conference on health education, the American Hospital Association took the position that it should act as the nationwide agency for stimulating the development of patient education programs. Their advocacy served as a milestone in the recognition of patient education within the health care system. Patient education was recommended as an integral part of patient care. This conference served as the impetus for *A Patient's Bill of Rights*,[5] which was approved by the Association's House of Delegates in 1973.

Both the National Cancer Institute's document entitled *Adult Patient Education in Cancer*[6] and the Oncology Nursing Society's *Outcome Standards in Cancer Patient Education*[7] identify a number of tasks for patient education. These include helping patients and family members adjust to the disease, participate in treatment, carry out treatment regimens, manage stress, recognize and control side effects, prevent social isolation and strengthen relationships with significant others, mobilize and manage resources, and adapt to a life of uncertainty.

In addition to these efforts are several other factors that contribute both to the historical development of patient education and to its role in the future.

1. As the population of older Americans increases, so will the number of individuals who have chronic diseases and disabilities. The emergence of chronic illness as a major health problem has provided much stimulus for the development of patient education services.[8]

2. The consumer rights movement has resulted in more patients asking for greater amounts of information and in *A Patient's Bill of Rights*. This document outlines the patient's right to know. It states that "the patient has the right to obtain . . . complete current information concerning his diagnosis, treatment, and prognosis in terms that he can be reasonably expected to understand . . ." and that "the patient has the right to refuse treatment to the extent permitted by law and to be informed of the medical consequences of his action . . . ."[5] In addition, legislation passed in Massachusetts, California, Minnesota, and Wisconsin mandates that patients be given information on treatment options for breast cancer (Massachusetts and California) or alternate modes of treatment for any disease (Minnesota and Wisconsin).

3. As a result of increasing health care costs and changing medical reimbursement policies, cost effectiveness of patient education has become a matter of concern.

4. Accountability by the health care provider has become more of a necessity and, as a result, issues related to informed consent are of greater concern. In addition, auditing of medical and nursing records, an attempt to document accountability, has become more of a routine practice.

Recent Literature

A review of articles on cancer patient education published between 1970 and 1985[9] cited growing evidence that cancer patient education can improve knowledge, attitudes, behavior, and health status. Specifically, Dodd's work with chemotherapy patients[10-13] provided evidence that planned patient education is capable of increasing self-care practices. In a study by Beck,[14] which looked at the effect of an oral care protocol on stomatitis after chemotherapy, patient education was credited with reducing infection and thus lowering financial as well as physiologic and psychologic costs of cancer. Other patient education programs have resulted in decreased anxiety and/or increased knowledge,[15-18] as well as improved self-concept and self-esteem.

On the basis of their review, Rimer and colleagues[9] suggest concise considerations for patient education programming that include the following:

- Use of a combination of education methods[11-14,17,19]

- Enhancement of educational methods by combining them with behavioral modalities such as relaxation, guided imagery, and/or hypnosis[20-23]

- Use of repetition to improve the generally compromised recall facilities of those with cancer[24]

- Preparation of informed consent forms at a reading level and in a format conducive to their use as educational vehicles

- Development of programs with the objective of teaching self-care as part of treatment regimens[10,11,25]

- Development of programs targeted at the special needs of the older patient as well as other high-risk patient audiences

An additional review of articles on cancer patient education based on a search of the Cancerlit data base, yielded more than 200 articles and abstracts published from 1979 to 1989. Subject areas receiving the greatest attention in terms of the number of publications during this time period were AIDS, patient information needs, self-care, and chemotherapy. The cancer that received the most attention in terms of patient education publications was breast cancer.

Program Priorities

Activities of the National Cancer Institute's (NCI) Patient Education Program[26] help shed light on extant national priorities in this area:

- A needs assessment conducted with hospital-based patient educators was conducted to determine what services their institutions provide, sources of educational materials used, and continuing education needs. Responses to the needs assessment will be used to provide direction for new Patient Education Program activities directed toward health professionals.

- A directory of patient education program contacts at clinical and comprehensive cancer centers nationwide has been prepared and distributed to encourage interaction and networking.

- A specific program area targeted to the special needs of older patients has been undertaken. A state-of-the-art paper describing the needs of this audience and services available for them has been developed. In addition, a working group of experts on cancer and aging has convened to help determine program priorities. Exhibits at meetings whose members are either representative of this audience or serve their needs are ongoing, as are the preparation of print advertisements for journals that cater to these two audiences.

- Collaboration with the National Coalition for Cancer Survivorship has been undertaken to create an information and education kit for cancer survivors.

- A project has been undertaken, in conjunction with NCI's Division of Cancer Treatment, with the hope of doubling patient participation in NCI-sponsored clinical trials by 1992. Called "Patients Helping Progress: Cancer Clinical Trials," activities include presentations and seminars at Oncology Nursing Society Congress meetings, development of a training program for Cancer Information Service telephone counselors, videotapes for patient and lay audiences, and a series of "updates" on clinical trials initiatives.

- NCI's International Cancer Information Center and the Office of Cancer Communications (OCC) have joined together to revise the current patient information file (PIF) component of the Physician Data Query (PDQ) cancer treatment data base. The PIF contains information about prognosis and treatment for different types and sites of cancer. Written in lay language, it is intended for use by patients and their families.

As more people live longer, and as more of those who have cancer experience long-term control or cure, the needs of two specific audiences—the elderly and cancer survivors—take on greater importance. Specific needs of older audiences must be considered, including their peculiar beliefs, myths, and misconceptions about the disease, information style preference,[27] and concomitant medications and diseases. Although these variables are necessary considerations in the education of any audience, older persons have needs and predispositions that are unique to them and should be considered in any effort to reach them.

Fitzhugh Mullan,[28] a physician and cancer survivor, brought new light to the definition of the terms *patient* and *survivor*. He maintains that the lives of all those living with cancer are similar in concept, if not always in form, and views their needs and concerns in a continuum that he has referred to as "seasons of survival."

There are specific implications for patient education in this updated definition of "patient" as one who should be considered a "survivor" from diagnosis onward. Educational needs of the "survivor," however, change according to the specific point in the continuum that the patient inhabits at a particular point in time.

The first season—the medical or acute stage—commences with diagnosis and is focused on efforts, both diagnostic and therapeutic, to contain the illness. Educational effort at this time should focus on the medical and psychosocial needs for information and self-care. The emphasis should be on maintenance of as good a quality of life as possible by fostering a "surviving" rather than a "getting by" attitude.

The next season begins when the patient has gone into remission or has completed the primary course of treatment. This period, aptly termed "watchful waiting," has as its governing force the fear of recurrence. During this phase, the person with cancer reintegrates into the community; medical personnel do not play the major role that they did during the previous phase. Educational efforts should address both the need for continuing medical surveillance and ways to live as normal a life as possible. Teaching strategies incorporate health-promotion behaviors and a wellness concept.

The final "season" is "permanent survival" or cure. Besides "victory over the disease," those who have entered this phase of the continuum have a very special comradeship with those in the previous "seasons of survival." This phase is characterized by concerns about employability, insurability, and long-term effects of treatment (see Chapter 19, Psychosocial Dimensions: Issues in Survivorship). Educational concerns are similar to those previously mentioned. Teaching people to be their own advocates is a means of empowering them to speak for their rights.

In recognition of the ever-growing network of cancer survivors, the American Cancer Society prepared a *Cancer Survivors' Bill of Rights* to call public attention to the 5 million Americans alive today who have a history of cancer.[1] The purpose of this document is to call attention to the specific needs of the cancer survivor in areas that include continued excellence in acute cancer care, as well as ongoing lifelong medical care, health insurance, job opportunities, and interpersonal happiness. In addition, 1986 saw the birth of the National Coalition for Cancer Survivorship, an organization dedicated to the needs of the survivor.

In summary, this new emphasis on the patient as a survivor should be a major theme in patient education programming. Considering all who are diagnosed with cancer as survivors, with needs peculiar to the specific "season" they inhabit, appears to be more timely than using the more traditional medical model to delineate patient needs in the educational arena.

DEFINITIONS

In an earlier article,[29] a composite definition of patient education was developed. Patient education is a series of structured or nonstructured experiences designed to help patients cope voluntarily with the immediate crisis response to their diagnosis, with long-term adjustments, and with symptoms; gain needed information about sources of prevention, diagnosis, and care; and develop needed skills, knowledge, and attitudes to maintain or regain health status.

Patient education is able to accomplish all of this by enabling patients and their families to plan strategies for change; interpret and integrate needed information for achieving the desired attitudes or behaviors; and meet patients' specific learning needs, interests, and capabilities.[30] Patient education through a combination of learning experiences derived from joint planning by patients, significant others, and health care professionals is considered part of total health care.[31]

RATIONALE FOR PATIENT EDUCATION

Teaching is integral to healing. It is a facet of cancer rehabilitation programs. Providing structured patient education courses and classes gives people an option for coping with their cancer diagnosis. The adaptation process is enhanced by patient education efforts.[32]

First, a structured patient education program ensures that important medical and psychosocial information is made available in a consistent manner. The key word is *consistency.* When procedures or treatments are being explained as part of routine care, interruptions are certain to occur that lead to disruption in teaching time and in-

advertent deletion of pieces of information. Distractions and lack of privacy inherent in the hospital environment also create a less than ideal learning environment. This can be remedied by providing a planned and scheduled time for patient education. This is not to say that the informal bedside exchange of information is not valuable. This approach should continue to be viewed as an integral part of patient care. Both approaches to providing patient education are incorporated into an overall plan. They work in concert, with each reinforcing information exchange.

Second, patient education addresses one of the major difficulties experienced by people with cancer—the loss of control over their disease and over their lives. In addition to providing information, patient education offers options, choices, and ways to engage self-care. It sets forth an expectation that people can be involved in their treatment decisions and obtain what they want and need from their health care providers. It promotes a proactive stance.

Patient education classes bring together people who have a common purpose or problem, providing opportunity for the exchange of ideas, problems, and solutions. Patients can learn from each other because of their similar situations. The educational setting is different from that of the neighborhood gathering or the doctor's waiting room. It provides a forum for exchange and a constructive guided direction for interaction between participants.

Finally, patient education broadens the opportunity for patient and provider to interact. Their roles in this setting are that of trainee and teacher. Patients gain a different perspective of their health care provider—that of facilitator and patient advocate. The relationship between patients and their health care providers can be strengthened by a broadening of the concept of partnership in health care.

DEVELOPING PATIENT EDUCATION MATERIALS AND PROGRAMS

Integral to the success of any patient education material or program is the extent to which the needs of the intended audience are met. Also called "social marketing," this perspective incorporates assessment of audience needs at particular points in the program/material development and implementation process.

Developing patient education materials and programs is viewed as a process whereby time and available resources are allocated in quantities sufficient to include concept, message, and actual resource development, along with attendant evaluations. This process is conceptualized in a six-part wheel (Figure 58-1)[33] whereby each section of the wheel represents a stage in a circular process in which the last stage feeds back to the first one in a continuous loop of replanning and improvement.

The key to the development process is pretesting, a qualitative research method executed during the development of materials and programs. The purpose of pre-

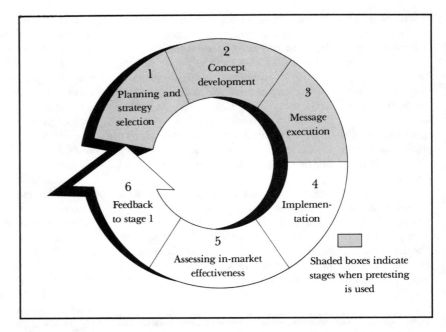

FIGURE 58-1 Stages in the development of patient education materials and resources. (Source: United States Department of Health and Human Services. Pretesting in Health Communications [NIH pub no. 84-1493]. Washington DC, US Government Printing Office, 1984.)

testing is to systematically gather target audience reactions to draft concepts and materials before final production and implementation. Pretesting is useful in determining which version of a concept, message, or material is most likely to meet stated objectives. In addition, pretesting is useful in identifying strengths and weaknesses of draft materials. Variables particularly amenable to pretesting are awareness and interest, comprehension, audience relevance, believability, acceptability, and gain in short-term knowledge.

Pretesting provides important diagnostic information that can lead to improvements in draft materials and programs before they are made widely available. It is important to recognize, however, that pretesting is a qualitative method and, as such, does not yield findings that are reportable in terms of their statistical significance. Results of pretesting are not absolutely predictive of potential success or failure of items in terms of variables pretested. Rather, pretesting provides direction on the basis of perception of needs of representative members of the target audience.

Pretesting Techniques

A host of research techniques can be usefully employed in pretesting. The particular method chosen depends on the target audience, the message or concepts being tested, objectives of the pretest, the best mode of access to the target audience, and time and resources available. In general, the techniques most conducive to pretesting of patient education materials and programs are the following:

readability testing, focus group interviews, individual in-depth interviews, self-administered questionnaires, and gatekeeper review.

Readability testing is an easily employed technique that is used to predict the level of reading comprehension necessary to understand a particular written piece. After extensive review of 12 selected formulas,[33] the Office of Cancer Communication of the National Cancer Institute chose the SMOG grading formula for readability testing of its public and patient education materials.[34] SMOG was chosen because of the ease of its use and its accuracy in determining readability. This formula considers the number of words of at least three syllables in determining the grade level needed for comprehension. Table 58-1[33] describes how to apply this formula.

Focus group interviews are guided group discussions with a group of 8 to 10 individuals who share specific target audience characteristics. Interviews are led by a facilitator who uses a list of open-ended questions to guide the discussion. This technique is particularly appropriate during the concept-development stage and provides insight into audience beliefs and perceptions. Adapted from group therapy, focus group discussion encourages participants to converse about specific topics. Frequently, direct or paraphrased dialogue from focus groups can be incorporated into educational materials, making them more realistic and readable. Reactions to artwork and logos can also be gathered through use of this pretesting technique.

Individual in-depth interviews or one-on-one discussions are carried out by an interviewer who uses a prepared questionnaire that consists of both open-ended and closed-end items. This technique is appropriate when

TABLE 58-1 The SMOG Readability Formula

To calculate the SMOG reading grade level, begin with the entire written work that is being assessed, and follow these four steps:

1. Count off 10 consecutive sentences near the beginning, in the middle, and near the end of the text.

2. From this sample of 30 sentences, circle all of the words containing three or more syllables (polysyllabic), including repetitions of the same word, and total the number of words circled.

3. Estimate the square root of the total number of polysyllabic words counted. This is done by finding the nearest perfect square, and taking its square root.

4. Finally, add a constant of three to the square root. This number gives the SMOG grade, or the reading grade level that a person must have reached if he or she is to fully understand the text being assessed.

A few additional guidelines will help to clarify these directions:

- A sentence is defined as a string of words punctuated with a period (.), an exclamation point (!) or a question mark (?).

- Hyphenated words are considered as one word.

- Numbers which are written out should also be considered, and if in numeric form in the text, they should be pronounced to determine if they are polysyllabic.

- Proper nouns, if polysyllabic, should be counted, too.

- Abbreviations should be read as unabbreviated to determine if they are polysyllabic.

Not all pamphlets, fact sheets, or other printed materials contain 30 sentences. To test a text that has fewer than 30 sentences:

1. Count all of the polysyllabic words in the text.

2. Count the number of sentences.

3. Find the average number of polysyllabic words per sentence as follows:

$$\text{Average} = \frac{\text{Total \# of polysyllabic words}}{\text{Total \# of sentences}}$$

4. Multiply that average by the number of sentences *short of 30*.

5. Add that figure on to the total number of polysyllabic words.

6. Find the square root and add the constant of 3.

Perhaps the quickest way to administer the SMOG grading test is by using the SMOG conversion table. Simply count the number of polysyllabic words in your chain of 30 sentences and look up the approximate grade level on the chart.

SMOG Conversion Table*

Total Polysyllabic Word Counts	Approximate Grade Level (+ 1.5 Grades)
0-2	4
3-6	5
7-12	6
13-20	7
21-30	8
31-42	9
43-56	10
57-72	11
73-90	12
91-110	13
111-132	14
133-156	15
157-182	16
183-210	17
211-240	18

*Developed by Harold C. McGraw, Office of Educational Research, Baltimore County Schools, Towson, Maryland.

Source: United States Department of Health and Human Services: Pretesting in Health Communications (NIH pub no. 84-1493). Washington DC, US Government Printing Office, 1984.

the subjects addressed are sensitive or require in-depth probing.

Self-administered questionnaires that can be completed by the subject without the assistance of an interviewer are more widely used in gathering reactions to draft materials. Use of short, closed-end questions and a data-collection technique that ensures return of completed questionnaires is advised when this technique is employed. Hand delivering and retrieving questionnaires, offering a small incentive for return of completed questionnaires, and/or including a postage-paid return envelope are techniques that have yielded higher return rates.

Since many health education materials and programs reach their audiences by way of a health professional, it is prudent to seek review and comment from such persons during the development of programs and materials. Because of their role in determining whether a particular material or program reaches its intended audience, such

health professionals are referred to as "gatekeepers." Review of draft materials by gatekeepers can be carried out through short self-administered questionnaires and can occur at the same time as the target audience review. If a discrepancy occurs between target audience needs and gatekeeper perception of these needs, deference should be made to the needs of the target audience. A memo announcing the availability of the program or material can summarize the extensive process and note that information ultimately included reflects the viewpoints of a number of persons.

The Development Process

Planning and strategy selection are the first activities in development of patient education materials and programs. During this period, a concise definition of what the material or program will address, objectives, and target audience identification are addressed. Planning and selection of educational strategies can be facilitated by conducting a needs assessment. Perusal of literature in the field and identification of other analogous materials and programs are undertaken. In addition, it may be useful to conduct a more formal assessment to determine education needs and strategies that have the greatest potential for meeting objectives.

Before development of the National Cancer Institute publication *What Are Clinical Trials All About?* a small-scale needs assessment survey was conducted, with patients, family members, and health professionals participating in clinical trials. This survey helped the staff determine that a booklet addressing specific topics would be most useful to the target audience, patient, and family members given the option of clinical trial participation.[35] Useful pretesting techniques during this stage are in-depth interviews, focus group interviews, and small-scale surveys.

During the concept-development stage, draft educational resources are developed on the basis of concepts that appear to have the greatest potential for educating the target audience. Drafts can take a variety of forms, ranging from short manuscripts with rough artwork, to slides or storyboards with accompanying dialogue, to draft posters. During the message-execution stage, draft educational resources are pretested before final production. Gatekeeper review takes place as part of pretesting to assure that those responsible for disseminating the education to the target audience are familiar with it and have had a chance to submit comments. Self-administered questionnaires are the most unobtrusive method of pretesting to employ during this stage. Pretesting comments can then be incorporated before final production.

During the next stage—implementation—the educational material or program is used with the target audience, with initial reaction monitored closely. With both informal comments and observations, along with more formal methods, initial use and usefulness of materials and programs can be assessed. Number of copies distributed, how often the program is carried out, and the value of short evaluation forms accompanying a material or program are all to be considered during this period of process evaluation.[36]

During the next stage—assessment of in-market effectiveness—the effectiveness of materials and programs in terms of meeting stated objectives is assessed. Self-administered questionnaires completed before and after exposure to the material or programs and assessment of behavioral change targeted by the material or program are sample means of outcome assessment.

The final stage in the development of educational materials and programs involves critical assessment of information gathered during pretesting, process, and outcome evaluations for the purpose of replanning. Problems incurred in use of the material or program, strengths of the material or program, and other feedback are assessed in terms of changes necessitated by actual implementation.

CLIMATE FOR LEARNING

Considerable time, energy, and money can be committed to providing quality patient education programs. However, unless peoples' health beliefs, attitudes, cultural backgrounds, and personal values are considered, patient education efforts may be less than successful.

Chaisson[37] reports on past patient education efforts from which the following mistakes were discovered by default:

1. Telling people what they should know rather than what they are ready and willing to learn.
2. Failure to individualize patient teaching content to accommodate the person's personal background, attitude, and motivation.
3. Failure to assess a person's knowledge before beginning the teaching process.
4. Lack of coordination of patient teaching efforts across the continuum of care.
5. Expecting people to be effective teachers when they are not knowledgeable about educational principles, methods, and evaluation.
6. Use of an incidental, informal approach as a basis for a patient education program.

In summary, studies of the clinical practice of health care show that more emphasis needs to be placed on the "how" of patient teaching.

Techniques of teaching are nearly as varied as people. Each person should be viewed as a special learner! There are a host of factors to be considered if a climate for learning is to be created.

> *H*uman
>> Interpersonal relations
>> Individual needs and wants
> *O*rganization
>> Policy
>> Structure
> *P*hysical
>> Environmental factors
> *E*ducational options
>> Methods
>> Materials

The first aspect is the human factor. There has to be interest and involvement on the part of both teacher and learner. The learners should be offered ways to participate actively throughout the entire educational process. To maximize readiness to learn, it is necessary to ascertain the concerns people have at that particular moment. Unless these concerns are addressed first, additional health teaching will not be heard.

A person's age will directly affect his or her ability to understand and master information and skills. Ability to learn depends on maturation. Growth and development of children is a crucial element of the teaching-learning process. Intellectual development moves from concrete to abstract. As children mature, they move toward a clearer distinction between what is internal and what is external to themselves.

Knowles[38] provides some valuable insights into the adult as a learner. He coined the word *andragogy*, the science of teaching adults, to distinguish the adult learner from the child. He proposes four assumptions about the adult learner. As people mature, (1) their self-concept moves from dependency to self-direction, (2) they accumulate life experiences that are an increasing resource for learning, (3) their readiness to learn is increasingly oriented to developmental tasks and social roles, and (4) time perspective changes and orientation to learning shifts to immediate application of knowledge and learning that is problem-centered rather than subject-centered.

Adult learners are motivated to learn when they recognize a gap between what they know and what they want to know. They accept a share of the responsibility for planning and carrying out a learning experience and therefore have a feeling of commitment toward it. The learning process capitalizes on their past experiences.[39]

Changes brought on by aging need to be acknowledged when the learner is an older adult. Intellectual ability does not necessarily diminish with age; rather, it changes. The speed of learning declines, not the ability! Thus, factors other than age are more likely to be barriers to learning for the older adult.[40] Alford[41] identifies the following changes:

1. Slowed processing time requires that older persons have more time to think through and absorb new information.
2. Stimulus persistence means that older persons must be given time to explore each concept in its entirety and to ask questions.
3. Decreased short-term memory causes older persons to have difficulty in remembering new information. Learning can easily become frustrating if learning requires recent recall. Ways can be devised to reinforce learning, such as linking it with past experiences or providing written data to supplement the verbal information.
4. Test anxiety occurs because older persons sense they cannot remember as well. Taking tests would prove this fact. If tests are necessary, verbal ones should be considered. Elderly learners need to be given a sense of confidence in their ability to maintain independence.

Material for older adults is printed in 10- or 11-point type on paper with a dull finish, and two-tone beige or green-tone colors are avoided. The print size used in written materials, the volume and speed of visual presentations, and the amount of information given at any one time are paced. Teaching is limited to 3 to 5 points. Older persons are accustomed to being in control, and teaching addresses this need whenever possible.

In addition to age, differences in culture, language, level of literacy, and physical impairment (for example, hearing and/or sight deficiencies) must be considered in providing the appropriate educational climate for each particular patient. Cultural differences significantly influence communication and subsequent education. Recognizing the importance of the person's family and even the immediate community as a support system is essential. Acknowledging culture-specific medical and religious beliefs and practices and attempting to incorporate them into educational opportunities is also advisable. Communicating in a language or dialect that is not the one most frequently used by a person can change both the expression of symptoms and the level of comprehension. When educating a patient with a different cultural background, it is wise to consider the use of a variety of methods to both convey and understand messages. For example, the use of pictures to illustrate instructions, and/or materials that have been translated into the person's primary language is helpful.[42]

In addition to cultural differences, level of literacy is an important consideration in the education of any patient. Although concise communication can enhance the education of any patient, those with poor reading or comprehension skills require special consideration concerning their educational needs. A major caveat in working with this audience is to simplify the language used. In addition, Chatham and Knapp[43] suggest the following: Speak and write in short sentences, conveying no more than one concept per sentence; use words of no more than two syllables as often as possible; use nontechnical language that the patient understands in offering explanations of medical terms; speak or write in the active voice. An excellent reference by Doak, Doak, and Root[44] entitled *Teaching Patients With Low Literacy Skills* provides a variety of additional suggestions.

A second aspect to consider when establishing a climate for learning is the need for support from the organization or institution. Squyres[45] proposes a foundation for health education services. It requires integration of a person's personal philosophy and goals with that of the organizations, along with the position statements of professional, legal, and accrediting bodies. Often patient education is given only lip service by an institution. Strategies for gaining support and recognition include knowing the state-of-the-art literature, supporting claims of effectiveness with research data, and presenting a cost-effective plan for implementing a program that addresses quality patient care. Patient education addresses accreditation standards, requirements for informed consent, self-care interests of consumers, and trends for earlier discharge with home care collaboration. Quality patient education is nurtured by a supportive administrative and medical staff. The physical component also must be considered in creation of a climate conducive to learning. The environment can be used to focus peoples' attention on what is to be learned. A learning resource center facilitates self-initiated learning. Visual aids, such as anatomic charts or a human torso, heighten peoples' interest in their own body parts. A positive learning environment offers mutual respect, acceptance of differences, and freedom of expression. If patient education is valued as an integral part of patient care, then time and space should be allocated for carrying it out. It is less than ideal to teach when there are frequent interruptions, a lack of privacy, and interference by hospital routines. For group classes, chairs and tables should be arranged in advance; lighting and microphones adequate for group size and the availability of group leaders who are knowledgeable about audiovisual equipment are important factors. Otherwise, distractions will interfere with class interaction and the group process.

A final factor to consider when establishing a climate conducive to learning is the choice of educational methods and materials. Consideration must be given to ways to best present the content to be taught. People learn better when more than one of their senses is involved in the learning process.[46] Hearing alone is a passive activity. Thus the use of only a lecture method to present information does not promote optimal learning. For each sense that is included, the more involved the learner and the more likely learning will occur.

Audiovisual materials are the tools of patient education programs. However, their use alone is not considered an adequate means for providing patient education.[47] Education is a process that requires human interaction. Appropriate materials enhance the teaching-learning process and are selected with that purpose in mind.

CONCLUSION

The rapid changes in health care technology as well as the complexities of the health care system present a challenge to both the health care professionals and the consumers within the health care system. People enter the system, become patients, and find themselves faced with a life-threatening illness that requires multiple changes. They need assistance in the form of guidance and information. Facilitating adaptation to these changes comes in the form of patient education. The process begins before an illness is diagnosed and continues long after the acute phase of an illness is over. Patient education has as its ultimate goal the restoration of a person to his or her highest state of wellness and reentry into society.

REFERENCES

1. American Cancer Society: Cancer Facts and Figures. Atlanta, American Cancer Society, Inc, 1988, p 3.
2. Green LW: The future of cancer patient education. Health Educ Q 10:102-110, 1984 (special suppl).
3. Brechon D: Highlights in the evolution of hospital-based patient education program. J Allied Health 3:35, 1976.
4. Shapiro I: The patient and control of quality in medical care. Proceedings Tenth Annual Group Health Association of America. Chicago, 1960.
5. American Hospital Association: A Patient's Bill of Rights. AHS Catalog No. 2415, Chicago, The Association, 1975.
6. National Cancer Institute: Adult Patient Education in Cancer. NIH pub no. 83-2601. Washington, DC, The Institute, 1983.
7. Oncology Nursing Society: Outcome Standards for Cancer Patient Education. Pittsburgh, Oncology Nursing Society, 1982.
8. Simonds S: Current Issues in Patient Education. New York, American Group Practice Association and Core Communications in Health, 1974.
9. Rimer B, Keintz MK, Glassman B: Cancer patient education: Reality and potential. Prev Med 14:801-818, 1985.
10. Dodd M: Assessing patient self-care for side effects of cancer chemotherapy. Part I. Cancer Nurs 5:263-268, 1982.
11. Dodd M: Cancer patients' knowledge of chemotherapy: Assessment and informational interventions. Oncol Nurs Forum 9:39-44, 1982.
12. Dodd M: Self-care for side effects in cancer chemotherapy: An assessment of nursing interventions. Part II. Cancer Nurs 6:63-67, 1983.
13. Dodd M, Mood D: Chemotherapy: Helping patients to know the drugs they are receiving and their possible side effects. Cancer Nurs 4:311-318, 1981.
14. Beck S: Impact of a systematic oral care protocol on stomatitis after chemotherapy. Cancer Nurs 2:185-199, 1979.
15. Cassileth BR, Heiberger RM, March V, et al: Effects of audiovisual cancer programs on patients and families. J Med Educ 57:54-59, 1982.
16. Jacobs C, Ross R, Walker IM, et al: Behavior of cancer patients: A randomized study of the effects of education and peer support groups. Am J Clin Oncol 6:347-350, 1983.
17. Johnson J: The effects of a patient education course on persons with a chronic disease. Cancer Nurs 5:117-123, 1982.
18. Watson PG: The effects of short-term postoperative counseling on cancer/ostomy patients. Cancer Nurs 6:21-29, 1983.
19. Green LW, Kreuter MW, Deeds SG, et al: Health Education Planning. Palo Alto, Calif, Mayfield, 1980.
20. Burish T, Lyles J: Effectiveness of relaxation training in reducing the aversiveness of chemotherapy in the treatment of cancer. Behav Ther Exp Psychiatry 10:357-361, 1979.
21. Burish T, Lyles J: Effectiveness of relaxation training in reducing adverse reaction to cancer chemotherapy. J Behav Med 14:65-78, 1981.
22. Redd W, Andresen G, Minagwa R: Hypnotic control of anticipatory emesis in patients receiving cancer chemotherapy. J Consult Clin Psychol 50:114-119, 1982.
23. Redd W, Hendler C: Learned aversions to chemotherapy treatment. Health Educ Q 10:57-64, 1984 (special suppl).
24. Ley P: Towards better doctor-patient communications, in Bennett AE (ed): Communication Between Doctors and Patients. London, Oxford University Press, 1976, pp 75-98.
25. Thomas NP, Cloak M, Crossan K, et al: Preparing cancer patients to administer medication. Patient Couns Health Educ 3:137-143, 1982.
26. National Cancer Institute, Office of Cancer Communication Patient Education Program: Overview of Current Activities, September 1988 (unpublished).
27. Wilson CM, Rimer B, Kane-Williams E, et al: Educating the older cancer patient: Obstacles and opportunities. Health Educ Q 10:76-87, 1984 (special suppl).
28. Mullan F: Seasons of survival: Reflections of a physician with cancer. N Engl J Med 313:270-273, 1985.
29. Johnson JL, Blumberg BD: A commentary on cancer patient education. Health Educ Q 10:7-18, 1984 (special suppl).
30. DeJoseph J: Writing and evaluating educational protocols, in Squyres W (ed): Patient Education: An Inquiry Into the State of the Art. New York, Springer, 1960.

31. Ulrich M, Kelley K: Patient care includes teaching. Hospitals 46:59-65, 1972.
32. Johnson J, Flaherty M: The nurse and cancer patient education. Semin Oncol 7 (March):63-70, 1980.
33. National Cancer Institute: Pretesting in Health Communications. NIH pub no. 84-1493, Washington, DC, The Institute, 1984.
34. Rader LA: The SMOG Grading Readability Formula. Michigan State University, 1980 (unpublished).
35. Blumberg B, Nealon E: Educational needs of the patient considering clinical trials. Paper presented at the Oncology Nursing Society Congress, Toronto, Canada, 1984.
36. Blumberg BD: Evaluating patient education programs. Oncol Nurs Forum 8(2):29-31, 1981.
37. Chaisson GM: Patient education: Whose responsibility is it and who should be doing it. Nurs Admin Q 4(2):1-11, 1980.
38. Knowles M: The Modern Practice of Adult Education, New York, Associated Press, 1975.
39. Woldum K, Ryan-Morrell V, Towson M, et al: Patient Education Foundations of Practice, Rockville, Md, Aspen, 1985.
40. Casserly D, Strock E: Educating the older patient. Caring 7(11):60-67, 1988.
41. Alford PM: Tips for Teaching Older Adults. Nurs Life 2:60-64, 1982.
42. American Hospital Association, Center for Health Promotion: Culture Bound and Sensory Barriers to Communication With Patient: Strategies and Resources for Health Education. Chicago, The Association, May 1982.
43. Chatham MAH, Knapp BL: Teaching patient with low literacy skills, in Patient Education Handbook. Bowie, Md, Robert J Brady, 1982, pp 145-150.
44. Doak CC, Doak LG, Root JH: Teaching Patients With Low Literacy Skills. Philadelphia, JB Lippincott, 1985.
45. Squyres W: Patient Education and Health Promotion in Medical Care. Palo Alto, Calif, Mayfield, 1985.
46. Bille DA: Practical Approaches to Patient Teaching. Boston, Little Brown, 1981.
47. Monaco RM, Salfen L, Spratt J: The patient as an education participant in health care. J Mo Med Assoc, 69(12):932-937, 1972.

Chapter 59

Cancer Nursing Education

Alice J. Longman, RN, EdD

INTRODUCTION

Cancer nursing as a specialized area of professional nursing practice has an important role in the decades ahead. The practice of cancer nursing has been influenced by "(1) national and international recognition of cancer as a major chronic health problem; (2) scientific and technological developments; (3) changes in professional and public perceptions of cancer, and (4) changes within the nursing profession."[1] These changes occurred as a result of a shift within nursing toward more extended and expanded roles. As these roles emerged, there was more emphasis on professionalism. The extension and expansion of cancer nursing practice have been related to organizational developments, educational developments, and research developments.[2]

The management of the care of individuals with cancer or at risk for the development of cancer is one of collaboration and coordination among various health professions. Changes in undergraduate nursing education have been marked by the gradual shift from hospital-based education to college-based education. More nurses practice nursing in a variety of settings, and practice is based increasingly on the use of findings from research.

CHARACTERISTICS OF CANCER NURSING PRACTICE

The Social Policy Statement issued by the American Nurses' Association in 1980 defined four characteristics of nursing: phenomena, theory application, nursing action, and evaluation of effects in relation to phenomena.[3]

Phenomena and Theory Application

The phenomena of concern in cancer nursing are multiple. Cancer no longer is regarded as one disease but rather "a group of diseases with clinically distinct presentations, and differing biologic behavior and clinical manifestations."[4] The impact of cancer on individuals has implications for numerous biologic, social, behavioral, and physical interventions. Furthermore, cancer can be described as a group of chronic diseases for which treatment is possible. Theoretic concepts for cancer nursing are drawn from biologic and social theories, as well as from systems, developmental, and change theories.

Improved observations that relate to levels of health and illness need to be stressed by nursing personnel. Individuals, families, and communities thus can be assisted in the early identification of potential or real problems. Of importance to the practice of cancer nursing are the facts that prevention and early detection of cancer are within the purview of nursing and that most cancers can be treated successfully at early stages.

Nursing Action

Actions in cancer nursing are based on a sound knowledge base to provide care for those individuals or groups at risk for the development of cancer or those who are being treated for cancer and its sequelae. A sound knowledge base is acquired in basic nursing education programs, continually updated through continuing education and expanded in graduate nursing education programs. Toward this end the major purpose of the Education Committee of the Oncology Nursing Society is to promote high-quality cancer education for nurses.[5] The Education Committee oversees and promotes the quality of all educational activities generated by the Oncology Nursing Society.

The complexity of care for individuals with cancer necessitated the development of a systematic process for nursing actions. The nursing process, including the formulation of nursing diagnoses, serves as an organizing framework for cancer nursing practice. In 1979 the American Nurses' Association and the Oncology Nursing Society published *Outcome Standards for Cancer Nursing Practice*.[6] Ten high-incidence problems were identified for individuals in primary, acute, or long-term care settings. The 10 areas were prevention and early detection, information, coping, comfort, nutrition, protective mechanisms, mobility, elimination, sexuality, and ventilation. Criteria for evaluation of nursing actions were provided.

Standards of Oncology Nursing Practice, published in 1987, presents professional practice standards and professional performance standards. The practice standards address theory, data collection, diagnosis, planning, intervention, and evaluation. Eleven high-incidence problem areas common to individuals with cancer are addressed. These are prevention and early detection, information, coping, comfort, nutrition, protective mechanisms, mobility, elimination, sexuality, ventilation, and circulation. The professional performance standards examine professional development, interdisciplinary collaboration, quality assurance, ethics, and research. Examples of nursing diagnoses in relation to the high-incidence problem areas are included in the document.

Care for individuals with cancer and their families is provided through the services of many health professions. These include but are not limited to diagnostic radiologists, nuclear medicine specialists, radiotherapists, surgeons, medical oncologists, hematologists, dietitians, social workers, physical therapists, and nurses. For individuals with the suspected or confirmed diagnosis of cancer and their families, the vast array of health care professionals may be overwhelming. Collaboration among health professionals is essential to assist individuals to achieve optimum health. Such collaboration provides consistency in the ongoing plan of treatment. Nurses often assume the role of coordinator in such collaboration.

Evaluation of Effects of Action

Evaluation of the effects of nursing actions suggests whether the actions have improved or resolved the conditions toward which they were directed. The knowledge base is continually examined and updated. The results of cancer nursing research provide evidence of the efficacy of nursing actions.

DEVELOPMENT OF CANCER NURSING PRACTICE

Recognition of cancer as a major health problem led to the development of the specialty of cancer nursing. A comprehensive approach to cancer care has contributed to the expansion of the boundaries of cancer nursing practice. Cancer nursing is practiced by nursing generalists and nursing specialists. Nursing generalists have conceptual knowledge and skills acquired through basic nursing education, clinical experience, and professional development. Nursing generalists meet the concerns of individuals with cancer and provide care in a variety of health care settings. Continuing education is a mechanism to update their knowledge of and skills in cancer care. Nursing specialists have substantial theoretic knowledge gained through preparation for the master's degree. Nursing specialists meet diversified concerns of individuals with cancer and their families and function in a discrete area of practice. The scope of cancer nursing practice includes clinical practice, education, administration, and research.

Oncology Nursing Society

In 1975 the Oncology Nursing Society was established to promote communication among cancer nurses, to generate new knowledge about cancer nursing, to promote cancer research in general, and to enhance the level of care being given to patients and families.[4] Activities of the Society include an annual congress to provide a forum for nurses to present and exchange information, major standing committees to foster the professional development of cancer nurses, a professional journal to disseminate scientific and clinical information, and a newsletter that reports on the activities of the Society. Formal and informal communication among and between individual nurses involved in cancer nursing has contributed to the impact of professional collaboration on cancer nursing. Yarbro[7] summarized the major accomplishments on the Oncology Nursing Society from 1975 to 1983.

Association of Pediatric Oncology Nurses

The Association of Pediatric Oncology Nurses was established in 1975 and became a nonprofit corporation in 1976.[8] A significant contribution of the Association has been the development of expanded nursing roles in pediatric cancer nursing. The organization has striven to provide a forum for mutual support, the exchange of

ideas, and the comparison of practice models through annual conferences and a professional journal. Close relationships are maintained with other specialty nursing organizations, in particular the Oncology Nursing Society.

National Cancer Institute

The National Cancer Act of 1971 has had a major impact on cancer and cancer control programs. The Act authorized a broad intensive program to reduce the incidence, morbidity, and mortality of cancer in human beings. The National Cancer Institute is a unique structure that systematically attacks the complex cancer problem.[9] Its mission is to support a network that provides information, distributes funding for research, and establishes research and treatment centers. Comprehensive cancer centers have been developed, and specialized clinical and research centers are in operation. Nursing generalists and nursing specialists are involved in the planning and development of specialized cancer units in general hospitals. The development of the Comprehensive Cancer Centers Outreach programs, community-based programs, and the Clinical Hospital Oncology programs also have involved nursing generalists and nursing specialists.

Individual predoctoral and postdoctoral research fellowships for cancer nurses are available from the National Cancer Institute. Nurses have had representation on the National Cancer Institute Cancer Control Grant Review Committee since the 1970s. In addition, with the assistance of a grant from the National Cancer Institute, the Oncology Nursing Society has offered a cancer nursing research short course at the Society's Congress for the past several years. A national forum for exchange between students and faculty is provided for those selected to participate in the research experience.[9]

American Cancer Society

The American Cancer Society appointed the first nursing consultant in 1948. The first Nursing Advisory Committee of the American Cancer Society was established in 1951, and its purpose was to offer advice on educational programs and materials.[10] Nurses were eligible to become members of all professional education and service committees at the divisional and local levels of the American Cancer Society. Since 1980 support for graduate students enrolled in master's degree programs that offer specialization in cancer nursing has been available. The scholarship program was expanded in 1986, and assistance also is available for those nurses engaged in doctoral studies. Through the efforts of the American Cancer Society a program was established for professorships in cancer nursing. By 1988 nine nurse educators were named professors in cancer nursing. These professors are actively involved in the education of graduate students and practicing nurses and in the activities of the Society.

PERSPECTIVES OF CANCER NURSING EDUCATION

The development of cancer nursing education reflects the changes in nursing practice, changes in nursing education, and rapid changes in cancer therapy and cancer care settings. In particular, two specific trends in cancer nursing education were noted by Tiffany[2]: the acceptance of the World Health Organization's definition of health as a state of complete physical, mental, and social well-being and not merely the absence of disease and infirmity and the recognition that patients and families should be active participants in their treatment and recovery process. The proliferation of roles that require definition and differentiation in cancer nursing also has influenced cancer nursing education. These roles have included the nurse specialist, the nurse clinician, the nurse oncologist, the oncology nurse practitioner, the oncology coordinator, and the clinical nurse specialist.[11-13]

General Cancer Nursing Education

Continuing education has been the most widely used method to increase the knowledge and skills of those engaged in cancer nursing. Because of the nature of educational preparation at the generalist level, that is, baccalaureate, associate degree, and diploma, nurses who required expertise in cancer nursing were unprepared. Thus continuing education programs were necessary to provide nurses with the opportunity to gain the knowledge essential for the practice of cancer nursing. Programs in cancer nursing in the early 1940s and 1950s, which were sponsored by the American Cancer Society in cooperation with professional nursing organizations, usually consisted of 1-day seminars.[10]

Many cancer nursing education programs were provided by cancer hospitals. Memorial Sloan-Kettering Cancer Center was a pioneer in offering educational programs in cancer nursing. The Center's activities included continuing education programs, in-service education, clinical practice for undergraduate and graduate students, and the development of teaching materials in cancer nursing.[14] Other cancer hospitals in the country, such as Roswell Park Memorial Hospital, Ellis Fischel State Cancer Center, City of Hope National Medical Center, and MD Anderson Hospital and Tumor Institute, also have provided continuing education for nurses through the years.[14]

The need for special training for nurses in cancer care was stressed in a report of the Division of Cancer Control Program.[15] In 1950 a 3-week institute on cancer nursing was conducted for 30 nurse instructors under the auspices of the National Cancer Institute.[14] After the completion of the institute, a Cancer Production Committee was formed and an outline developed to demonstrate how cancer nursing could be incorporated into basic nursing programs.[16]

Through the years the Nursing Advisory Committee of the American Cancer Society has been concerned with the preparation and publication of educational resources for nurses. The first *Cancer Source Book for Nurses* was published in 1950; subsequent revisions have been published through the years.

The incorporation of cancer content in baccalaureate nursing programs was addressed in the early 1950s. The National Cancer Institute awarded grants to four baccalaureate nursing programs to integrate cancer nursing content into the nursing courses.[15] Tools were developed to measure knowledge about cancer among students within existing baccalaureate nursing programs.[17,18] The tools served to interest other faculty members in cancer content. Instruments for use by nursing instructors then were designed to evaluate cancer nursing education.[19] Courses for public health nurses, institutional nurses, and nursing faculty also were in progress in various states.[20]

In 1971 the National Cancer Institute contributed seed funding for a 10-week work-study program for students enrolled in baccalaureate nursing programs. Students were provided the opportunity to increase their knowledge and skills in caring for individuals with cancer in the areas of prevention, detection, diagnosis, treatment, and rehabilitation.[21] The program was successful in recruiting nurses for cancer nursing practice.

Currently, the National Cancer Institute offers a Cancer Nurse Training Program, which is a 9-month clinical traineeship for new baccalaureate nursing graduates.[22] The program offers a comprehensive review of current cancer practice and its implications for nursing. A monthly stipend is given to participants in the program.

Another project funded by the National Cancer Institute in recent years was the evaluation of the current essential cancer content in an undergraduate nursing program.[23] Five activities were included in the project: measurement of students' attitudes toward cancer patients and cancer knowledge of students, research experiences for selected students, research symposia related to cancer nursing, an update on cancer treatment for nursing faculty, and the development and implementation of an interdisciplinary elective course. As a result the content was integrated more logically into the program. Two instruments, Ideas About Oncology Patient Care and a Knowledge Inventory, were developed and tested.

Graduate Cancer Nursing Education

Teachers College of Columbia University offered the first academic courses in cancer nursing at the graduate level.[10,14] Two eight-credit courses were offered over two semesters. The theoretic content included the nature of cancer as a biologic phenomenon, the theoretic basis for specific nursing care measures, and the community health aspects of cancer for individuals and their families. The course included a clinical practicum, which was conducted at Memorial Sloan-Kettering Cancer Center. Through the efforts of the director of nursing at the hospital, a grant of $30,000 was received from the American Cancer Society, New York Division, for support of the program.[14]

When funding was discontinued, the courses were dropped.

The earliest reported survey of graduate programs to determine those that offered cancer nursing was conducted in 1958 by the American Cancer Society. Representatives of 30 graduate programs were contacted; 22 responded and only two programs indicated that cancer nursing was included in their programs.[10] Nursing guidelines, entitled "Assessing Graduate Education in Oncology Nursing,"[24] were published by the Education Committee of the Oncology Nursing Society to assist those nurses interested in graduate education with a specialty in cancer nursing. By 1988 more than 45 graduate programs offered specialization in cancer nursing. An annual listing of such programs is prepared by the Education Committee of the Oncology Nursing Society and published in the *Oncology Nursing Forum*. Additional information about graduate education content is available from the Oncology Nursing Society in the publication, *The Master's Degree with a Specialty in Oncology Nursing: Role Definition and Curriculum Guide*.[25]

Two programs that prepare graduates of master's programs as teachers of cancer nursing were supported by the National Cancer Institute for 5 years (1979-1984). The dissemination of the model curriculum and evaluation results were important parts of the project.[26]

Support for graduate students enrolled in master's degree programs specializing in cancer nursing has been available since 1980 through the efforts of the American Cancer Society.[27] Graduate scholarships for those pursuing additional preparation also are awarded by the Oncology Nursing Foundation. Five doctoral programs offer specialization in cancer nursing. Support also is available from the American Cancer Society for those engaged in doctoral studies. One program offers a postdoctoral fellowship in cancer nursing.

Certificate programs are available for those who specialize in cancer nursing. Preparation in the management of care for selected individuals with cancer and their families is provided. Advanced practitioner skills related to taking health histories, performing physical examinations, and monitoring laboratory results are included.

Educational Needs of Nurses

The educational needs of cancer nurses have been studied. An early study identified the need for further education in assisting patients to meet their psychosocial needs.[28] Grant and Padilla[29] reviewed the status of cancer nursing research and categorized the studies into two groups, those on cancer nursing knowledge and those on oncology nurses. The studies on cancer nurses concerned nurses' attitudes toward cancer patients, death, cancer nursing care, and cancer care. The Western Consortium for Cancer Nursing Research, a regional collaborative research group in Canada, conducted a Delphi study to establish priorities for cancer nursing research.[30] The top-ranked topic with respect to nursing practice was to determine strategies to promote morale and prevent burnout among oncology nurses.

The Education Committee of the Oncology Nursing Society developed educational standards to provide guidelines for cancer nursing education.[31-33] *Outcome Standards for Cancer Nursing Education: Fundamental Level*[31] delineated the knowledge needed to provide cancer nursing care consistent with *Outcome Standards for Cancer Nursing Practice*.[6] The latter was developed to delineate the knowledge needed by those with cancer.[32] *Outcome Standards for Public Cancer Education*[33] was developed to provide information on prevention, early detection, rehabilitation, and living with cancer. To address the implementation of the education standards, examples were published in the *Oncology Nursing Forum*. The first example described the development of a clinical elective for senior nursing students using the education standards[34] whereas the second example was the development of a program for nurses to integrate into clinical practice current knowledge and research results related to antineoplastic drug treatment of cancer.[35] The determination of readiness for learning in cancer care was addressed in the third example.[36] A model for cancer patient education was proposed in terms of the cancer patient education standards. The final example described an approach to provide the public with information on cancer prevention, detection, and treatment.[37] A Cancer Information Day was planned and proved to be a valuable and worthwhile enterprise. The public cancer education standards were used to guide the program.

EDUCATION FOR CANCER NURSING PRACTICE

Because of the high incidence of cancer, most practicing nurses become involved in the care of individuals with cancer and their families. As a result of the basic education in nursing, however, the knowledge and skills nurses have about cancer nursing vary. It is incumbent on nurses who care for individuals with cancer to become knowledgeable about current cancer care practices so that they can provide optimal nursing care to these patients and their families.

To determine the status of cancer nursing education in the United States, a descriptive study was conducted by the Oncology Nursing Society.[38] The impetus of the study, which was supported by the American Cancer Society, was the concern that the basic education of nurses in cancer care may be inadequate.

Questionnaires were sent to 982 professional schools in the United States that were accredited by the National League for Nursing. The total number of returned questionnaires was 672 (68%). The results indicated that some content areas received considerable attention, whereas others did not. Content areas inadequately covered were prevention and detection; acute problems; late effects of treatment; unorthodox treatments; attitudes toward cancer; home care; social and political issues; resources for patients, families, and nurses; and legal implications in cancer nursing practice. The most frequent amount of time designated for cancer nursing content was 14½ hours.

The results of the survey indicated the need to maximize the time designated for cancer nursing content in basic nursing programs. There was a need for educational resources that are current and readily available. Suggestions were made to improve the knowledge necessary for cancer nursing practice.

The Education Committee of the Oncology Nursing Society proposed an organizing framework and approach for the education of nurses in cancer nursing practice.[39] Two levels were proposed: fundamental and advanced education. Education at the fundamental level provides the basic knowledge, skill, and attitudes for cancer nursing practice whereas the advanced level provides in-depth knowledge, skills, and attitudes. To reflect the changes within the profession, as well as the changes within cancer nursing, the terms *generalist* and *specialist* currently are used.

Conceptual Framework

A conceptual framework for cancer nursing education was developed that was consistent with those in *Outcome Standards for Cancer Nursing Practice*.[6] Four concepts were included in the framework: individual-family, health-illness continuum, health care system, and community-environment.[31] The four concepts interact with one another as they apply to caring for individuals with cancer and their families. The individual-family concept is the central focus of cancer nursing practice. The health-illness concept is defined as adaptation of the individual and family along a continuum. The health care system concept is the setting

for the practice of cancer nursing, and the community-environment concept refers to the resources and support necessary for those with cancer. The nursing process and the research process are the methods used for the organization of knowledge for cancer nursing practice.

Generalist Level

The generalist level of cancer nursing education encompasses basic education for nurses, continuing education to improve current nursing practice, and professional development. With the use of the concepts of individual-family, health-illness continuum, health care system, and community-environment, an outline of content for cancer nursing education is presented in Table 59-1.

Individual-family

Individuals are viewed as having biologic, psychologic, spiritual, cultural, developmental, and economic dimensions. These dimensions should be considered in assessing the impact of the diagnosis of cancer on individuals and their families. The strengths and limitations of each individual can be determined, and they provide direction for nursing actions.

Three strategies are important in managing the care of individuals and families dealing with the impact of cancer. Communication strategies employed by individuals and families should be assessed and used in planning nursing care. Basic communication strategies are obtained in preservice preparation and then are expanded in nursing curricula. The sophistication of the strategies depends on the organization of the nursing program, but most faculty

TABLE 59-1 Outline of Content for Cancer Nursing Education

Individual and Family	Health-Illness Continuum	Health Care System	Community-Environment
Impact of cancer: biologic, psychologic, spiritual, cultural, developmental, economic	Cancer epidemiology terminology	Organizational design: primary care, acute care, ambulatory care, long-term care	Cancer-related resources: local, regional, national
	Incidence: trends, patterns of occurrence, cancer risk factors		Community: economic, legal, political, employability/insurability
Communication strategies	Prevention and early detection	Accessibility/availability of health care services	
Decision-making strategies	Diagnosis and staging		Environment: occupational, physical
Stress management strategies	Pathophysiology of cancer	Continuity of health care services	
Individual and family resources	Treatment: surgery, radiation therapy, chemotherapy	Utilization of health care services	
	Other modalities: immunotherapy, hyperthermia, biologic response modifiers	Accountability (standards for practice)	
	Rehabilitation: economic, physical, psychosocial, life cycle		

members would agree that graduates of basic nursing programs need to have acquired a variety of communication strategies. Decision-making strategies employed by individuals and their families are important in planning interventions to meet identified short- and long-term needs. Content related to these strategies usually is offered in preservice courses and further expanded in successive nursing courses. Various stressors are brought about by the nature of cancer and its treatment. Stress management strategies are numerous and are provided in both preservice courses and nursing courses.

The resources that individuals and families use to assist them in their life activities need to be identified because they often can be mobilized to assist them during the course of the disease. Accurate information about cancer, treatment options, consequences of treatment, potential problems, and alternative care settings is necessary for individuals and their families. The need for adequate preparation based on sound knowledge and experience is evident.

Health-illness continuum

The health-illness continuum is defined as the adaptation individuals and families undergo during the cancer experience. Because cancer is a major and prevalent disease, information about the epidemiology of cancer is provided and includes national, regional, and local incidence rates. Trends in the incidence of cancer in certain populations, as well as the patterns of occurrence, are addressed. Cancer risk factors and prevention and early detection of cancer are discussed at several levels in nursing programs. In addition, the causes of cancer, as well as the cellular biology of cancer, are addressed. The epidemiology of cancer and cell growth processes often are provided in science courses in most nursing programs. Additional information then is given as major cancers are described. Although information on the characteristics of major cancers may vary from program to program, content related to lung cancer, breast cancer, colon cancer, genitourinary cancer, gynecologic cancer, and the leukemias is included. Other cancers related to specific populations may or may not be added, depending on the region of the country. Content related to common diagnostic tests is included in nursing courses. The importance of diagnostic and staging procedures is best discussed in relation to the characteristics of major cancers.

The rationale for and principles of the major treatment modalities should be included, along with the specific skills appropriate to the treatment modalities. Management of comfort, nutrition, mobility, elimination, sexuality, ventilation, and circulation is necessary to assist individuals in dealing with their treatment regimens. The final consideration in the health-illness continuum is rehabilitation, which includes economic, physical, and psychosocial needs of individuals and their families. Life cycle considerations and the level of functioning each person had achieved or is capable of achieving are of utmost importance.

Health care system

Cancer nursing is practiced in multiple settings. Primary care settings provide a range of services required by individuals and their families during initial diagnostic examinations. Acute care settings also provide multiple services necessary for individuals with cancer. The organizational design of community hospitals, major medical centers, and major cancer centers should be well understood by those who practice in them. The roles of the members of the health care team need to be defined and understood by the other members so that assistance can be rendered most appropriately to the patients served by the institution. Ambulatory care settings are becoming increasingly important in the care of patients with cancer. The resources needed by individuals and their families are important for satisfactory delivery of care in these settings. Long-term care settings such as hospice also provide services required by individuals with cancer.

Mutual understanding of each of the systems should be well known by those who practice cancer nursing. Individuals with cancer and their families need to be assisted to search for the appropriate components of the health care system available to them. Accountability for nursing actions is an integral part of this concept.

Community-environment

Cancer-related resources at the local, regional, and national levels are available. Students are apprised of the services offered by the American Cancer Society at each level. Home care services and bereavement services in each community are included in the content of courses.

Content related to the economic impact of cancer often is included in preservice preparation and expanded in the nursing courses. Political factors that influence cancer care, legal implications of cancer nursing practice, issues of employability and insurability, the identification of environmental carcinogens, and knowledge of safety measures related to hazards of cancer treatment are necessary components of curricula that prepare individuals for cancer nursing practice.

The fostering of the development of empathy in those who will care for individuals with cancer and their families is important in basic nursing education programs. It is recommended that the promotion of empathy be incorporated at the beginning of nursing programs.[40] Attitudes and feelings of students toward caring for patients with cancer need to be assessed. A clinically useful instrument to evaluate nursing students' attitudes toward caring for patients with cancer has been designed and tested.[41] This instrument, Ideas About Oncology Patient Care, measures the multidimensional nature of attitudes toward caring for cancer patients.

Strategies for increasing undergraduate nursing students' knowledge about cancer have been proposed. These include the development of a clinical elective for students[34]; the use of an independent study option for selected students[42]; the use of alternate methods of obtaining information beyond assigned textbook readings[43]; and an annual nursing student cancer workshop.[44] These strategies were developed in response to the amount of information necessary to practice cancer nursing.

Clinical experience

The relationship of theory to practice is crucial to cancer nursing. Students are given the opportunity to practice their skills in multiple care settings. Through the use of the nursing process, including nursing diagnosis, acquired clinical skills can be used in meeting individual and family needs. Physical and psychosocial assessment is necessary in the provision of direct care. Technical skills need to be carefully and meticulously integrated into each student's program.

In the past several years numerous resources have become available to educators. These have included journals devoted exclusively to cancer nursing, audiovisual resources that detail specific aspects of cancer prevention and detection, diagnosis, and treatment, and textbooks that include content on cancer nursing care.

For students enrolled in baccalaureate nursing programs the Cancer Work-Study Program sponsored by the National Institutes of Health is another option. Students must have completed their junior year toward a baccalaureate degree in nursing. Twenty students are selected, paid a stipend, and complete a 10-week program. Opportunity is provided for enhancement of knowledge and skills in caring for individuals with cancer in the areas of prevention, detection, diagnosis, treatment, and rehabilitation.

The "Position Statement on Nursing Roles—Scope and Preparation"[45] addressed the necessity to improve the quality of nursing education programs and described the range of nursing practice roles. *Standards for Professional Nursing Education*[46] was designed to help the nursing profession meet the changing needs of society. Both documents stated that professional nursing practice requires the minimum of a baccalaureate degree with a major in nursing, and technical nursing practice requires an associate degree or a diploma in nursing.

Continuing education

For nurses who are consistently involved in cancer nursing practice and have been prepared at the baccalaureate level, associate degree level, or diploma level, continuing education becomes a practical necessity. Educational opportunities are provided by universities, nursing organizations, hospitals, and health departments and may be offered either on a short- or on a long-term basis. The Oncology Nursing Society was granted accreditation as an approver and provider of continuing education for nurses by the American Nurses' Association in 1988. As an approver of continuing education the Oncology Nursing Society reviews applications for educational programs, offerings, and independent studies. Contact hours are awarded to registered nurses who attend programs. As a provider of continuing education the Oncology Nursing Society is committed to planning and implementing continuing education according to the standards of the American Nurses' Association.

Standards of Oncology Nursing Practice[1] provides guidelines for continuing education programs. That practicing nurses are eager to acquire further knowledge and skill is evident in the attendance at conferences throughout the country. Since 1973 the American Cancer Society has sponsored a national conference on cancer nursing every 4 years. At the first conference in 1973, more than 2500 nurses participated in the activities, and successive conferences have been equally well attended.

The Department of Nursing Education at Memorial Sloan-Kettering Cancer Center presents an Overview of Cancer Nursing four times annually. Content includes information related to the major modalities of cancer treatment, content on the major cancers, and implications for nursing care in terms of individual needs. Observational experiences are available throughout the program. The University of Texas System Cancer Center, MD Anderson Hospital and Tumor Institute, sponsors cancer prevention and detection programs for nurses. The offerings vary from 1 day to 3 weeks in length. Scripps Memorial Hospital Cancer Center sponsors an annual cancer symposium for nurses. The conference is 3 days in length and attracts participants from all across the country.

The Institute of Continuing Education for Nurses at the University of Southern California sponsors an annual cancer nursing seminar. Workshops during the seminar are planned to suit individual learning needs. The opportunity to meet other cancer nurses from across the country is an important outcome of the conference.

To assist nurses with the development of continuing education programs in cancer nursing, the Education Committee of the Oncology Nursing Society presented an instructional session at the 11th Annual Congress.[47] The session was based on the assumption that consumers of continuing education programs in cancer nursing are adult learners. How to conduct a learning needs assessment with examples was presented in the first paper.[48] Formulating educational objectives was the focus of the second paper.[49] Examples of objectives for continuing education programs were given. In the third paper the need for congruency between content and methodology and program objectives was discussed.[50] Examples were given to illustrate the material. The benefits of specific methods were described. Finally, program evaluation was addressed, with a discussion of the process, as well as the components, of the programs.[51]

The efficacy of the benefits of short-term programs has been a subject of interest to educators. The advantages of the acquisition of knowledge in a short period of time are debatable. For many practicing nurses, however, short-term programs offer information that they might not otherwise obtain. To determine the effects of an intensive 3-day cancer nursing workshop on nurses' attitudes toward patients and cancer nurses, 36 participants were evaluated before and 6 weeks after the completion of the course.[52] The Activity Vector Analysis, an adjective check-list of 81 nonderogatory adjectives to describe human behavior, was used. The results suggested that perhaps no one type of nurse is attracted to cancer nursing and that nurses in the specialty of cancer nursing need to develop realistic expectations about their roles.

Long-term continuing education programs have been offered to provide a broad overview of cancer nursing and specific knowledge in the different types of cancer. Most of these courses include advanced physical assessment skills, supervised clinical practice, and the awarding of a certificate at the completion of the program. *Standards of Oncology Nursing Practice* presents useful guidelines for the implementation of these programs. Because of the length of these programs, a more comprehensive offering is possible. An annual listing of long-term continuing education programs is prepared by the Education Committee of the Oncology Nursing Society and published in the *Oncology Nursing Forum.*

Meeting the needs of individuals with cancer and their families continues to be a challenge for those engaged in cancer nursing. By organizing the necessary knowledge, practicing nurses can continue to increase their expertise in cancer nursing.

To assist in the planning and evaluation of generalist level education, *Standards of Oncology Nursing Education: Generalist and Advanced Practice Levels*[53] is useful. Designed to guide the achievement of quality education for nurses, these standards reflect structure, process, and outcomes of educational offerings. Another publication, *Standards of Oncology Education: Patient/Family and Public,*[54] is available to assist in the planning and evaluation of formal and informal patient and family teaching and public education programs. Descriptive statements guide the achievement of quality education for these populations. Additionally, materials related to patient, family, and public education are available from the American Cancer Society, the Leukemia Society of America, and the National Cancer Institute.

Specialist Level

The specialist level of cancer nursing education encompasses graduate education for nurses to develop a broader scope of practice, as well as the development of resources and an increased emphasis on coordination, continuity, and evaluation of care.[39] Specialists require substantial theoretic knowledge in cancer nursing and proficient use of this knowledge in providing expert care to individuals with cancer and their families.[1]

A cancer nursing workshop, Curriculum Construction and Role Definition, was convened by the American Cancer Society in 1978. The purpose was to reach a consensus about the educational preparation for nursing specialists in cancer nursing.[14] Content for preparation as a clinical nurse specialist was outlined and has proved beneficial inasmuch as programs have continued to offer specialization in cancer nursing at the master's level. The publication, *Master's Degree with a Specialty in Oncology Nursing:*

Role Definition and Curriculum Guide,[25] is useful for nurse educators in planning graduate cancer nursing education. Its content, which is based on the current body of knowledge in advanced cancer nursing practice, is organized by role components, that is, clinical practice, education, consultation, administration, research and professionalism, and steps of the nursing process.

Individual-family

The dimensions ascribed to individuals at the generalist level are considered in the delineation of content at the graduate level. Courses should be available that address the recurrent phenomena related to cancer such as depression, pain, anxiety, body image, and coping. Courses often are available in other departments of a university or may be available in the graduate program in nursing.

Communication strategies are included and specifically related to individuals with cancer and their families. These may include self-help groups, support groups, or group work that addresses counseling needs of individuals and their families. Decision-making strategies are most effectively taught as they relate to role preparation in graduate education. Ethical implications of cancer is an area that is included in many graduate programs; thus the decisions made by individuals and their families related to cancer treatment and its consequences can be supported. Stress management theories are incorporated into the major courses of the program. These theories can be related to stressors that individuals encounter as they adapt to living with cancer. Nurses prepared at the specialist level are in a position to act as advocates for individuals with cancer and their families. Those who assume this role must of course be trained to do so. Specialists in cancer nursing have the ability to integrate and evaluate the factors that have an impact on coping with the disease.[13]

The identification of resources available to individuals and their families is crucial to their care. Content related to health care agencies and community resources should be included to assist students in early and rapid identification of available assistance. Specialists need to be knowledgeable in the identification of high-risk individuals in terms of complications resulting inside and outside of the health care system. The problems of long-term survival also need to be addressed.

Health-illness continuum

Determination of the individual's position on the health-illness continuum is a major emphasis in graduate programs. Building on the basic sciences of undergraduate programs, graduate education broadens this foundation. Courses in advanced physiology and pathophysiology are recommended for students interested in cancer. Special attention is given to the acquisition of knowledge related to cellular biology, cellular kinetics, radiation biology, and immunology. Courses often are offered in other departments of the universities, and every effort should be made to have students participate in these courses.

Analysis of the cancer problem in terms of the application of epidemiologic techniques is an important component of the curriculum. Indications for prevention and early detection, identification of high-risk populations, and diagnostic techniques are crucial for understanding the continuum. Emphasis in graduate programs often is placed on the pathophysiology of malignant processes. The goals and general principles of therapy, including cure, control, and palliation, are discussed. Surgery, radiotherapy, chemotherapy, and other treatment modalities then are discussed in relation to the physiologic aberrations that have occurred. Unproved methods and their implications are described. The relationship of medical management to nursing management then is analyzed. Research that has been conducted or is being conducted is an integral part of the content.

Not all graduate programs have as their major focus the management of the acute manifestations of cancer. Some may be concerned with the management of advanced disease or the rehabilitative aspects of care. Nonetheless, medical management and nursing management are necessary for cancer nursing practice at the specialist level. Indications for supportive management such as nutritional support, pain control, infection control, and blood component therapy also are studied. Other content areas include acute problems related to cancer, such as cardiac tamponade, disseminated intravascular coagulation, hypercalcemia, inappropriate antidiuretic hormone syndrome, sepsis, spinal cord compression, superior vena cava syndrome, and tumor lysis syndrome.

Health care system

Role preparation is an integral component of graduate education at the master's degree level and includes clinical specialist, practitioner, educator, and administrator.[55,56] Because most students enrolled in graduate programs have practiced in the health care system before returning for further education, their experiences should be considered. The organization of each of the major health care systems is discussed in relation to the functional area in which the student is or will be practicing. Ideally, students may be able to practice in ambulatory care settings, home care settings, or hospice settings during their graduate program. Although this may not always be possible, it certainly is desirable. Continuity of health care service can thus be described and implementation ensured. Utilization of health care services can be clearly explained in relation to continuity of health care services. Professional, legal, and ethical issues in the management of the care of individuals with cancer and their families are inherent in practice accountability. Content related to informed consent, human investigation, legal aspects of cancer nursing practice, cancer economics, and employability and insurability is presented.

Community-environment

Resources that are available for individuals and their families should be investigated and understood by cancer nurses. The expertise of the members of the cancer health team provides assistance with problem solving. The political implications of cancer care is one other area that should be addressed in graduate education. In the future the politics of cancer care will play an increasing role in cancer nursing.

Clinical experience

The application of theory to practice is crucial to graduate preparation in cancer nursing. Clinical experience for graduate students is directed by the overall program objectives. The objectives generally specify performance in clinical specialization, functional roles, and research.[57,58]

By means of organized approaches to nursing care problems, the objectives of the clinical components of the program can be met. The approaches most widely used involve the nursing process, including nursing diagnosis, and the research process. Both approaches enable students to accomplish the objectives of the program.

Physical and psychosocial assessment skills are necessary for the provision of direct care and are acquired before admission to the program or concurrent with attendance. Technical skills are reinforced during the course of the program. The rationale for the use of technical skills is explained, and students need to investigate the basis for the use of technical skills. The need to acquire teaching skills is important in graduate education because graduates are involved in the teaching of other nurses, patients and their families, and community personnel.

Three different groups of personnel interact with graduate students as they engage in clinical practice during their program. These groups—faculty members, practicing clinical nurse specialists, and nursing service administrators in health care settings—all influence the students as they progress in the program.[59,60] Ample time should be allowed for students to integrate the expectations of these professionals.

The role of the clinical nurse specialist in cancer nursing has received considerable attention in the last few years. Consistency in preparation has been alluded to, but to date few studies have been conducted to verify the role of the clinical nurse specialist in practice. A national invitational conference entitled "The Oncology Clinical Nurse Specialist-Role Analysis and Future Projections" was held in 1984. The conference, sponsored by the Cancer Nursing Service at the Clinical Center, National Institutes of Health, was held for the purpose of providing guidelines for currently practicing cancer clinical nurse specialists to optimize current practice and to provide goals for future development. Most would agree that the role of the clinical nurse specialist encompasses direct patient care, teaching nursing personnel, role modeling for other nursing personnel, consultation, and research.[11,13,58,61]

The characteristics of the clinical nurse specialist in cancer nursing are summarized in Table 59-2. Achieving this role in nursing practice remains a challenge, and problems have been cited in relation to role implementation.[62,63] A survey conducted by Yasko[64] described the characteristics and perceptions of nurses with a master's degree in

TABLE 59-2 Characteristics of Clinical Nurse Specialist in Cancer Nursing

Clinical competence
Direct nursing care
Coordinate patient care services
Patient/family advocate

Teaching
Patient/family
In-service education
Basic, continuing, and graduate education
Public education

Research
Conduct of research
Clinical trials
Research protocols
Experimental regimens

Consultation
Resource for nursing personnel
Intraprofessional resource
Evaluation of health programs
Evaluation of health delivery

nursing, who were currently employed as clinical nurse specialists in cancer nursing; 185 nurses with master's degrees participated in the study. Variations in master's level curricula were apparent, as well as variations in the implementation of the role. A modified Delphi survey with 47 participants, conducted by McGee et al,[65] identified 363 competencies required of cancer clinical nursing specialists. Attitudes and human traits received the highest mean ratings of the competency categories identified. Findings indicated a consistent ranking of knowledge and skill categories. Moore et al[66] reported on a longitudinal evaluation of students' abilities to apply new knowledge to clinical behaviors. The Appraisal of Practice Behaviors Instrument was developed to measure cancer nursing practice and tested on 38 enrollees in a master's program.

Trends that affect the future role of the clinical nurse specialist have been examined and include those related to societal changes, new developments in health care, and professional directions. It will be up to the clinical nurse specialist to describe the changes in practice, to identify new arenas for practice, and to continue to evaluate the impact of the role.

Continuing education

For those nurses prepared at the master's degree level and consistently involved in cancer nursing, continuing education is a practical consideration. The direction this education takes depends on the position and the setting in which nursing specialists practice. Often clinical nurse specialists are engaged in numerous teaching activities. These may include but are not limited to patient/family education, in-service education, public education, and ed-

ucation at the generalist or specialist level. Further preparation in teaching strategies and methods may be sought and is available through university programs and professional organizations.

Standards of Oncology Nursing Practice,[1] *Standards of Oncology Nursing Education: Generalist and Advanced Practice Levels*[53] and *Standards of Oncology Education: Patient/Family and Public*[54] provide useful guidelines for promoting continuing education for practicing nursing specialists. Conferences often are arranged around such themes as symptom management, management of pain, and strategies used by individuals with cancer. Interdisciplinary conferences also are available for cancer nursing specialists.

The International Union Against Cancer was established in 1934 to provide leadership and an international forum for the exchange of information in the fight against cancer.[67] Meetings are held every 4 years in various parts of the world and offer an opportunity for nurses to participate in the sessions or to present papers. A permanent activity of the UICC is the Nurses' Cancer Education Project. The first International Conference on Cancer Nursing, sponsored by the Royal Marsden Hospital, London, was held in 1978, and the second took place in 1980. A commitment was then made to conduct an international conference every 2 years beginning in 1984. These conferences offer an opportunity for nurses to present clinical findings at international conferences.

ISSUES IN CANCER NURSING EDUCATION

Education of Ancillary Health Workers

As more individuals with cancer are cared for at home, the preparation of family members and other health workers will assume greater importance. Cancer nurses are in a position to offer assistance and education for both family members and ancillary health workers. Continuing education has a role to play in the offering of programs to meet community needs.

Certification and Recertification

For the past few decades many nursing specialty organizations have developed certification programs. Soon after World War II, the American Association of Nursing Anesthetists developed its certification program. The American Nurses' Association established its certification program in 1973 to provide recognition of professional achievement in a defined clinical or functional area of nursing. The American Nurses' Association's definition of certification is that it is the process by which the Association's Committee of Examiners validates, on the basis of predetermined standards, an individual nurse's qualifications, knowledge, and practice in a defined functional or clinical area in nursing.[68] The American Nurses' Association offers more than 17 programs in nursing administration certification. Most nursing specialty organizations offer certification.

The definition of certification most widely used is that stated in the report entitled *The Study of Credentialing in Nursing: A New Approach*:[69]

> Certification is a process by which a non-governmental agency or association certifies that an individual licensed to practice a profession has met certain predetermined standards specified by that profession for specialty practice. Its purpose is to assure various publics that an individual has mastered a body of knowledge and acquired skills in a particular specialty.

The principal advantage of certification is that it provides an additional measure of quality nursing care for the consumer. More important, certification assists the entire nursing profession in upgrading its performance and provides individual nurses with tangible acknowledgment of professional achievement in nursing. Through a system of peer review, recognition of expertise in both current knowledge and in clinical practice is provided.

A survey of the Oncology Nursing Society members indicated a strong interest in certification for cancer nursing.[70] In 1981 the Board of Directors of the Oncology Nursing Society voted to explore the possibility of a certification program. A Task Force on Certification in Oncology Nursing was established to explore the methodology for a certification program and to determine the cost of such a program.[71] A survey of the members of the Oncology Nursing Society was undertaken in 1982 to determine the commitment to certification in cancer nursing. The questionnaire was sent to 4365 nurses; 693 returns, or 15.9%, were used as the study base of the survey.[72]

The response indicated support of a certification program, as well as a sense of commitment to the process. The results of the survey were presented to the members at the 1983 Oncology Nursing Society Congress through an instructional session and an open forum.[72] The task force recommended that a certification program be considered for members and be directed first at the generalist level. Plans for subspecialization and specialist level were to be considered in the future.

The Core Curriculum Task Force of the Oncology Nursing Society prepared a core curriculum and a bibliography for the development of the certification examination, a study guide for those preparing for the examination, and a format for workshops.[73] The Oncology Nursing Certification Corporation (ONCC) was established for the development, administration, and evaluation of the certification program. The ONCC contracted with the Educational Testing Services for the development of the certification examination. Members of the Test Specification Committee developed test items for inclusion in the examination. Before the test administration, rigorous procedures were used to determine the examination's cut score.[74] The cut score represents the lowest score qualifying a candidate for certification. The test development was supported by the Oncology Nursing Society and in part by a grant from the American Cancer Society.

Nurses with an RN license, 3 years' experience as a registered nurse within the last 5 years, and a minimum of 1000 hours of cancer nursing practice within the last 3 years are eligible for certification. Nursing experience may be in the areas of nursing administration, education, clinical practice, or research. The first examination was offered in 1986, and subsequent examinations have been offered twice yearly since. Successful candidates receive a certificate from ONCC and use the designation of Oncology Certified Nurse (OCN). Certification for cancer nursing is valid for 4 years. The total number of OCNs in 1989 was 5116, and a task force was formed to address recertification issues.[75] Recommendations were that the renewal of certification should be a voluntary credentialing process similar to the initial process. Candidates must meet the same criteria as before, and an examination will constitute the requirements for recertification. OCNs certified in 1986 are eligible for recertification in 1990.

A bulletin is prepared each year for candidates. The bulletin includes information regarding the examination process, core curriculum for the certification examination, selected references, and sample questions.[76] Additionally, a textbook has been developed for use by those preparing for certification.[77] A role delineation study is under way to identify critical indicators to help determine the content of future examinations of cancer nursing. Issues being considered by the ONCC are identifying the focus of educational efforts and providing a body of knowledge for the development of a specialist core curriculum and a baseline to describe specialist practice.

Research

The research process is an integral component of cancer nursing education. Nursing education at the generalist level, particularly in baccalaureate programs, fosters a beginning knowledge of the research process. Students are encouraged to use research findings, both in the theoretic portion of the program and in their practice. For practicing nurses the identification of nursing practice problems is an ongoing process. Assistance should be sought from those qualified to engage in the investigation of these problems.

For those engaged in graduate education the research process is applied in most courses of the program. Nursing practice problems are identified and analyzed on the basis of systematic use of the process. A thesis or research project often is required for completion of the program. For those engaged in doctoral education the conduct of research is required and the application to nursing practice mandated.

Using the criteria of *Outcome Standards for Cancer Nursing Education: Fundamental Level*,[31] Grant and Padilla[29] undertook a review of the current status of cancer nursing research. More than 300 studies were reviewed and categorized. Suggestions for the future development of clinical nursing research were made. Fernsler et al[78] conducted a study of cancer nursing research from 1975 to 1982. The findings described the quantity and nature of cancer nursing research and affirmed that patient needs were the focus of most of these studies. The Oncology Nursing Society has conducted two surveys of research priorities.[79,80] Both these studies used the educational standards as the framework for the categorization of the studies. Research priorities were symptom management, including pain control, patient education, coping and stress management, and prevention and early detection. The results of the 1988 survey were submitted to the National Center for Nursing Research as the organization's top research priorities. To guide the development of cancer nursing research in western Canada, five priority topics were identified by a regional collaborative group.[30] Collaborative approaches hold promise for generating solutions to researchable problems.

Funds are required for the conduct of research, and qualifying for funds will be a challenge in the decade ahead. Sound research proposals that address cancer morbidity and mortality will have to be developed.

CONCLUSION

Nursing as a professional discipline has a unique place in society. Cancer nursing as a component of this professional discipline must meet the challenges of society, and its practice must continue to be based on a sound theoretic and clinical base.

REFERENCES

1. American Nurses' Association and Oncology Nursing Society: Standards of Oncology Nursing Practice. Kansas City, Mo, American Nurses' Association, 1987.
2. Tiffany R: The development of cancer nursing as a specialty. Int Nurs Rev 34:35-39, 1987.
3. Nursing: A Social Policy Statement. Kansas City, Mo, American Nurses' Association, 1980.
4. Marino LB: Cancer Nursing. St Louis, CV Mosby, 1981.
5. Oncology nursing society education committee. Oncol Nurs Forum 6:20-21, 1979.
6. American Nurses' Association and Oncology Nursing Society: Outcome Standards for Cancer Nursing Practice. Kansas City, Mo, American Nurses' Association, 1979.
7. Yarbro CH: The early days: Four smiles and a post office box. Oncol Nurs Forum 11:79-85, 1984.
8. Greene PE: The association of pediatric oncology nurses: The first ten years. Oncol Nurs Forum 10:59-63, 1983.
9. ONS salutes NCI on its 50th anniversary. Oncol Nurs Forum 14:14-16, 1987.
10. Hilkemeyer R: A historical perspective in cancer nursing. Oncol Nurs Forum 9:47-55, 1982.
11. Siehl S: The clinical nurse specialist in oncology. Nurs Clin North Am 17:753-761, 1982.
12. Spross J: An overview of the oncology clinical nurse specialist role. Oncol Nurs Forum 10:54-58, 1983.
13. Welch-McCaffrey D: Role performance issues for oncology clinical nurse specialists. Cancer Nurs 9:287-294, 1986.
14. Craytor JK: Highlights in education for cancer nursing. Oncol Nurs Forum 9:51-59, 1982.
15. Peterson R: Federal grants for education in cancer nursing. Nurs Outlook 4:103-105, 1956.
16. Peterson R, Soller G: Cancer nursing in the basic professional nursing curriculum. Washington, DC, US Government Printing Office, 1951.
17. Peterson R, Heil L: Tools for the evaluation of cancer nursing for nursing instructors. Washington, DC, US Government Printing Office, 1957.
18. Diller D: An Investigation of Cancer Learning in Ninety-One Selected Schools of Nursing. Saratoga Springs, NY, Skidmore College, 1955.
19. Diller D: An Investigation of Cancer Learning in Ninety Selected Schools of Nursing. Third Report. Saratoga Springs, NY, Skidmore College, 1957.
20. Hilkemeyer R, Kinney H: Teaching cancer nursing. Nurs Outlook 4:177-180, 1956.
21. Barckley V: Work study program in cancer nursing. Nurs Outlook 19:447-452, 1971.
22. National Cancer Institute: Cancer Nurse Training Program. Washington, DC, National Institutes of Health, 1987.
23. Longman AJ, Verran JA, Clark M: Improving oncology nursing content in an undergraduate program. J Nurs Ed 27:42-44, 1988.
24. Education Committee, Oncology Nursing Society: Assessing graduate education in oncology nursing. Oncol Nurs Forum 7:37-38, 1980.
25. The Master's Degree with a Specialty in Oncology Nursing: Role Definition and Curriculum Guide. Pittsburgh, Pa, Oncology Nursing Society, 1988.
26. Seigele D: Longitudinal evaluation of a model post-master's program in oncology nursing. Oncol Nurs Forum 11:61-71, 1984.
27. Frerichs M, Yasko JM: The American Cancer Society's scholarship program. Oncol Nurs Forum 12:62-64, 1985.
28. Craytor JK, Brown JK, Morrow GR: Assessing learning needs of nurses who care for persons with cancer. Cancer Nurs 1:211-220, 1978.
29. Grant M, Padilla G: An overview of cancer nursing research. Oncol Nurs Forum 10:58-69, 1983.
30. Priorities for cancer nursing research: A Canadian replication. Cancer Nurs 10:319-326, 1987.
31. Oncology Nursing Society: Outcome Standards for Cancer Nursing Education: Fundamental Level. Pittsburgh, Pa, The Society, 1982.
32. Oncology Nursing Society: Outcome Standards for Cancer Patient Education. Pittsburgh, Pa, The Society, 1982.
33. Oncology Nursing Society: Outcome Standards for Public Cancer Education. Pittsburgh, Pa, Oncology Nursing Society, 1983.
34. Nevidjon B, Deatrich J: An oncology clinical elective. Oncol Nurs Forum 12:57-59, 1985.
35. Kimball DD, Heft PL: The development of an antineoplastic drug education program. Oncol Nurs Forum 12:59-62, 1985.
36. Welch-McCaffrey D: Evolving patient education needs in cancer. Oncol Nurs Forum 12:62-66, 1985.
37. Vega T: Outcome standards for public cancer education: The foundation for community education programs. Oncol Nurs Forum 12:66-67, 1985.
38. Brown J, Johnson J, Groenwald S: Survey of cancer nursing education in US schools of nursing. Oncol Nurs Forum 10:82-83, 1983.
39. Given B: Education of the oncology nurse: The key to excellent patient care. Semin Oncol 7:71-79, 1980.

40. Welch-McCaffrey D: Promoting the empathetic development of nursing students in the care of the patient with cancer. J Nurs Ed 23:73-75, 1984.

41. Verran JA, Longman A, Clark M: Development of a scale to measure undergraduate students' attitudes about caring for patients with cancer. Oncol Nurs Forum 14(5):51-55, 1987.

42. Mooney M, Dudas S: Undergraduate independent study in cancer nursing. Oncol Nurs Forum 14(1):51-53, 1987.

43. Daly JM, Erdmann WS: Oncology search: An innovative teaching method. Nurs Ed 13:28-30, 1988.

44. Quinn-Casper P, Holmgren C: Enhancing nursing concepts in undergraduate curricula. Cancer Nurs 10:274-278, 1987.

45. Position statement on nursing roles—scope and preparation. Nurs & Health Care 3:212-213, 1982.

46. Standards for professional nursing education. Kansas City, Mo, American Nurses' Association, 1984.

47. Fernsler J: An overview. Oncol Nurs Forum 14:59-60, 1987.

48. Volker DL: Learning needs assessment. Oncol Nurs Forum 14:60-62, 1987.

49. Itano J: Developing educational objectives. Oncol Nurs Forum 14:62-65, 1987.

50. Belcher AE: Defining content and methods. Oncol Nurs Forum 14:65-67, 1987.

51. McMillan SC: Program evaluation. Oncol Nurs Forum 14:67-70, 1987.

52. Johnson J, Mosier MA, Johnson C: Registered nurses: Perceptions of patients, cancer nurses and themselves. Oncol Nurs Forum 9:27-31, 1982.

53. Oncology Nursing Society: Standards of Oncology Nursing Education: Generalist and Advanced Practice Levels. Pittsburgh, Pa, The Society, 1989.

54. Oncology Nursing Society: Standards of Oncology Education: Patient/Family and Public. Pittsburgh, Pa, The Society, 1989.

55. Holzemer WL: Quality in graduate nursing education. Nurs & Health Care 3:536-542, 1982.

56. Piemme JA: Oncology clinical nurse specialist education. Oncol Nurs Forum 12:45-48, 1985.

57. Hodges LC, Poteet GW, Edlund BJ: Teaching clinical nurse specialists to lead and to succeed. Nurs & Health Care 6:192-196, 1985.

58. Paulen A: Practice issues for the oncology clinical nurse specialist. Oncol Nurs Forum 12:37-39, 1985.

59. Cason CL, Beck CM: Clinical nurse specialist role development. Nurs & Health Care 3:25-38, 1982.

60. Wyers MEA, Grove SK, Pastorino C: Clinical nurse specialist: In search of the right role. Nurs and Health Care 6:202-207, 1985.

61. Kwong M, Manning MP, Koetters TL: The role of the on-cology nurse specialist: Three personal views. Cancer Nurs 5:427-434, 1982.

62. Starck P: Factors influencing the role of the oncology clinical nurse specialist. Oncol Nurs Forum 10:54-58, 1983.

63. Spross J, Donoghue M: The future of the oncology clinical nurse specialist. Oncol Nurs Forum 11:74-78, 1984.

64. Yasko JM: A survey of oncology clinical nursing specialists. Oncol Nurs Forum 10:25-30, 1983.

65. McGee RF, Powell ML, Broadwell DC, et al: A Delphi survey of oncology clinical nurse specialist competencies. Oncol Nurs Forum 14:29-34, 1987.

66. Moore IM, Piper B, Dodd MJ, et al: Measuring oncology nursing practice: Results from one graduate program. Oncol Nurs Forum 14:45-49, 1987.

67. Ash CR: Cancer nursing: An international perspective. Cancer Nurs 9:172-177, 1986.

68. American Nurses' Association 1988 Certification Catalog. Kansas City, Mo, American Nurses' Association, 1988.

69. The study of credentialing in nursing: A new approach, vol 1: The Report of the Committee. Kansas City, Mo, American Nurses' Association, 1979.

70. Cobb ME, Maier P: Informational needs of the oncology nursing society membership. Oncol Nurs Forum 8:58-61, 1981.

71. Moore P, Hogan C, Longman A, et al: Report of the task force on certification in oncology nursing. Oncol Nurs Forum 9:75-80, 1982.

72. Longman A, Hogan C, McNally J, et al: Report of the task force on certification in oncology nursing. Oncol Nurs Forum 10:84-88, 1983.

73. Certification committee. Oncol Nurs Forum 11:77-79, 1984.

74. Ewing T: Determining examination cut scores. Oncol Nurs Forum 14:88, 1987.

75. Piper BF, Longman A, Protho P, et al: Certification renewal task force and recommendations. Oncol Nurs Forum 13:97-98, 103-105, 1986.

76. Oncology Nursing Certification Corporation Bulletin and Application 1989. Pittsburgh, Pa, Oncology Nursing Certification Corporation, 1989.

77. Ziegfeld CR: Core curriculum for oncology nursing. Philadelphia, Pa, WB Saunders, 1987.

78. Fernsler J, Holcombe J, Pulliam L: A survey of cancer nursing research January 1975-June 1982. Oncol Nurs Forum 11:46-52, 1984.

79. McGuire D, Frank M, Varricchio C: 1984 ONS research committee survey of membership's research interests and involvement. Oncol Nurs Forum 12:99-103, 1985.

80. Funkhouser SW, Grant MM: 1988 ONS survey of research priorities. Oncol Nurs Forum 16:413-416, 1989.

Chapter 60

Cancer Nursing Research

Marcia M. Grant, RN, DNSc, OCN

Geraldine V. Padilla, PhD

INTRODUCTION

Research has provided critical knowledge concerning the care of cancer patients. Basic science, medical science, and nursing science all form the foundation important in the prevention, detection, treatment, and management of cancer. The focus of this chapter is the role of the cancer nurse in the implementation of medical research and in the development, implementation, dissemination, and application of cancer nursing research. An examination of the role of the nurse in each of these activities provides a basis for understanding the rapid development of nursing research in the provision of care for today's cancer patient.

RESEARCH DEFINED

Research involves a structured approach to answering questions or discovering new knowledge.[1] It is conducted for the broad purpose of increasing scientific knowledge. Research can be considered valid only when it is replicated. The process of research involves an orderly and standardized series of steps. These steps can be compared to the steps in the nursing process; that is, both processes are specialized forms of problem solving.[2] Differences between the two processes involve amount of detail and accuracy of measurement. In addition, research focuses on a group of patients and includes the obligation to disseminate the results for critique by others. A comparison of the research and nursing processes is found in Table 60-1.

DEVELOPMENT OF MEDICAL RESEARCH IN CANCER

The focus of medical research and nursing research differs. In the development of cancer treatment, medical research is used to describe the natural history of the diseases, to test new treatment approaches and evaluate the value of singular and multimodal approaches to cancer treatment. Through these endeavors have developed surgical, chemotherapeutic, radiation, and biologic response-modifier approaches to the treatment of cancer, as well as supportive care measures.

Until the 1950s surgery was the primary approach to the treatment of cancer.[3] After World War II, radiation therapy began to develop as an offshoot of diagnostic radiation activities.[4] As radiation therapy improved and doses and schedules were adapted to specific cancers such as those of the skin, oral cavity, larynx, and breast, it became available as both a singular treatment for some diseases (eg, Hodgkin's disease) and in combination with surgery for other diseases (eg, breast and cervical cancer).

TABLE 60-1 Comparison of Clinical Nursing and Research Processes

Steps Involved	Clinical Nursing	Nursing Research
Defining the problem	Individual patient assessment	Identify area of concern
	Nursing diagnosis	Review literature and select a conceptual or theoretical framework
		Conduct preliminary studies
		Define methods
		Select population
		Define designs
		Define samples
		Operationally define variables
		Describe procedures
		Identify data analysis
Carrying out the action	Intervention implementation	Implement study
		Accrue consenting subjects
		Administer standardized tools
		Check reliability of data collection
Evaluating the results	Outcome evaluation	Code and analyze data
		Interpret findings
		Publish results

The development of chemotherapy for cancers (eg, leukemia) that were not amenable or responsive to either surgery or radiation gave the nurse a primary role in implementation of medical research.[5] The chemotherapeutic agents were administered intravenously over a course of therapy given on a regular (daily, weekly, etc) basis.

The Chemotherapy Research Nurse

The chemotherapy nurse assumed one of the first specialty roles in the development of cancer nursing practice. These nurses were responsible for the administration and monitoring of chemotherapy. They accrued patients for medical protocols, administered medications, counseled patients on management of side effects, collected data, and kept the physician informed of the patient's condition. Because of the complex nature of the medications and the potentially lethal side effects, chemotherapy nurses sought out and developed an extensive knowledge base about chemotherapeutic principles. Their involvement with accruing, monitoring, and teaching chemotherapy patients increased their familiarity with the research process as used in clinical chemotherapy research. These nurses were among the first nurses to participate as collaborators in cancer research. With their research skills as background, many of them sought further education and developed into primary researchers interested in either medical or nursing aspects of cancer care.

The first survey of research skills of Oncology Nursing Society (ONS) members conducted by the ONS Research Committee revealed that a large proportion of oncology nurses had participated in a variety of steps in the research process.[6] The continued participation of oncology nurses in the implementation of medical research is considered in further detail in our discussion of the members of the clinical research team and their roles.

The Clinical Trials Approach

The medical research approach to clinical investigation of cancer treatment methods has resulted in a specialized approach to clinical research called the clinical trials approach.[7] Developed and encouraged under the influence of studies funded by the National Cancer Institute (NCI), this approach involves several phases of study, each designed to answer specific clinical questions at a different time in the development of applied scientific knowledge. Each study or research protocol includes a well written and detailed guide which serves as the procedure for implementation of the study.

Clinical trials are divided into phase 1, 2, and 3 studies.[7] Each has a different purpose and design. After testing of medical treatment approaches (surgical, chemotherapeutic, or radiation) with appropriate animal or cell models, phase 1 studies are implemented as the first clinical tests of new treatments on human patients. The purpose of a phase 1 study is the determination of dose schedules and toxicities. Because new drugs and treatments are used, the population eligible to participate in phase 1 clinical trials includes patients for whom standard therapy has failed. Since the determination of how to use a drug or treatment in a phase 1 clinical trial has not yet been made, patients for whom standard treatments can be issued are *not* eligible or enrolled in phase 1 studies.

Data in phase 1 clinical trials include determination of the maximum tolerated dose (MTD), drug toxicities, and the response of tumors. Pharmacokinetic data on the medication being tested may be conducted as well. Thus the collection of timed specimens is common and requires precision by the nursing staff implementing the protocol. An example of a current phase 1 trial is the use of new investigational drugs for patients in whom standard chemotherapy has failed and who are not eligible for other treatments, such as radiation therapy. A phase 1 clinical trial requires accrual of the smallest number of patients to determine at what dose or schedule of treatments toxicities occur. Frequently the only benefit to a phase 1 patient is the satisfaction of having contributed to scientific knowledge for treatment of other cancer patients. However, patients often view participation in a phase 1 study from a hopeful perspective—prolongation of life for themselves or for other patients.

In phase 2 trials, the focus shifts to specific tumor types for which the treatment appears promising.[7] To be eligible for phase 2 trials, patients must either be not able to participate in standard therapy or have failed standard therapy. Specific tumors are selected that have shown some positive responses in preclinical or phase 1 trials. An example of a current phase 2 trial is the use of LAK and IL2 for patients with colorectal cancer and renal cell carcinoma. Toxicities during phase 2 trials are frequently profound, and close monitoring of patients is necessary to provide data for evaluation of patient response and early detection of toxicities.

The focus shifts again for phase 3 studies.[7] These studies determine (1) the effects of a treatment relative to the natural history of the disease, (2) whether a new treatment is more effective than a standard therapy, and (3) whether a new treatment is as effective as a standard therapy but is associated with less morbidity. In phase 3 trials, the focus is on comparison of a new treatment with the standard treatment. These studies involve randomization of patients to the experimental or the standard treatment.

Phase 1 clinical trials are implemented only at NCI-designated cancer centers (see Yellow Pages for list of these centers). This specification is done to assure the full spectrum of clinical support needed in studies in which toxicities are not predictable and close monitoring of patients is critical. Depending on the nature of the treatment being tested, phase 2 trials may also be conducted in NCI-designated cancer centers. Phase 3 trials, which require the greatest number of subjects to answer the research question, are conducted in large medical centers, university hospitals, and community centers with qualified cancer researchers and needed clinical support resources. Participation of cancer patients in all three kinds of clinical trial has been the critical element in the rapid development of current cancer treatment options. Through clinical trials we have developed options for primary breast cancer treatment involving either radiation therapy or surgery and options for Hodgkin's disease involving either chemotherapy or radiation. An interesting corollary to this approach to medical research is the increased participation and involvement of the patient in the selection of medical treatment. Today an informed citizen may read about a new cancer treatment in the newspaper and seek out a physician who is able to provide that approach to treatment.

The Medical Research Team

Implementation of clinical trials for cancer is carried out by a research team composed of a variety of multidisciplinary members: principal investigator, coinvestigator, research or protocol nurse, data manager, investigational pharmacist, statistician, and clinical nursing staff. Clinical nurses are important members of this team. The principal investigator is generally a physician and is responsible for the scientific integrity of the study. Responsibilities include development of the protocol, presentation of the study to the Institutional Review Board for review of appropriate informed consent procedures, and implementation of the study. Coinvestigators may include other physicians whose patients may be eligible for the study and other scientists (eg, molecular biologists or psychologists) interested in other aspects of cancer patients' responses.

The research nurse is responsible for patient accrual, implementing the physician's orders as described in the protocol, and observing patient responses and toxicities. In implementing the role, the nurse is involved in informed consent issues, astute clinical care, and education of supporting nursing staff.

While the principal investigator is legally responsible for obtaining informed consent from the patient, all members of the research team share this responsibility.[5] The research nurse ensures that patients understand what has been defined as the treatment, what the risks and benefits are, what alternative treatment approaches are available, and what the probability is that the patient will receive personal benefit from the treatment. This is especially important if the patient is participating in phase 1 or phase 2 clinical trials, wherein personal benefit to the individual patient is infrequent or nonexistent. Since many patients are reluctant to ask questions of the physician, the nurse is frequently in a position to answer patients' questions, explain further, define more clearly, and generally help the patient understand the research. Identification of patients who obviously do not understand the treatment approach being administered or the implications of the research in relation to personal benefits requires that the principal investigator be notified, so that before any treatment is administered further clarification of the patient's concerns is provided and any possibility of coercion is eliminated.

The nurse also carries out astute clinical care in implementing the study for the research patient. Since many of the patients involved in phase 1 and phase 2 trials may have profound toxicities, the observation and reporting of these toxic effects are critical for safe patient care. The nurse is in a key position to monitor the patient's symptoms and report toxicities that are a threat to the patient's comfort. For some studies, toxicities are unknown, and life-threatening complications are a possibility. Both anticipated and nonanticipated toxicities occur and make it essential for the nurse to observe patients frequently and thoroughly.

The observation and evaluation of toxic responses to the research protocol are important priorities in clinical research trials. When the research or protocol nurse is not present, responsibilities must be delegated to someone else. Thus a major responsibility of the protocol nurse is the education of the patient's caregiver. Education may involve the clinical nursing staff, the patient, and/or the family or significant other. Depending on the protocol, observations for specific reactions may be necessary. For example, the occurrence of nausea and vomiting may be an expected toxic response but needs to be monitored and treated so that nutritional depletion does not occur. The patient and the caregiver need to know when to notify the physician or the research nurse of side effects. The use of one-to-one teaching followed by discussion of standard educational materials is a common and effective way to provide the patient with the information needed to recognize and report significant toxic effects.

The role of the data manager is to collect the information on toxicities from the chart and to enter these data into the computer for statistical analysis. Various forms in the chart are used. Laboratory responses, pathology reports, and physician's progress notes are frequent sources of data. The toxicity data are usually collected from standardized forms, which include a grading system for rating various symptoms. The data manager does not have to be a nurse, and thus the job description does not generally include any clinical observations for which clinical nursing skills are needed.

The investigational pharmacist is a part of the team when the focus of the clinical trial is chemotherapy. Many phase 1 and 2 trials involve investigational drugs, which are not available for public use, and for which specific records need to be kept. The investigational pharmacist is responsible for dispensing these medications, making sure that the records on the drugs are in order. This person also is usually the first to learn about changes in drug administration, dosage changes, problems reported by other research institutions, and reclassification of the medications. Once a drug moves from an investigational drug to a medication available for general use (usually with a physician's prescription), the drug is no longer available free of charge. This change may have a major impact on the patient's ability to continue the protocol.

The statistician is responsible for a variety of activities in relation to a clinical trial. These include determination of initial sample size, study design and protocol review, data evaluation and analysis, interpretation of findings, and preparation of manuscripts. Frequently data managers report to the statistician, and protocol tracking, randomization, data entry, and statistical analysis are carried out in the department of biostatistics. This support is vital to maintenance of the integrity of the study design.

Members of the clinical nursing staff make up the remainder of the research team. While most of the patients in medical research protocols are hospitalized, other settings may be involved as well. Thus, staff includes nurses in hospital units, ambulatory care settings, physicians' offices, and home care agencies. The protocol nurse is frequently involved in the education of clinical nursing staff, ensuring that patient assessments are relevant and charted. Introduction and explanation of toxicity rating forms are frequently needed. The clinical nursing staff has a major contribution to make in terms of patients' responses to the research therapy.

SETTINGS FOR MEDICAL RESEARCH

Medical research related to cancer treatment may be conducted in a number of settings. Four types of cancer centers are defined by the NCI. While all four types are required to have a broad foundation of peer-reviewed research activities, they differ from each other in the type of research that is conducted. Basic science centers conduct laboratory research (for example, research on the biology of cancer). Clinical cancer centers conduct a combination of basic and clinical research. Comprehensive cancer centers include the same research as clinical cancer centers, plus cancer-control research. Consortium centers involve clinical and cancer control research, plus cancer-control activities. Cancer-control research focuses on the reduction in incidence of cancer by primary and secondary disease-prevention activities. Medical research related to cancer treatment may be conducted at any of these settings. Oncology nurses have been involved in all aspects, ranging from extravasation studies that use animal models, to clinical trials of experimental therapies, to research and activities on cancer prevention and early detection.

The conduct of phase 1 clinical trials is restricted to NCI-designated cancer centers. However, because of the low number of all cancer patients proportionately treated at cancer centers, programs have been developed to allow patients at community agencies to participate in cancer treatment research. Phase 2 and 3 clinical trials are thus conducted at institutions with cooperative arrangements with NCI-designated cancer centers. This not only provides for a larger number of patients available for research accrual; it also provides patients with options that are not available in the practices of their own private physicians. As increased numbers of patients are accrued into phase 2 and 3 trials, results will accumulate more rapidly and new, successful treatments may be demonstrated earlier and made available to a wider spectrum of patients.

Studies on cancer treatment are also conducted by principal investigators who are not located at NCI-designated centers. Thus nurses from a variety of settings may be involved in medical research and learn a variety of research skills useful in nursing studies as well.

DEVELOPMENT OF NURSING RESEARCH IN CANCER

The focus of nursing research differs from that of medical research. Nursing research is defined as the systematic investigation of the responses of patients to actual or potential health problems.[8] Nursing research focuses on the patient rather than on the disease and may encompass biologic, psychologic, and social aspects.

Because of the profound effect of cancer and cancer treatment on the patient, cancer nursing care has provided a rich source of questions and problems for nursing research investigators. The inclusion of a large proportion of data-based articles in the primary cancer nursing journals (ie, *Oncology Nursing Forum* and *Cancer Nursing*) attests to the flourishing amount of nursing research relevant to cancer care. In the first edition of this book, it was possible to catalog cancer nursing research and identify areas of diverse activity, beginning investigations, and areas of no activity.[9] Since then, expansion in the number of cancer nursing studies makes such a review unrealistic. This discussion will examine the development of cancer nursing research by focusing on the role of the nurse in clinical

research, emphasizing the increasing participation in research, the resources available for cancer nurses, and the priorities for research questions as identified by cancer nurses. A summary of cancer nursing research is used to exemplify recent activity.

The Role of the Nurse in Clinical Research

Currently the nurse has several roles in the implementation of research for cancer patients. For a protocol nurse or a clinical staff nurse, the role is that of a member of the research team conducting medical research. Another role is that of initiator of a study conducted along with a medical protocol. This arrangement has been useful in the testing of a variety of nursing approaches. Advantages include the participation of patients already being accrued to another study and the provision of many of the basic demographic and treatment variables needed for study analysis. Cotanch's work on relaxation for chemotherapy-related nausea and vomiting provides a good example of such a study.[10]

The nurse may also act as a principal investigator, initiating the study, writing up the protocol, selecting the subjects, and evaluating the results. The shift to increased numbers of nurses participating as principal investigators is evident from the latest Research Committee survey.[11] The advantage of this shift is that study results can expand the knowledge basic to the development of nursing science. Several recent developments have made the expansion of cancer nursing research possible. Resources for nursing research have increased and include financial as well as knowledge-dissemination opportunities.

Resources for Oncology Nursing Research

Financial support for oncology nursing research has expanded in the last few years and is a major resource for the growth of cancer nursing research activities. While some research can be carried out with a minimum of expense, most research requires financial support for literature searches, proposal development time, supplies, space, data management, secretarial assistance, statistical analysis, and manuscript preparation. Support is available in both educational and clinical settings.

One source that is increasingly available to nurses is internal support at one's own institution. This is an especially valuable resource for the investigator with limited or no grant-writing experience. In educational institutions, seed money is frequently available through the school or college of nursing, as well as the general institution budget. These funds are specifically focused toward increasing research productivity in faculty. Senior faculty or faculty members with other financial resources for research are frequently not eligible for these seed funds, unless a major change in research focus is being attempted. Funds may also be available from an alumni association.[12]

Biomedical support grants from the federal government are available for both educational and clinical institutions that have already achieved a specific level of research support from the government. These biomedical support funds are used to fund beginning or pilot studies that are expected to develop into large-scale projects submitted for outside funding. Each institution establishes criteria by which these funds are distributed. The application process is usually relatively simple, involving a one- to three-page proposal.

External funds are available for individual investigators and can be divided into those available from the government and those available from private foundations. For cancer nursing research, two major sources for federal funds are the National Center for Nursing Research and the National Cancer Institute. Federal funds for research support are by far the biggest resource, and are distributed through a well-defined application and review process. One of the most valuable resources for cancer nurses looking for federal funds is the publication entitled *NIH Guide for Grants and Contracts*. Published by the National Institutes of Health, this document is mailed at regular intervals and lists grant programs and deadline dates for grants and contracts administered by the National Institutes of Health. This free publication can be ordered from NIH Guide, Distribution Center, National Institutes of Health, Room B4B-N-08, Building 31, Bethesda, MD 20892. This publication provides program descriptions and calls for research proposals in specific problem areas.

Private funds for cancer nursing research have expanded and are found in both oncology nursing organizations and outside groups. The Oncology Nursing Foundation funds a variety of research projects yearly. Sigma Theta Tau, both the national organization and local chapters, funds many research projects. Multidisciplinary private groups that fund oncology nursing research include the American Cancer Society and the Robert Wood Johnson Foundation. Addresses for some of these resources are found in Table 60-2. This financial support has increased through the last few years as the educational background and experience of cancer nurses has increased and the demand for research support has risen.

Changing characteristics of oncology nurses can be viewed as an additional resource. According to J. Kinzler (personal communication, June 13, 1989), the number of nurses has increased tremendously, as illustrated by an increase in membership of the Oncology Nursing Society to 15,198 members in 1989. This membership represents an increase of 2578 members from 1988 to 1989. Two surveys of this membership illustrate the changes in research focus that have occurred in the membership. Grant and Stromborg[6] reported findings of a survey conducted by the ONS Research Committee. This mailed survey was sent to the total 1980 membership of ONS (N = 2205) and was returned by 988 members, a response rate of 45%. The respondents reported a high degree of interest in participating in research, with 42% giving research a large or highest priority, 41% giving it a moderate priority, and 17% giving it a lower or no priority. A majority of the respondents (52%) had participated in research as part of

TABLE 60-2 Contacts for Cancer Nursing Research Support

Service	Contact Person/Address
American Cancer Society	Trish Greene, RN, MS Vice-President for Cancer Nursing American Cancer Society 1599 Clifton Rd., NE Atlanta, GA 30029
American Nurses' Foundation	Pauline Brimmier, RN, PhD Director, Center for Nursing Research America Nurses' Foundation 2420 Pershing Rd. Kansas City, MO 64100
National Cancer Institute	Ann Bavier, RN, MN Program Director Community Oncology and Rehabilitation Program Division of Cancer Prevention & Control Blair Bldg. Room 7A-05 National Cancer Institute Bethesda, MD 20892
National Center for Nursing Research	Ada Sue Hinshaw, RN, PhD Director, National Center for Nursing Research Building 31, Rm. B1-C02 National Institutes of Health Bethesda, MD 20892
National Institute of Aging	National Institute of Aging Building 31, Rm. 5C05 National Institutes of Health Bethesda, MD 20892
Oncology Nursing Foundation	Pearl Moore, RN, MS Executive Director Oncology Nursing Foundation 1016 Greentree Rd. Pittsburgh, PA 15220
Sigma Theta Tau	Sigma Theta Tau International Honor Society of Nursing 1200 Waterway Blvd. Indianapolis, IN 46202

their education experiences; 40% reported participation in one to three projects after completion of their last educational experience. Participation involved a variety of tasks associated with research implementation. Data collection was by far the most common activity, with 75% of the respondents reporting this as part of their nursing role. Implementation of clinical protocol was done by 42%, data analysis by 37%, writing up project results by 36%, and development of a research protocol by 35%. A reported 10% of the respondents had published research results.

Education preparation is likely to influence participation in various research activities, and respondents also illustrated a level of education that paralleled their reported research activities. A comparison of the educational preparation of the members of the American Nurses' Association with that of members of the Oncology Nursing Society revealed that ONS members had a higher percentage of nurses with baccalaureate preparation (39% versus 25%) and with master's preparation (24% versus 16%).[6]

A second survey revealed changes in the characteristics of oncology nurses relevant to today's increased productivity in research activities. Participants in this second survey responded to a questionnaire published in the *Oncology Nursing Forum*.[13] The 350 respondents represented 46 states. The typical respondent (1) had either a baccalaureate or a master's degree, (2) had been in nursing under 10 years and in oncology nursing less than 6 years, (3) worked in a hospital setting or a school of nursing, and (4) was employed as either a clinical specialist or an educator. A major difference reported in this survey was the increase in the number and variety of research roles in which participation was reported. Findings that contrast with the 1981 survey revealed that between 1981 and 1985 the primary role changed from that of data collector to a variety of more independent research roles, including proposal development, individual investigation, and statistical analysis, as well as data collection. These expanding roles in research reflect a growing sophistication in ability to conduct oncology nursing research.

A third resource for development in cancer nursing research is support from nursing administration in both educational and clinical settings. In educational settings, more and more faculty members are prepared at the doctoral level and are expected to conduct research on a regular basis and within a program of research interests. Students frequently work with faculty in their programs of research. As doctoral programs for nurses have increased, dissertation research involving cancer patients' clinical problems has increased. Because of these research expectations, educational settings have developed additional resources for researchers. Computer facilities are common; statistical consultation is generally available and at reasonable rates for students; data coding and management assistance are provided.

In clinical settings, the expectations for conducting research are less frequent. An initial institutional commitment to research is exemplified by a statement in the clinical nurse specialist job description that specifies that research is a job expectation.[14] Such commitment may be found in institutions that have no specific individual or department with a designated nursing research focus. For clinical nurses in these settings to conduct research, success is related to the enthusiasm and tenacity of the individual nurse. A trend that has become evident recently is the increased frequency of establishment of a specific position or department for nursing research.[15] This position or department may be a separate department, or it may be combined with either education and/or quality-assurance departments. The kind of research carried out by investigators in clinical settings differs from that carried out by investigators in educational settings. In the clinical setting a larger percentage of investigators plan and conduct evaluation research specific to the institution and its problems.[16] Such research may emerge from quality-assurance studies. For example, vascular access devices show an increased occurrence of infection. A study comparing currently used but different dressing techniques for these devices may be launched in response to the quality-assurance findings.

Resources for oncology nursing research have changed over the last few years, and these changes have been positive. Increased financial support has become available. The education and experience of oncology nurses reflect increased academic preparation for research and increased involvement in a variety of research activities. These resources will continue to expand the knowledge base of cancer nursing care as studies become more sophisticated and are replicated.

Priorities for Cancer Nursing Research

One method that has proved useful in the development of depth in the scientific foundation for nursing practice has been a systematic targeting of researchers and resources to areas of needed knowledge. The identification of priorities for studies has provided information useful in the development of a program for nursing research that leads to well-tested areas of study. With such an approach, the accurate information needed for development of clinical nursing practice is possible. The National Center for Nursing Research has been involved in identification of clinical nursing research priorities through the development of a national nursing agenda.[17] One aspect of this endeavor has been to seek out research priorities identified by various nursing groups.

Cancer nursing research priorities have been identified and revised over the years. One of the first reports was published by Oberst.[18] This list of priorities was developed through a Delphi survey technique in which 254 oncology nurses participated. The following five top priority areas were identified:

1. Relieving nausea/vomiting induced by chemotherapy/radiation
2. Pain management
3. Discharge planning and follow-up
4. Grief and death
5. Stomatitis

This study was followed by several other studies conducted through the Oncology Nursing Society, the Canadian Consortium, and the National Cancer Institute.[6,13,19,20] The most recent survey is that by Funkhouser and Grant.[11] This survey was sent to 700 ONS members who had previously identified research as their major focus, members who had participated as research faculty in ONS short courses, and/or members who had functioned in leadership positions in ONS. A total of 213 respondents returned the survey. Respondents had practiced nursing for an average of 15 years and had specialized in oncologic nursing for an average of 9 years. Distribution of highest educational degrees was as follows: doctoral degree, 30%; master's de-

TABLE 60-3   1988 Cancer Nursing Research Priorities

1 Prevention and early detection	23 Hospice care
2 Symptom management	24 Oncologic emergencies
3 Pain control and management	25 Characteristics of oncology nurses
4 Patient or health education	26 Role of specialist
5 Coping and stress management	27 Bereavement
6 Home care	28 Comfort
7 Economic influences on oncology	29 Physiologic aspects
8 Cancer rehabilitation	30 Epidemiology
9 AIDS	31 Quality of life
10 Compliance with treatment	32 Pediatric oncology
11 Self-care	33 Body image
12 Early detection activities	34 Protective mechanisms
13 Nurse burn-out	35 Labor costs
14 Cancer in the elderly	36 Cancer survival
15 Cost containment	37 Stomatitis
16 Spiritual aspects/religiosity	38 Family issues
17 Counseling	39 Primary nursing
18 Nutrition	40 Acuity/staffing
19 Sexuality	41 Health care delivery systems
20 Implementation of ONS standards	42 Outcome measures for interventions
21 Quality assurance	43 Occupational hazards
22 Smoke cessation	44 Mobility
	45 Elimination
	46 Ethnic/cultural issues

gree in nursing, 24%; bachelor's degree in nursing, 30%. Of the 213 respondents, 150 reported that their current position included research expectations. Table 60-3 contains a listing of the research topics rank-ordered between 1 and 5 by respondents.

Why changes in priorities have occurred over the years is not clear. One interpretation is that some research activity has been completed and findings are being implemented in the management of patient care. One area in which considerable medical and nursing research activity has occurred is that of nausea and vomiting associated with chemotherapy or radiation therapy. It is interesting to note that symptom management and pain persist in the top-priorty positions and that prevention and early detection is No. 1. This listing may be of assistance to nurses who are interested in developing a focus for a research program or even a specific research project. The breadth of topics reflects the extent of nursing care problems and researchers' interests.

Examples of Recent Cancer Nursing Research Publications

To provide examples of the progress in cancer nursing research, Padilla[11] analyzed the 1986 issues of *Cancer, Nursing, Oncology Nursing Forum, Nursing Research, Research in Nursing and Health, Western Journal of Nursing Research,* and *Advances in Nursing Science.* The three research journals published 120 scientific articles, excluding features, editorials, and the like. Of these 120 articles, 8 (6.6%) were considered to concern cancer nursing research since they dealt with oncology patients, oncology nursing problems, or hospice care. The two cancer journals published 79 articles, excluding features, editorials, etc. Of these, 40 (50.6%) were identified as scientific investigations.

The 48 cancer nursing research articles published in the five journals included 4 instruments-development studies; 3 descriptive program-evaluation studies; 27 one-group descriptive studies and 9 two- or three-group comparison descriptive studies with infrequent use of a random selection procedure; and 5 experimental or quasi-experimental studies. Data collection covered periods of 6 months or less. Units of analysis were patients (27 studies), families or care givers (4 studies), nurses (15 studies), healthy subjects (5), and agencies (2). Some studies included more than one type of unit of analysis. Number of subjects ranged from one agency[22] whose "day hospital for cancer patients" was being evaluated, to 823 nurses[23] who returned a mailed survey questionnaire on prevalence and quit rates of smoking-related behaviors. Diagnoses of patients participating in these research studies were not always stated. Mail-out/mail-return surveys were conducted as part of five studies. The return rate for these surveys was quite good, ranging from 46%[24] to 88%,[25] with the mean at 63%.

The nursing research studies were classified, according to Padilla and Grant,[9] into five categories. The categories were population descriptors,[23-35] impact of the diagnosis,[36-46] impact of cancer treatment,[47-58] impact of cancer prognosis,[22,59-63] and education regarding cancer and death.[64-66]

FUTURE DIRECTIONS FOR CANCER NURSING RESEARCH

By comparing the results of the review of cancer nursing research[21] with the recommendations made by Grant and Padilla in the first edition of this book, areas of continued concern can be identified. These areas can be viewed as the authors' personal observations of where studies will occur and are still needed. (1) Descriptive studies of patient care questions continue to form the bulk of cancer nursing efforts and are likely to continue. (2) Recommended population descriptor studies on nurse needs and incidence of patient care problems have been published. (3) Recommended studies on the impact of the cancer diagnosis in relation to pain control and adjustment have been published. However, studies on blame and guilt are still needed, as are studies on nutrition, weight loss, and physical activity. (4) Recommended investigations related to the impact of treatment have included hospitalization and cognitive, physical, and emotional side effects of therapy and standards of care. Lacking are studies on disruptions in sleep and sexual activity and neglect of cancer patients. (5) Recommended studies on the impact of cancer prognosis in relation to needs of dying patients and alternative care systems for these patients have been published. There continues to be a paucity of information on physiologic aspects of the dying process, related care, and quality of life. (6) Only three studies relating to education about cancer and death were identified in the 1986 cancer nursing research publications.

There continues to be a need for investigations of the cost of oncology nurse and patient education programs in relation to cancer prevention, hospitalization, self-care, and adaptation to illness. Also needed are studies that investigate the impact of patient and nurse education programs on desired patient and nurse behavioral outcomes.

CONCLUSION

Research continues to be an important aspect of the cancer nursing specialty. Both medical and nursing research activities are important in improving the care, treatment, and quality of life for patients with cancer. A review of the nature of medical research in cancer care and of nursing research activities provides ample evidence of the essential role that nurses play in this aspect of care. Recent review of cancer nursing research publications reveals a rapidly growing collection of valuable studies. Nurses have made and will continue to make important contributions through research endeavors.

• • •

Partial support was provided by NIH Cancer Support Grant CA 33572.

REFERENCES

1. Polit D, Hungler B: Nursing Research: Principles and Methods. Philadelphia, JB Lippincott, 1987.
2. Padilla GV: Incorporating research in a service setting. J Nurse Admin 9:44-49, 1979.
3. Eilber FR: Principles of cancer surgery, in Haskell CM (ed): Cancer Treatment (ed 2). Philadlephia, WB Saunders, 1985, pp 7-13.
4. Rubin P: The emergence of radiation oncology as a distinct medical specialty. Int J Radiat Oncol Biol Phys 2:1247-1270, 1985.
5. Hubbard SM: Cancer treatment research: The role of the nurse clinical trials of cancer therapy. Nurs Clin North Am 17:763-783, 1982.
6. Grant M, Stromborg M: Promoting research collaboration: ONS research committee survey. Oncol Nurs Forum 8(2):48-53, 1981.
7. Fisher B: Clinical trials for the evaluation of cancer therapy. Cancer 54:2609-2617, 1984.
8. American Nurses' Association: Nursing—A social policy statement. Kansas City, Mo, American Nurses' Association, 1980.
9. Padilla GV, Grant MM: Cancer nursing research, in Groenwald SL (ed): Cancer Nursing: Principles and Practice. Boston, Jones & Bartlett, 1987, pp 827-853.
10. Cotanch PH: Relaxation training for control of nausea and vomiting in patients receiving chemotherapy. Cancer Nurs 6:277-283, 1983.
11. Funkhouser SW, Grant MM: 1988 ONS survey of research priorities. Oncol Nurs Forum 16:413-416, 1989.
12. Schmitt MH, Chapman MK: Alumni involvement in nursing research development. Nurs Outlook 28:572-574, 1980.
13. McGuire D, Frank-Stromborg M, Varricchio C: 1984 ONS research committee survey of membership's research interest and involvement. Oncol Nurs Forum 12:99-103, 1985.
14. Varricchio C, Mikos D: Research: Determining feasibility in clinical setting. Oncol Nurs Forum 14(1):89-90, 1987.
15. Pranulis M, Gortner S: Researchmanship: Characteristics of productive research environments in nursing. West J Nurs Res 7:127-131, 1985.
16. McArt E: Research facilitation in academic and practice settings. J Prof Nurs 3(2):84-91, 1987.
17. Hinshaw AS, Heinrich J, Bloch D: Evolving clinical nursing research priorities: A national endeavor. J Prof Nurs 4:398, 458-459, 1988.
18. Oberst M: Priorities in cancer nursing research. Cancer Nurs 1:281-290, 1978.
19. Degner L, Arcand R, Chekryn J, et al: Priorities for cancer nursing research. Cancer Nurs 10:319-326, 1987.
20. Dodd M: Problem approaches and priorities in oncology nursing research. AARN Newsletter 43(2):13-14, 1987.
21. Padilla GV: Progress in cancer nursing research, in Grant MM, Padilla GV (eds): Cancer Nursing Research: A Practical Approach. New York, Appleton-Lange, 1990, pp 14-18.
22. Clark M: A day hospital for cancer patients: Clinical and economic feasibility. Oncol Nurs Forum 13(6):41-45, 1986.
23. Feldman BM, Richard E: Prevalence of nurse smokers and variables identified with successful and unsuccessful smoking cessation. Res Nurs Health 9:131-138, 1986.
24. Dalton JA, Swenson I: Nurses and smoking: Role modeling and counseling behaviors. Oncol Nurs Forum 13(2):45-48, 1986.
25. Gritz ER, Kanim L: Do fewer oncology nurses smoke? Oncol Nurs Forum 13(3):61-64, 1986.
26. Kesselring A, Lindsey AM, Dodd MJ, et al: Social network and support perceived by Swiss cancer patients. Cancer Nurs 9:156-163, 1986.
27. Blesch KS: Health beliefs about testicular cancer self-examination among professional men. Oncol Nurs Forum 13(1):29-33, 1986.
28. Massey V: Perceived susceptibility to breast cancer and practice of breast self-examination. Nurs Res 35:183-185, 1986.
29. Weinrich SP, Weinrich MC: Cancer knowledge among elderly individuals. Cancer Nurs 9:301-307, 1986.
30. Karani D, Wiltshaw E: How well informed? Cancer Nurs 9:238-242, 1986.
31. Martin BA, Belcher JV: Influence of cultural background on nurses' attitudes and care of the oncology patient. Cancer Nurs 9:230-237, 1986.
32. Larson PJ: Cancer nurses' perceptions of caring. Cancer Nurs 9:86-91, 1986.
33. Trygstad L: Professional friends: The inclusion of the personal into the professional. Cancer Nurs 9:326-332, 1986.
34. Jenkins JF, Ostchega Y: Evaluation of burnout in oncology nurses. Cancer Nurs 9:108-116, 1986.

35. Williams HA, Wilson ME, Hongladarom, et al: Nurses attitudes toward sexuality in cancer patients. Oncol Nurs Forum 13(2):39-43, 1986.

36. Solodky M, Mikos K, Bordieri J, et al: Nurses' prognosis for oncology and coronary heart disease patients. Cancer Nurs 9:243-247, 1986.

37. Derdiarian AK: Informational needs of recently diagnosed cancer patients. Nurs Res 35:276-281, 1986.

38. Tringali CA: The needs of family members of cancer patients. Oncol Nurs Forum 13(4):65-70, 1986.

39. Kesselring A, Dodd MJ, Lindsey AM, et al: Attitudes of patients living in Switzerland about cancer and its treatment. Cancer Nurs 9:77-85, 1986.

40. Waterhouse J, Metcalfe MC: Development of the sexual adjustment questionnaire. Oncol Nurs Forum 13(3):53-59, 1986.

41. Longman AJ, Graham KY: Living with melanoma: Content analysis of interviews. Oncol Nurs Forum 13(4):58-64, 1986.

42. Brown ML, Carrieri V, Janson-Bjerklie S, et al: Lung cancer and dyspnea: The patient's perception. Oncol Nurs Forum 13(5):19-24, 1986.

43. Bressler LR, Hange PA, McGuire DB: Characterization of the pain experience in a sample of cancer outpatients. Oncol Nurs Forum 13(6):51-55, 1986.

44. Austin C, Eyres PJ, Hefferin EA, et al: Hospice home care pain management: Four critical variables. Cancer Nurs 9:58-65, 1986.

45. Barbour LA, McGuire DB, Kirchhoff KT: Nonanalgesic methods of pain control used by cancer outpatients. Oncol Nurs Forum 13(6):56-60, 1986.

46. Coyle N, Mauskip A, Maggard J, et al: Continuous subcutaneous infusions of opiates in cancer patients with pain. Oncol Nurs Forum 13(4):53-57, 1986.

47. Lovejoy NC: Family responses to cancer hospitalization. Oncol Nurs Forum 13(2):33-37, 1986.

48. Fernsler J: A comparison of patient and nurse perceptions of patients self-care deficits associated with cancer chemotherapy. Cancer Nurs 9:50-57, 1986.

49. Hopkins MB: Information-seeking and adaptational outcomes in women receiving chemotherapy for breast cancer. Cancer Nurs 9:256-262, 1986.

50. Moore IM, Kramer J, Ablin A: Late effects of central nervous system prophylactic leukemia therapy on cognitive functioning. Oncol Nurs Forum 13(4):45-51, 1986.

51. Post-White J: Glucocorticosteroid-induced depression in the patient with leukemia or lymphoma. Cancer Nurs 9:15-22, 1986.

52. Scott DW, Donahue DC, Mastrovito RC, et al: Comparative trial of clinical relaxation and an antiemetic drug regimen in reducing chemotherapy-related nausea and vomiting. Cancer Nurs 9:178-187, 1986.

54. Stajich GV, Barnett CW, Turner SV, et al: Protective measures used by oncologic office nurses handling parenteral antineoplastic agents. Oncol Nurs Forum 13(6):47-49, 1986.

55. Strauman JJ: Symptom distress in patients receiving phase I chemotherapy with taxol. Oncol Nurs Forum 13(5):40-43, 1986.

56. Huldij A, Giesbers A, Poelhuis EHK, et al: Alterations in taste appreciation in cancer patients during treatment. Cancer Nurs 9:38-52, 1986.

57. Shell JA, Stanutz F, Grimm J: Comparison of moisture vapor permeable (MVP) dressings to conventional dressings for managment of radiation skin reactions. Oncol Nurs Forum 13(1):11-16, 1986.

58. La Monica EL, Oberst MT, Madea AR, et al: Development of a patient satisfaction scale. Res Nurs Health 9:43-50, 1986.

59. Sawyer PF: Breast self-examination: Hospital-based nurses aren't assessing their clients. Oncol Nurs Forum 13(5):44-48, 1986.

60. Holing EV: The primary caregiver's perception of the dying trajectory: An exploratory study. Cancer Nurs 9:29-37, 1986.

61. Francis MR: Concerns of terminally ill adult Hindu cancer patients. Cancer Nurs 9:164-171, 1986.

62. Reed PG: Religiousness among terminally ill and healthy adults. Res Nurs Health 9:35-41, 1986.

63. Lauer ME, Mulhern RK, Hoffmann RG, et al: Utilization of hospice/home care in pediatric oncology. Cancer Nurs 9:102-107, 1986.

64. Martinson IM, Moldow DG, Armstrong GD, et al: Home care for children dying of cancer. Res Nurs Health 9:11-16, 1986.

65. Hauck SL: Pain: Problem for the person with cancer. Cancer Nurs 9:66-76, 1986.

66. Fredette SL, Beattie HM: Living with cancer: A patient education program. Cancer Nurs 9:308-316, 1986.

67. Brailey LJ: Effects of health teaching in the workplace on women's knowledge, beliefs, and practices regarding breast self-examination. Res Nurs Health 9:233-231, 1986.

PART IX

YELLOW PAGES FOR THE CANCER NURSE

Marilyn Frank-Stromborg, RN, EdD, NP, FAAN

Beth Savela, RN, BSN

AUDIOVISUAL

Audiovisual Sources

The past few years have witnessed a dramatic growth in the use of video technology in all areas of professional health care education. Many institutions such as schools and hospitals are finding audiovisual material to be a highly efficient information and training medium. The number of available audiovisual programs (software) continues to increase substantially each year. Several directories or catalogs that index software may be rented or purchased. These indexes list the following for each entry: physical description (including format, width, and mode of videotape and length of program), indication of additional materials, audience level, costs to rent or purchase, year of production, producer/distributor, subject headings, and a brief summary of the contents of the program.

1. American Cancer Society
   Tower Place
   3340 Peachtree Road NE
   Atlanta, GA 30026
   (404) 320-3333

   The American Cancer Society (ACS) has films, videos, filmstrips, slides, and audiotapes available for free loan. Contact the national office or your local ACS unit for a catalog on the available audiovisual materials.

2. American Hospital Association
   Catalog of Publications and Audiovisual Products
   840 North Lake Shore Drive
   Chicago, IL 60611
   (312) 645-9400

   Free Catalog

3. National Audiovisual Center
   Information Services SF
   Washington, DC 20409
   (301) 763-1896/763-4385 (TDD)

   This center distributes over 13,000 US government–sponsored productions at low prices. Contact the center for your specific area of interest and request free catalogs. Example of listings in the catalog are as follows: *Diet and Cancer Prevention*, 1986, 58 min., videocassette, Dr. Peter Greenwald, Director, Division of Cancer Prevention and Control, NCI explores the effects of fat on breast and colon cancer.

4. NLN Directory of Educational Software for Nursing
   Christine Bolwell
   National League for Nursing
   350 Hudson Street
   New York, NY 10014
   (800) 669-1656
   Pub no. 41-2215

   This directory provides information for anyone interested in using the microcomputer to teach nursing. Each program listed in this directory was reviewed and described along with ratings of the software and the educators' comments that accompany each computer-assisted instruction. There are complete descriptions and purchasing information for over 300 programs, program ratings by a pool of more than 730 health care professionals, and sections on how to evaluate computer-assisted instruction. There are several oncology-related programs listed in this directory.

5. Media Review Digest
   Lesley Orlin (ed)
   The Pierian Press
   Ann Arbor, MI 48104

   This reference book is an annual index to and digest of reviews, evaluations, and descriptions of all forms of nonbook media. This text reviews films, videotapes, filmstrips, records, and tapes.

6. Many universities and medical centers produce audiovisual material that can be purchased. Contact your local university to see if they produce audiovisuals that can be loaned or if the film library contains cancer-related audiovisuals that you could borrow. Several examples are listed below:

   The University of Michigan Media Library
   Department of Postgraduate Medicine and Health Professionals' Education
   R4440 Kresge
   Box 0518
   Ann Arbor, MI 48109-0518
   (313) 763-2074

   You can request a free catalog of medical and nursing audiovisuals.

   Carle Medical Communications
   510 West Main
   Urbana, IL 61801
   (217) 384-4838

   This company produces several cancer-related films/videotapes. One example is *Controlling the Behavioral Side Effects of Chemotherapy*.

Cancer Communications Pretesting

The NCI's Office of Cancer Communications has been experimenting with various pretesting techniques and has gained experience with a number of approaches among a variety of individuals. It has published three booklets that provide information and guidance about measuring the effectiveness of the health message. All three booklets are provided free of charge and can be obtained by calling the **1-800-4-CANCER** telephone number.

1. Making Health Communication Programs Work: A Planner's Guide
   NIH pub no. 89-1493, 1989

   Originally published in 1984 and revised in 1988, *Making Health Communication Programs Work: A Planner's Guide* discusses the purpose of pretesting, planning the health message, conducting pretesting research, conducting the pretest, and measuring the readability of the health message. It also provides an extensive bibliography about pretesting as well as suggestions on how to write the message and determine its readability.

2. Pretesting Television PSAs
   NIH pub no. 85-2670, 1985

   Pretesting Television PSAs is a guidebook developed to assist in designing, implementing, analyzing, and interpreting television public service announcements. The booklet provides specific step-by-step directions for the pretesting process and provides examples of how to handle communication with the pretesting audience. There is also a discussion of what the pretest results should mean to the individual planning the public service announcement.

3. Making PSAs Work—TV and Radio. A Handbook for Health Communication Professionals
NIH pub no. 83-2485, 1983

Making PSAs Work—TV and Radio. A Handbook for Health Communication Professionals is the third booklet designed to provide assistance in planning health messages. The booklet offers guidelines for producing effective messages and for planning, pretesting, implementing, and evaluating a PSA campaign. There is a discussion of how to define the campaign objectives, who the target audience is, selecting an appropriate medium format and length, and what is involved in the technical aspects of filming and recording the PSA. This booklet, like the other two, also provides the user with a helpful bibliography and appropriate appendixes.

ACADEMIC PROGRAMS AND CONTINUING EDUCATION OPPORTUNITIES

Master's Degree Oncology Nursing Programs

Several nursing schools offer graduate education in oncology, and the potential student can choose from several types of programs. Some programs offer separate, distinct, oncology clinical specialist master's curricula, whereas others offer the oncology component within the graduate program in medical-surgical nursing. Because curricula and programs change, the reader is advised to contact local universities to determine if the school of nursing offers a master's program in oncology nursing. In addition, the Oncology Nursing Society publication, "The Master's Degree With a Specialty in Oncology Nursing: Role Definition and Curriculum Guide" (1988), serves a dual purpose as a guide for (1) nursing educators in establishing new oncology programs or evaluating current ones and for (2) prospective students in selecting a program. Another excellent source is the article "Survey of Graduate Programs in Cancer Nursing" in *Oncology Nursing Forum* 15:825-831, 1988. This article details specific information about each program (clinical focus, program length, application deadline, NLN accreditation, etc.).

Graduate Oncology Nursing Programs

Alabama
University of Alabama
School of Nursing
Judy Holcombe, RN, DSN
Associate Professor
University of Alabama at Birmingham
University Station
Birmingham, AL 35294

Arizona
University of Arizona
Alice J. Longman, RN, EdD
Associate Professor
College of Nursing
Tucson, AZ 85721

California
University of California, Los Angeles
School of Nursing
Ada Lindsey
Dean
Los Angeles, CA 90024

University of California, San Francisco
Co-Program Directors
Marylin Dodd, RN, PhD
Patricia Larson, RN, DNSc
School of Nursing
Department of Physiological Nursing
San Francisco, CA 94143

Connecticut
Yale University
School of Nursing
Dorothy Sexton, RN, EdD
Associate Professor and Chairperson
Medical-Surgical Nursing Program
New Haven, CT 06520

Delaware
University of Delaware
Jayne Fernsler, RN, DSN
Assistant Professor
College of Nursing
University of Delaware
Newark, DE 19716

District of Columbia
Catholic University of America
Janice Hallal, RN, DNSc
Coordinator—Graduate Oncology Nursing
School of Nursing
Washington, DC 20064

Florida
University of Miami
School of Nursing
Beverly Nielsen, RN, EdD
Oncology Nursing
Miami, FL 33124

University of South Florida
College of Nursing
Susan McMillan, RN, PhD
Chairperson, Oncology Nursing
Tampa, FL 33612

Georgia
Emory University
Rose F. McGee, RN, PhD
Professor
Oncology Nursing
Atlanta, GA 30322

Illinois
Loyola University of Chicago
Niehoff School of Nursing
Claudette Varricchio, RN, DSN
Associate Professor
Medical-Surgical Nursing
Chicago, IL 60626

Northern Illinois University
School of Nursing
Marilyn Stromborg, RN, EdD
Professor, Adult Oncology
DeKalb, IL 60115

Northwestern University
Center for Nursing
Janet A. Deatrick, RN, PhD
Associate Director, Graduate Program in Nursing
750 North Lake Shore Drive
Chicago, IL 60611

Rush University
College of Nursing
Judith Paice, RN, MS
Acting Coordinator, Graduate Program in Oncology Nursing
Chicago, IL 60612

University of Illinois at Chicago
College of Nursing
Susan Dudas, RN, MSN
Associate Professor
Chicago, IL 60612

Indiana
Indiana University
Judy Lambert, RN, MSN
Assistant Professor
School of Nursing
Indianapolis, IN 46223

Massachusetts
Massachusetts General Hospital Institute of Health Professions
Sylvia Drake Page, RN, DNSc
Coordinator, Oncology
Boston, MA 02108-9990

Missouri
St. Louis University
School of Nursing
Ramona M. Wessler, RN, PhD
St. Louis, MO 63104

University of Missouri, Columbia
Ann Rosenow, RN, PhD
Associate Dean for Research
Director, Graduate Studies
Columbia, MO 65211

New York
Columbia University
School of Nursing
Anne Hubbard, MS, MPH
Director, Master's Program in Oncology Nursing
New York, NY 10032

Russell Sage College
Marjory Keenan, EdD
Professor of Nursing
Troy, NY 12180

State University of New York, Buffalo
Yvonne Sherer, RN, EdD
School of Nursing
Department of Graduate Education
Faculty of Health Sciences
Buffalo, NY 14214

University of Rochester
School of Nursing
Jean Johnson, RN, PhD
Cancer Center Nursing
Rochester, NY 14642

North Carolina
Duke University
School of Nursing

Dorothy Brundage, RN, PhD
Interim Dean
Durham, NC 27710

University of North Carolina at Chapel Hill
Inge Corless, PhD, FAAN
Chairman, Secondary Care Nursing
School of Nursing
Chapel Hill, NC 27514

Ohio
Frances Payne Bolton
School of Nursing
Case Western Reserve University
Ellen Rudy, RN, PhD
Chairperson
Cleveland, OH 44106

Medical College of Ohio
School of Nursing
Sharon Utz, RN, PhD
Associate Professor
Medical-Surgical Nursing
Toledo, OH 43699

University of Cincinnati
M. Linda Workman, RN, PhD
Assistant Professor
College of Nursing and Health
Cincinnati, OH 45221

Pennsylvania
Gwynedd-Mercy College
Patricia Bennett, RN, MA
Oncological Nursing
Graduate Nursing Division
Gwynedd Valley, PA 19437

University of Pennsylvania
Ruth McCorkle, RN, PhD, FAAN
Nursing Education Building
School of Nursing
Philadelphia, PA 19104

University of Pittsburgh
School of Nursing
Catherine Bender, RN, MN
Assistant Professor
Graduate Program Oncology Nursing
Pittsburgh, PA 15261

Widener University
Jean Fergusson, RN, MSN (Pediatrics)
Susan Cobb, RN, MSN, CS, OCN (Adult)
Graduate Program
School of Nursing
Chester, PA 19013

South Carolina
University of South Carolina
College of Nursing
Janet F. Nussbaum, RN, EdD
Oncology Nursing
Columbia, SC 29208

Tennessee
University of Tennessee
College of Nursing
Dianne Greenhill, RN, EdD
Associate Dean
Memphis, TN 38163

Vanderbilt University
James Pace, RN, DSN

Dana Rutledge, RN, PhD
Oncology Specialty Coordinators
Nashville, TN 37240

Texas

University of Texas
Health Science Center
Patricia Bohannan, RN, PhD
Program Coordinator
School of Nursing
Houston, TX 77030

Utah

Brigham Young University
Camilla Wood, RN, PhD
Professor and Oncology Nursing Program Coordinator
College of Nursing
Provo, UT 84602

Virginia

George Mason University
Graceann Ehlke, RN, DNSc
Coordinator, Advanced Clinical Nursing
Fairfax, VA 22030

Virginia Commonwealth University
Medical College of Virginia
Ethelyn Exley, RN, EdD
Assistant Dean of Academic Affairs
Richmond, VA 23298

Washington

University of Washington
Betty Gallucci, RN, PhD
Professor, Department of Physiological Nursing
Seattle, WA 98195

University of Washington
Marion Rose, RN, PhD
Professor, Department of Parent and Child Nursing SC-74
Seattle, WA 98195

Wisconsin

University of Wisconsin
Marilyn Oberst, RN, EdD
School of Nursing
Clinical Science Center
Madison, WI 53792

IAET-accredited ET Nurse Education Programs are listed below:

Abbott Northwestern ET Nursing Education Program
800 East 28th Street at Chicago Avenue
Minneapolis, MN 55407
(612) 863-4601

Emory University ET Nursing Education Program
1365 Clifton Road, NE, Room 360, Emory Clinic
Atlanta, GA 30322
(404) 321-0111 ext. 3321

Harrisburg Hospital School of Enterostomal Therapy
South Front Street
Harrisburg, PA 17101
(717) 782-5565

M. D. Anderson Hospital and Tumor Institute
Department of Nursing
6723 Bertner
Houston, TX 77030
(713) 792-7132

Northwest Community Hospital
ET Education Program of the Department of
Continuing Education
800 West Central Road
Arlington Heights, IL 60005
(312) 259-1000 ext. 5161

R. B. Turnbull Jr. School of ET
Cleveland Clinic Foundation
9500 Euclid Avenue 3L20
Cleveland, OH 44106
(216) 444-5966

Tucson Medical Center
c/o Restorative Services
ET Nurse Education Program
5301 East Grant Road
Box 42195
Tucson, AZ 85733
(602) 327-5461 ext. 5400

University of Southern California
c/o MSN Program
Leavey Hall
320 West 15th Street
Los Angeles, CA 90015
(213) 743-2362

Enterostomal Therapy Programs

Enterostomal therapy (ET) is an allied healthcare field specializing in the care of patients with all types of abdominal stomas
as well as the management of patients with a wide variety of
draining sinus tracts and fistulas. This nurse specialist is called
an enterostomal therapist. Currently, an applicant must be an RN
with a baccalaureate degree in nursing with 1 year of recent
(within 5 years) clinical experience in medical-surgical nursing.
Tuition varies among programs. Scholarships are available
through the International Association for Enterostomal Therapy,
Inc. (IAET), ACS, United Ostomy Association, and many of the
individual ET nurse programs.

It is best to first obtain a list of IAET-approved professional
education programs from:

IAET
2081 Business Center Drive
Suite 290
Irvine, CA 92715
(714) 476-0268

PRINT SOURCES

Library Retrieval Services

For those readers who are not familiar with the benefits of mech-
anized literature search or the "how-to's," the following articles
will supply this information. In addition, you are advised to consult your local librarian or the closest college or university library
near you. Most higher education libraries now have public access
terminals for students and the public to conduct their own computer search.

1. Treece E, Treece J: The library and computer-based literature
   searches, in *Elements of Research in Nursing* (ed 4). St Louis,
   CV Mosby, 1986, pp 91-112. This chapter discusses how to
   use the MEDLARS retrieval service.

2. Nieswiadomy R: Review of the literature, *Foundations of Nursing Research*. Norwalk, Conn, Appleton-Lange, 1987, pp 73-89. This chapter details the multiple computer-assisted literature searches that are available to the nurse desiring to do a literature review.

3. Polit D, Hungler B: Locating and summarizing existing information on a problem, *Nursing Research. Principles and Methods* (ed 2). Philadelphia, JB Lippincott, 1987, pp 62-78. This chapter provides a guide to selected abstracts and indexes for nursing and related subjects and relationship to computer searches and databases.

4. Woodbury M: Computerized retrieval services, *A Guide to Sources of Educational Information*. Washington, DC, Information Resources Press, 1982. This chapter gives an in-depth description of computerized retrieval services—location, information stored, cost, and availability.

In addition, the following catalog contains extensive information on data banks and computerized retrieval services.

1. *Dialog Database Catalog 1988*, Dialog Information Services, Inc., a subsidiary of Lockheed Corporation, contains a description of all available databases, including years the database covers, number of records in the database, when the database is routinely updated, who provides the database, and costs to access the database.

A partial list of computerized retrieval services follows, with an emphasis on medically oriented systems.

1. MEDLARS: MEDLARS is a computer-based bibliographic processing system operated by the National Library of Medicine (NLM) at Bethesda, MD. It has been designed to achieve rapid bibliographic access to over 3000 international journals published in the United States and 70 other countries. Included is all the material in *Index Medicus, International Nursing Index,* and *Index to Dental Literature* from 1966 to the present. MEDLARS is identical to MEDLINE (MEDLARS ON-LINE), but MEDLINE makes it possible for the researcher to obtain the bibliographic retrieval faster. Over 40% of records added since 1975 contain author abstracts taken directly from the published articles. Over 250,000 records are needed each year, of which over 70% are English language. Cost as of 1989 is $36 each hour of computer connect time, $0.20 for a full record printed offline, and $0.05 for a full record typed or displayed online.

2. AVLINE: AVLINE (audiovisuals-on-line) is a computer information service available through the MEDLARS system of the NLM. The AVLINE database is searchable through any MEDLARS terminal by using the classification established in the medical subject headings of the *Index Medicus*. AVLINE is a clearinghouse of nontextbook educational materials to assist the health science community. All audiovisual material is catalogued, indexed, abstracted, and described according to physical characteristics and rated (highly recommended, recommended, or not recommended). It is updated weekly, with approximately 100 records added per month.

3. CHEMLINE: A chemical dictionary, it is used primarily to aid in searching other databases. It is produced by *Chemical Abstracts* and the NLM.

4. TOXLINE: All aspects of toxicology are on this computer tape, including material from *Chemical Abstracts, Toxicity Bibliography, Bio Research Index, Health Effects of Environmental Pollutants,* etc. The database covers from 1930 to the present. It is part of the NLM database.

5. HEALTH (Health planning and administration): Bibliographic citations covering nonclinical aspects of health care delivery. Subject areas emphasized include the administration and planning of health facilities, services and personnel, health insurance, health policy, aspects of financial management, etc. Citations are prepared by the NLM, the American Hospital Association (AHA), and the National Health Planning Information Center.

6. CATLINE: This database is available through the NLM (as are MEDLINE, HEALTH, TOXLINE, CHEMLINE, CANCERLINE, and AVLINE). It contains a listing of over 600,000 books and serials acquired since 1965 by the NLM. The cost of doing a MEDLINE search is based on the actual cost of searching the database. For example, a 5-minute search on MEDLINE may cost $3 (based on the average cost of $36 an hour). You can print citations on your printer or have them printed elsewhere and sent to you ("offline").

7. Smoking and Health: Smoking and Health contains bibliographic citations and abstracts to journal articles, reports, and other literature that discuss the effects of smoking on health. The files contain information from 1960 to the present and are updated every 2 months. Presently Smoking and Health contains over 37,000 records. This database corresponds to the printed government publication "Smoking and Health Bulletin." It is operated by the NIH, Office of Smoking and Health, Rockville, MD. Cost is $45 for each hour of computer connect time and $0.20 for a full-record printed offline.

8. CANCERLINE: A computer-based system for on-line retrieval of abstracts derived from published results of cancer research. Includes material from *Carcinogenesis Abstracts* and *Cancer Therapy* (1963 to present). CANCERLINE is available at all terminals linked to the computer system at the NLM in Bethesda, MD. This service is available to scientists, physicians, nurses, and other health care professionals and educators. Terminals for the NLM are located at more than 700 medical library locations throughout the United States and in 12 foreign countries. The CANCERLINE system is composed of three separate computer databases:

  a. CANCERLIT (CANCERLITerature): This database contains more than 617,812 records and is updated monthly. CANCERLIT contains abstracts that appeared in *Carcinogenesis Abstracts* from 1963 to 1969 and in *Cancer Therapy Abstracts* from 1967 to 1979. In 1977 the database was enlarged to include cancer-related articles from a variety of sources.

  b. CLINPROT (CLINICAL PROTOCOLS): CLINPROT, sponsored by the NCI, has been designed to disseminate information to clinical oncologists engaged in the development and testing of clinical protocols. It is also useful to other clinicians who wish to learn about new cancer treatment methods currently being evaluated in controlled clinical trials. It provides descriptions of the clinical trials, including patient entry criteria, the therapy regimen, and special study parameters.

  c. PDQ (PHYSICIAN DATA QUERY): The PDQ database has three major files: (1) a file that summarizes the most current approaches to cancer treatment, (2) a file of research treatment protocols that are open to patient entry, and (3) a directory of physicians that provide cancer treatment and health care organizations that have programs of cancer care. At any time, the PDQ protocol file contains approximately 1000 treatment protocols, 20% of which have been voluntarily submitted. Each protocol is indexed according to disease and stage-specific eligibility criteria, as well as details of treatment, to allow users to narrow down geographically classified information on participating investigators.

PDQ, CANCERLIT, and CLINPROT are available through the NLM's MEDLARS computer system at U.S. medical libraries and health care organizations. For more information contact:

MEDLARS Management Section
National Library of Medicine
Building 38, Room 4 N 421
8600 Rockville Pike
Bethesda, MD 20894
301-496-6193
800-638-8480 (toll free)

The staff of NCI's Cancer Information Service network (toll free 1-800-4-CANCER) will also provide information on PDQ.

9. Nursing and Allied Health: This database provides access to more than 300 English-language nursing journals, publications of the American Nurses' Association and the National League for Nursing. It also includes citations from approximately 3200 biomedical journals in *Index Medicus* and from the psychological, management, and popular literature. It contains over 72,764 records and is updated bimonthly. Beginning with 1986 issues, abstracts from approximately 45 nursing journals were added to the database. The cost is $54 per computer connect hour and $0.25 for a full-record printed offline.

10. Education Resources Information Center (ERIC): The ERIC system is a network of clearinghouses, each devoted to collecting, evaluating, storing, abstracting, and disseminating resource material in its own area of specialization. Materials included are research projects, theses, speeches, books, proceedings, and project reports. ERIC corresponds to two printed indexes: *Resources in Education,* which is concerned with identifying the most significant and timely education research reports, and *Current Index to Journals in Education,* an index of more than 700 periodicals of interest to every segment of the education profession. Consult the university library, state department of education, or state library system nearest you for the availability of this service and the specific procedures to be followed at that institution, or write:

ERIC Processing and Reference Facility
4350 East-West Highway
Suite 1100
Bethesda, MD 20814-4475

11. EMBASE (formerly EXCERPTA MEDICA): EMBASE is one of the leading sources for searching the biomedical literature. It consists of abstracts and citations of articles from over 4000 biomedical journals published throughout the world. Updated every 2 weeks, EMBASE contains over 3,021,722 records on file that correspond to the 43-specialty abstract journals and 2 literature indexes that make up the printed EXCERPTA MEDICA. More information can be obtained from:

EMBASE
Elsevier Science Publishing Co., Inc.
North American Data Base Department
52 Vanderbilt Avenue
New York, NY 10017

12. Dissertation Abstracts Online: Dissertation Abstracts Online is a definitive subject, title, and author guide to every American dissertation accepted at an accredited institution since 1861. This is a computerized bibliographic file of abstracts of doctoral theses originally listed in *Dissertation Abstracts* and

Dissertation Abstracts International. Abstracts are included for a large majority of the degrees granted after January 1980. It is updated every month and contains over 955,147 records. The database also contains citations to master's theses appearing in the quarterly "Masters Abstracts" published by University Microfilms International since 1962. For more information contact:

University Microfilms International
A Bell and Howell Information Company
300 North Zeeb Road
Ann Arbor, MI 48106

13. Psyc INFO: Worldwide literature in psychology and the related disciplines of psychiatry, sociology, anthropology, education, linguistics, and pharmacology are covered in this database. This database corresponds to the printed *Psychological Abstracts* and covers 1967 to the present. Write to the following for information on costs and location of terminals:

American Psychological Association
1400 N. Uhle Street
Arlington, VA 22201

14. Clinical Abstracts: Clinical Abstracts is designed to meet the needs of the practicing clinician. The database provides access to more than 300 leading English-language medical journals. Major subject areas include pediatrics, family practice, internal medicine, general surgery, and cardiovascular surgery. Material from 1981 to the present is included, and the database is updated monthly. Contact:

Medical Information Systems
Reference and Index Services
Indianapolis, IN 46223

15. SCISEARCH: SCISEARCH is a multidisciplinary index to the literature of science and technology prepared by the Institute for Scientific Information (ISI). It contains all the records published in *Science Citation Index.* The ISI staff indexes all significant items from about 2600 major scientific and technical journals. This database contains over 8,000,000 records and is updated biweekly.

Oncology Periodicals

An excellent resource for a discussion of cancer journals and serials is *Cancer Journals and Serials. An Analytical Guide,* compiled by Pauline Vaillancourt (New York, Greenwood Press, 1988). The content of each journal is discussed along with costs, where published, price, frequency of the journal, and number of cancer-related articles usually found in each issue.

Acta Haematologica
Acta Oncologica
Advances in Cancer Research
American Journal of Clinical Oncology
American Journal of Hematology
Anticancer Research
Australian Cancer Society
Breast Cancer and Research Treatment
Breast/Diseases of the Breast
British Journal of Cancer
British Journal of Haematology
British Journal of Preventive and Society Medicine
Ca—A Cancer Journal for Clinicians
Canadian Cancer Society
Cancer Cells
Cancer: A Journal of the American Cancer Society
Cancer Chemotherapy Reports
Cancer Detection and Prevention: International Study Group for Detection and Prevention of Cancer

Cancer Federation, Inc.
Cancer Forum
Cancer Genetics and Cytogenetics
Cancergram (abstracts of selected cancer-related articles): Breast Cancer, Cancer Detection and Management, Cancer Research: Techniques and Applications, Cell Biology, Dietary Aspects of Carcinogenesis, Environmental and Occupational Carcinogenesis, Metastasis, Molecular Biology, Organ Site Carcinogenesis (Liver), Organ Site Carcinogenesis (Skin), Pediatric Oncology
Cancer Immunology and Immunotherapy
Cancer Letters
Cancer Metastasis Review
Cancer Nursing: An International Journal for Cancer Care
Cancer Review
Cancer Treatment Reports
Cancer Treatment Reviews
Cancer Update
Carcinogenesis
Clinical Cancer Letter
Clinical Oncology: The Journal of the British Association of Surgical Oncology
Clinics in Oncology
Current Problems in Cancer
Cancer Victors Association
European Journal of Cancer
European Journal of Gynaecological Oncology
European Journal of Nuclear Medicine
Fox Chase Cancer Center
Gynecologic Oncology: An International Journal
Important Advances in Oncology
Indian Cancer Society
International Journal of Cancer
International Journal of Radiation Oncology, Biology, Physics
International Union Against Cancer
Journal of Cancer Education
Journal of the British Association of Surgical Oncology
Journal of Clinical Hematology and Oncology
Journal of Clinical Oncology
Journal of the National Cancer Institute
Journal of Psychosocial Oncology
Journal of Surgical Oncology
Journal of Tumor Marker Oncology
Lancet
Leukemia Research
Medical and Pediatric Oncology
National Cancer Institute Monographs
Neoplasma
Oncology
Oncology: International Journal of Cancer Research and Treatment
Oncology: Journal of Clinical and Experimental Cancer Research
Oncology Nursing Forum
Preventive Medicine: An International Journal Devoted to Practice and Theory
Proceedings of the American Association for Cancer Research
Progress in Clinical Research
Radiotherapy and Oncology
Recent Results in Cancer Research
Seminars in Oncology
Seminars in Oncology Nursing
Yearbooks in Cancer
UCLA Cancer Center

Oncology Patient Education Material

Many of the self-help organizations offer literature that emphasizes their organization, and the reader is advised to contact these groups for special-interest material. There are many excellent sources for patient education material, and a partial list follows:

1. American Academy of Dermatology
    PO Box 3116
    Evanston, IL 60204-3116

    The American Academy of Dermatology offers brochures, audiovisuals, and posters. Information is available to the public by writing the above address and enclosing a self-addressed stamped envelope; it is free of charge unless requested in quantities. The Academy gives referrals to physicians in the patient's area.
    Brochures:
    The Sun and Your Skin
    Melanoma/Skin Cancer
    Posters:
    Be Sun Smart
    Ban the Burn
    Lighten Up—Cover Up
2. American Cancer Society
    Tower Place
    3340 Peachtree Road, NE
    Atlanta, GA 30026
    (404) 320-3333

    The reader is urged first to contact the American Cancer Society in his or her area. The Society has an extensive collection of material for both the public and the professional. The material covers all aspects of cancer and is available as books, films, reprints, posters, audiotapes, programs, and proceedings.
    Patient education rehabilitation pamphlets (partial listing):
    Care of Your Sigmoid Colostomy
    First Aid for Laryngectomees
    Helping Words (for Laryngectomees)
    Reach to Recovery—After Mastectomy: A Patient Guide
    Sex and the Male Ostomate; Sex and the Female Ostomate; Sex, Courtship and the Single Ostomate
    What is Reach to Recovery
    Your New Voice
    Breast Reconstruction—After Mastectomy
    Emergency Info for Tracheo-Esophageal Fistula Users
    Help for the Patient Going Home
    Another Spring: The Diary of a Radiation Patient
    Patient education site pamphlets (partial listing):
    Cancer of the Breast
    Cancer of the Colon
    Cancer of the Larynx
    Cancer of the Lung
    Cancer of the Mouth
    Cancer of the Prostate
    Cancer of the Skin
    Cancer of the Stomach
    Cancer of the Uterus
    Childhood Cancers
    Hodgkin's Disease
    Testicular Cancer
    Patient education pamphlets (partial listing):
    Finding a Lump in Your Breast
    The Last Day in April (the story of a child with leukemia, written by her mother)

Cancer Facts for Men

Cancer Facts for Women

Parents' Handbook on Leukemia

Sexuality and Cancer for the Woman who has Cancer and Her Partner

Sexuality and Cancer for the Man who has Cancer and His Partner

Facts on Cancer Treatment

3. American Lung Association
   1740 Broadway
   New York, NY 10019
   (212) 315-8700

The reader is encouraged to contact his or her local American Lung Association for a free catalog of public education materials. *The following is a partial list of available materials:*

Asbestos: Lung Hazards on the Job

Lung Hazards in the Workplace

Occupational Lung Cancer

Lung Cancer—You Need to Know the Facts

Your Lung Facts

Carcinogens and Synonyms

About Smoking and Cancer

4. *Candelighters Childhood Cancer Foundation Youth Newsletter*
   Candelighters Childhood Cancer Foundation
   Suite 1001
   1901 Pennsylvania Avenue
   Washington, DC 20006
   (202) 659-5136

Candelighters Childhood Cancer Foundation Youth Newsletter is written by and for adolescent cancer patients and teenage siblings.

5. *Coping*
   Pulse Publications, Inc.
   377 Riverside Drive
   PO Box 1677
   Franklin, TN 37065-1677
   (615) 791-5900

The magazine *Coping* is published quarterly for cancer patients and their families. It includes such categories as education, support, life-style, treatment, research, and progress reports. Cost is $14 for 1 year (outside the United States it is $22) and $24 for 2 years.

6. Ellis Fischel State Cancer Hospital
   Business 70 and Garth Avenue
   Columbia, MO 65201
   (314) 875-2100

Several pamphlets are available designed specifically to answer the questions of cancer patients undergoing chemotherapy, radiation, and surgery.

Pamphlets (partial list):

Chemotherapy

Radiotherapy Information and Hints for You

Radium Implant Booklet

7. Office of Cancer Communications
   National Cancer Institute
   Building 31, Room 10A24
   Bethesda, MD 20892
   1-800-4-CANCER

A variety of pamphlets and booklets are available that discuss symptoms, diagnosis, and treatment of different cancer sites as well as research. In addition, there are pamphlets designed to help the parents of children with cancer.

Partial list of materials available (these are frequently updated):

Breast Exams: What You Should Know

Diet, Nutrition and Cancer Prevention: The Good News

Help Yourself: Tips for Teenagers with Cancer

Progress Against Cancer of the Skin

Progress Against Cancer of the Larynx

Questions and Answers About Breast Lumps

Research Report Series (includes many sites such as kidney, bladder, pancreas, stomach, uterus, etc)

Services Available to Cancer Patients

What You Need to Know About Cancer Series (includes many sites such as brain, breast, lung, etc)

Booklets:

Chemotherapy and You

Eating Hints

Questions and Answers About DES Exposure During Pregnancy and Before Birth

Radiation Therapy and You

What are Clinical Trials All About?

Young People with Cancer

8. National Alliance of Breast Cancer Organizations
   1180 Avenue of the Americas
   2nd Floor
   New York, NY 10036
   (212) 719-0154

NABCO is a central resource of information on breast cancer. The Breast Cancer Resource List compiled by NABCO in 1988 is shown on p. 1290. The list includes resources available from the NCI and other sources.

9. Patient Education Center
   The North Carolina Memorial Hospital
   Manning Drive
   Chapel Hill, NC 27514
   (919) 966-4131

Series of patient education booklets are available that cover a variety of topics. For example, the *Series of Home Health Care Procedures* includes booklets on wound drainage, tracheostomy care, intracavity radiation therapy, biliary catheter care, and turning and positioning a patient. Each booklet is illustrated, uses simple language, and has questions throughout to test the patient's understanding of the material. The catalog is currently being revised, but a list of series and booklets is available. Each booklet costs $2.

10. The Skin Cancer Foundation
    245 Fifth Avenue, Suite 2402
    New York, NY 10016
    (212) 725-5176

On request, the Skin Cancer Foundation will provide samples and an ordering form for brochures, leaflets, booklets, and posters. A contribution of $25 or more entitles the contributor to a 1-year subscription of *Sun and Skin News* and *The Melanoma Letter*, four issues each.

The following is a limited list of materials available:

It's Never Too Early to Stop Skin Cancer . . . Or Too Late

Skin Cancer Booklet

Types and Descriptions of Skin Cancers

The ABCD's of Moles and Melanomas

The Many Faces of Malignant Melanoma

For Every Child Under the Sun, A Guide to Sensible Sun Protection

Basal Cell Carcinoma, The Most Common Cancer

Simple Guidelines on Sun Protection

Malignant Melanoma—Guidelines and Early Warning System

Dysplastic Nevi and Malignant Melanoma

Breast Cancer Resources
Overview Information and Treatment Choices

Title	Author	Source	Catalogue Number or Publisher	Number of Pages	Charge
What You Need To Know About Breast Cancer		NCI	88-1556	33	None
Breast Cancer: We're Making Progress Every Day		NCI	86-2409	12	None
The Breast Cancer Digest: A Guide To Medical Care, Emotional Support, Educational Programs and Resources		NCI	84-1691	212	None
Alternatives	R. Kushner	Bookstores	Warner Books, 1986	438	$5.95
If You've Thought About Breast Cancer (1987 edition)	R. Kushner	Women's Breast Cancer Advisory Center, PO Box 224, Kensington, MD 20895			$3.00
Every Woman's Guide To Breast Cancer	V.L. Seltzer, MD	Bookstores	Viking Books, 1987	209	$17.95
A Real Choice	R. Moss	Bookstores	St. Martin's Press, 1984	249	$13.95
Breast Biopsy: What You Should Know		NCI	87-657	12	Free
Breast Cancer: Understanding Treatment Options		NCI	87-2675	19	Free
Mastectomy: A Treatment For Breast Cancer		NCI	87-658	24	Free
Radiation Therapy: A Treatment For Early Stage Breast Cancer		NCI	87-659	20	Free
Radiation Therapy and You: A Guide To Self-Help During Treatment		NCI	88-2227	39	Free
Breast Reconstruction: A Matter Of Choice		NCI	88-2151	19	Free
Breast Reconstruction After Mastectomy		ACS	4630-PS	20	Free
An Informed Decision: Understanding Breast Reconstruction	M. Snyder	Bookstores	Little, Brown, 1989	201	$10.95

The following books are excellent resources for cancer patients and their families. There is a great deal of useful information that can help with care and decision making. Further resources also may be found within these books addressing many aspects of diagnosis, treatment, and care.

Benjamin H, Trubo R: *From Victim to Victor*. New York, Dell, 1987.

Bergman T: *One Day at a Time: Children Living with Cancer*. Milwaukee, Gareth Stevens, 1989.

Bloch A, Bloch R: *Cancer . . . There's Hope*. Kansas City, Mo, Cancer Connection, 1987.

Bloch A, Bloch R: *Fighting Cancer*. Kansas City, Mo, Cancer Connection, 1988.

Borysenko J: *Minding the Body, Mending the Mind*. New York, Bantam, 1988.

Bruning N: *Coping with Chemotherapy*. New York, Ballantine, 1985.

Cousins N: *Anatomy of an Illness*. New York, Bantam, 1983.

Doan Nayes D, Mellody P: *Beauty & Cancer: A Woman's Guide to Looking Great while Experiencing the Side Effects of Cancer Therapy*. Los Angeles, AC Press, 1988.

Gaes J: *My Book for Kids with Cansur*. Aberdeen, SD, Melius Peterson, 1988.

Grollman E: *Talking about Death: A Dialogue between Parent and Child*. Boston, Beacon Press, 1976.

Harwell A: *When Your Friend Gets Cancer*. Wheaton, Ill, Harold Shaw, 1987.

Holleb A (ed): *The American Cancer Society Cancer Book*. New York, Doubleday, 1986.

Le Shan L: *Cancer as a Turning Point: A Handbook for People with Cancer, their Families, and Health Professionals*. New York, Dutton, 1989.

Matthews-Simonton S: *The Healing Family*. New York, Bantam, 1984.

Morra M, Potts E: *Choices: Realistic Alternatives in Cancer Treatment*. New York, Avon, 1987.

Muraa A, Stewart B: *Man to Man: When the Woman You Love Has Breast Cancer*. New York, St. Martin's Press, 1989.

O'Toole D: *Aarvy Aardvark Finds Hope*. Burnsville, NC, The Rainbow Connection, 1988.

Patterson JT: *The Dread Disease: Cancer and Modern American Culture*. Cambridge, Mass, Harvard University Press, 1987.

Rosenfeld I: *Second Opinion: Your Guide to Alternative Treatment*. New York, Bantam, 1988.

Sattilaro A: *Recalled by Life*. New York, Avon, 1984.

Shook RL: *Survivors: Living with Cancer*. New York, Harper & Row, 1983.

Siegel B: *Love, Medicine & Miracles*. New York, Harper & Row, 1988.

Simonton C, Matthews-Simonton S, Creighton J: *Getting Well Again*. New York, Bantam, 1988.

ORGANIZATIONS: PROFESSIONAL AND CLIENT SELF-HELP

Nonsmokers Organizations

Between 1964 and 1975, a dramatic change occurred in adult smoking behavior; more than 29 million Americans quit smoking during this period. A growing concern for the rights and health of nonsmokers has resulted in social and legislative pressures on smokers, and new antismoking education and information materials and programs have been introduced in local communities around the country. The following is a list of some national organizations for the rights of nonsmokers. This list was obtained from The Action on Smoking and Health (ASH) Organization.

1. Action on Smoking and Health (ASH)
   2013 H Street, NW
   Washington, DC 20006
   (202) 659-4310

   ASH is a national nonprofit legal-action organization fighting for the rights of nonsmokers everywhere and helping nonsmoking passengers to protect their rights. ASH is the organization primarily responsible for the airline nonsmoking rules and their enforcement. ASH also publishes a bimonthly newsletter on smoking and nonsmokers' rights, has available a variety of other educational materials, and sells signs, buttons, stickers, etc. to help nonsmokers speak out. ASH has compiled a list of nonsmoking organizations (updated January 1989) in every state that can be requested. A partial listing is given below.

2. Group Against Smokers' Pollution (GASP)
   PO Box 632
   College Park, MD 20740
   (301) 577-6427

   Provides information about activities in support of non-smokers' rights. GASP chapters are found throughout the United States.

3. Non-smokers Travel Club
   8929 Bradmoor Drive
   Bethesda, MD 20034
   (301) 530-1664

   Arranges smoke-free tours—both domestic and international.

4. Citizens Against Tobacco Smoke (CATS)
   PO Box 2232
   Rockville, MD 20852
   (301) 369-1473

   A national organization with chapters throughout the United States.

5. Stop Teenage Addiction to Tobacco (STAT)
   PO Box 60658
   Longmeadow, MA 01116
   (413) 567-7587

   Chapters of STAT are found throughout the United States.

Smoking Cessation Information

I have frequently urged people to stop smoking but have difficulty really substantiating why they should stop. Where can I obtain scientific information on the hazards of smoking? Also, what types of programs are available for the person who desires to stop smoking? Many different approaches to smoking cessation are being offered around the country. These approaches include group therapy, individual counseling, physician messages, and self-help guides. Methods of therapy include the use of drugs, electric shock, hypnosis, and acupuncture. The following is a discussion of the various types of smoking cessation methods, educational materials that can be obtained, health organizations, and professional material that discusses all aspects of smoking (psychological, economic, social, and physiologic).

1. The Health Consequences of Smoking (1988)
   DHHS pub no. (CDC) 88-8406

   May be ordered from the Superintendent of Documents, US Government Printing Office, Washington, DC 20402. Updated annually, presenting new topics each year (ie, addiction of nicotine).

2. The Health Consequences of Involuntary Smoking (1986)
   DHHS pub. no. (CDC) 87-8398

   May be ordered from the Superintendent of Documents, US Government Printing Office, Washington, DC 20402. Definitive presentation of the hazards of smoking to nonsmokers.

3. Smoking and Health Bulletin
   US Department of Health and Human Services
   Public Health Service
   Centers for Disease Control
   Center for Health Promotion and Education
   Office on Smoking and Health

   The Smoking and Health Bulletin is a bimonthly publication from the Technical Information Center of the Office on Smoking and Health. The Bulletin presents abstracts from the medical, nursing, sociology, public health, political, biological, and psychological literature on smoking, tobacco, and tobacco use. The yearly cumulation of the Smoking and Health Bulletin is titled *Bibliography on Smoking and Health*.

4. National Cancer Institute
   Office of Cancer Communications
   Building 31, Room 10A30
   Bethesda, MD 20892

Materials for health care professionals.

"Quit for Good" kit—a complete packet of materials designed specifically for health care professionals to assist their smoking patients to quit. Each kit contains enough materials for 50 patients. There is a similar kit for pharmacists, and the pharmacist kits contain enough material for 25 patients.

"Smoking Programs for Youth" (81-2156)—this paperback book (92 pages) is a comprehensive state-of-the-art report covering demographics of youth smoking in the United States, smoking regulations in schools and examples of how specific school systems are dealing with the problem, past approaches to smoking education and how these approaches have changed, factors likely to influence smoking among young people, and descriptions of innovative smoking solutions for youth today.

Public information:

Quit for Good
Why Do You Smoke?
Clearing the Air. A Guide to Quitting Smoking
Life as a Nonsmoker
How to Quit Smoking
Chew or Snuff is Real Bad Stuff

5. American Cancer Society

Some examples of available pamphlets, booklets, posters, buttons, and films are listed below. Contact your local ACS for more information.

Pamphlets:

Quit Cigarettes—Live Longer (in Spanish)
Quit Smoking—Live Longer (for black Americans)
Danger
The Smoke Around You: Risk of Involuntary Smoking
Decision Maker's Guide (workplace smoking booklet)
Why Start Life Under a Cloud?
Can They Stop Smoking (for black women)
How to Quit Cigarettes
The Decision is Yours
Don't Bite Off More Than You Can Chew
The Dangers of Smoking—Benefits of Quitting
Smokeless Tobacco: Cause for Concern?
Just a Pinch Between Your Cheek and Gum (Ohio Division)
Everything You Wanted to Know About Chewing and Dipping—But Were Afraid to Ask (Texas Division)

Regular Films and Video Tapes:

Women and Smoking (film and videotape)
Let's Call it Quits
Breaking Free (film and videotape)
The Feminine Mistake (film and videotape)—powerful film showing the effects of smoking. Although the film is geared to women, it is effective for men.
Taking Control (slide/tape and video)—provides an introduction to a healthy, enjoyable lifestyle that may prevent cancer. The program gives an overview of five "protective factors" against cancer and five preventable "risk factors."
Smokeless Tobacco (slide/tape and video)—presents all the health hazards related to smokeless tobacco.
Breaking Free—a film designed to promote smoking cessation especially among students who concentrate on vocational/career classes (film and video)

Posters and Buttons:

Smoking is Very Glamorous (poster)
Sean Marsee Poster
Best Tip Yet, Don't Start (poster)
Quite Smoking, Lives You Could Save (poster)
Thank You for Not Smoking

Kiss a Non-smoker, Taste the Difference (poster)
Smoking Stinks (buttons)
Are You a Draggin' Lady? (poster)
Archie, Smoke-Free Young America (poster)
His Spittin' Image (poster)

6. American Lung Association

Some of the smoking literature, posters, buttons, and smoking cessation materials are listed below. Contact your local American Lung Association.

Pamphlets:

How Not To Love Your Kids (English and Spanish)
Emphysema—The Facts About Your Lungs
Cigarette Smoking—The Facts About Your Lungs
Marijuana: A Second Look at Health Hazards
Is There a Safe Tobacco?
Facts About Second-Hand Smoke
A Guide to Smokeless Tobacco
A No-Smoking Coloring Book (coloring booklet for children)
Help a Friend Stop Smoking
Nonsmokers' Rights, What You Can Do
Me Quit Smoking? How?

Posters:

This Is a Smoke-Free Workspace
Thanks For Not Smoking
Almost 35 Million Americans Quit Smoking
Brooke Shields: Smoking Spoils Your Looks
Be Kind to Nonsmokers

Films:

Breathing Easy Film—film for 5th and 8th graders.
As We See It—made for pre-teens.
Everything You Always Wanted to Know About How to Stop Smokers But Were Afraid to Try—interviews with non-smokers, filled with humor and imagination.

Anti-smoking programs:

Freedom From Smoking Booklets—Freedom From Smoking in 20 Days—self-help book shows you how to quit smoking in 20 days
Freedom From Smoking Home Video Program "In Control"
Freedom From Smoking T-Shirt Iron-Ons
Freedom From Smoking The Workplace Booklets
Freedom From Smoking buttons and posters and tent cards

Puzzles:

Have Fun!! Figure Out the Smoking Puzzle

7. Narcotics Education, Inc.
6830 Laurel Street, NW
Washington, DC 20012-9979
(1-800-548-8700)

This organization has multiple pamphlets, booklets, films, videos, posters, and teaching aids that stress smoking cessation as well as advocating not starting to smoke. Request a free catalog of their materials. A sample of a few items are given below:

Pamphlets:

How to Stop Smoking and Breathe Free ($8.95 per 25)
Your Health: What Smoking May Do
One Strike Against You

Booklets:

I Love Not Smoking—coloring book (grades 1 to 3) ($12.50 per 25)
To Smoke Or Not (grade 7 to adult) ($0.95 each)

Audiovisuals:

Death in the West. (Grade 7 to adult)—can be purchased or rented. A British television documentary showing six real-life cowboys who are dying of disease caused by their smoking (in contrast to the Marlboro man).

Smokeless Tobacco—It Can Snuff You Out (grade 7 to adult)—can be purchased or rented. Young people tell their own experiences, including their difficulties in quitting, and one young man's death emphasizes the hazards of smokeless tobacco.

Teaching aids:

Real Human Lung Sections (grade 5 to adult) ($128.75 per item)

Mr. Gross Mouth (grade 1 to adult) ($65.00 for model that accurately shows the oral effects of chewing and dipping tobacco, including cancers)

8. American Cancer Society
   Local Units

   Assists hospitals and organizations in establishing Fresh Start or I Quit Clinics where participants attempt to learn why they smoke, identify ways to quit, and are motivated and encouraged by the leader, usually an ex-smoker, and other group members. The ACS provides all materials for the sessions, including films and books, free of charge, but the institutions usually charge for the clinic itself.

9. Narcotics Education Division
   6840 Eastern Avenue, NW
   Washington, DC 20012

   They offer a smoking cessation program called "The Breathe-Free Plan to Stop Smoking." A Director's Kit can be purchased at a cost of $59.95. This kit includes (1) The Director's Manual—How-to explanation of the entire program includes a planning and advertising guide for attracting people to the program, (2) Program Scripts—These scripts are so complete that when the traditional physician-minister team is not available, other health care professionals, counselors, and experienced laypersons may competently conduct the plan, and (3) Handout Masters—one-time activity sheets. Buttons, diplomas, personal plan booklet, and matchless pens/lighter plugs can be purchased for the program, as can pamphlets, posters, advertising materials and films, and videos and slide-tape programs.

10. Schick Laboratories
    Los Angeles, CA
    (213) 553-9771 or 1-800-CRAVING

    Schick Laboratories operates 13 smoking cessation centers in the western part of the United States, which conduct individual therapy sessions for 1 hour on 5 consecutive days. The centers' goal is behavior modification, and aversion therapy is stressed. Methods include a rapid smoking (quick puff) and an "electrostimulus" applied to the participant's arm. Schick charges participants $625 for the 5-day program. There is also a 6-week support phase following the 5-day program, with weekly telephone calls from a counselor and one "booster" session in the second week. For more information see Smith J: Long term outcomes of clients treated in a commercial stop smoking program. *Journal of Substance Abuse Treatment* 5:33-36, 1988.

11. Office on Smoking and Health
    Department of Health and Human Services
    Public Health Service
    Rockville, MD 20857
    (301) 443-1575

    The following materials can be obtained from this government office:

    Public Information:

    Two Reasons to Quit (English and Spanish poster and brochure)

    If Your Kids Think Everyone Smokes

No More Butts

Adult Self Test

A Self Test for Teenagers

Why People Smoke Cigarettes

A Decision Maker's Guide to Reducing Smoking at the Worksite

Passive Pamphlet

Technical Information:

Review and Evaluation of Smoking Cessation Methods

Smokeless Tobacco Report

Smoking and Health—A National Status Report

Smoking and Health Bulletin

Surgeon General's Report:

1985—Cancer and Chronic Lung Disease in the Workplace

1986—Involuntary Smoking

1988—Nicotine Addiction (GPO Stock #017-001-00468-5)

1989—25 Years of Progress (Summary)

Self-Help Organizations

1. American Cancer Society: CanSurmount

   This program is composed of the patient, family member, trained volunteer (also a cancer patient), and health care professional. The program is designed to have volunteers visit cancer patients in the hospital and home and to provide patient and family education, information, and emotional support.

2. American Cancer Society: I Can Cope

   I Can Cope is a formal educational program designed to provide information (treatment, side effects, nutrition, resources, etc.) and support to people with cancer and their families. Contact your local ACS for details about this program in your area.

3. American Cancer Society: Loan Closets and Transportation Services

   Many ACS units have loan closets that supply sickroom equipment for home cancer patients. Equipment may include wheelchairs, walkers, surgical dressings, bedpans, hospital beds, shower chairs, etc. This equipment can be borrowed for as long as needed. Contact your local unit for this free service. In some communities the ACS offers patient transportation to physicians' offices, hospitals, or clinics for diagnosis and treatment. This service is run by ACS volunteers.

4. American Cancer Society: Reach to Recovery

   This is one of the best-known self-help groups. It was founded in 1952 by Terese Lasser and has been part of the ACS since 1969. Reach to Recovery works through its volunteer visitors, who have adjusted successfully to their own mastectomies. Once the patient's physician has given permission, the volunteer makes a hospital visit a few days after surgery. She brings a kit containing a manual of information about rehabilitation exercises and exercise equipment and a temporary breast form. Volunteers have up-to-date lists of prostheses and bathing suits available locally, which may be given to patients along with lists of national manufacturers. Volunteers who have had reconstructive surgery are available to visit women who are deciding about this type of surgery. Some units have women volunteers who have had chemotherapy or radiation meet with women before surgery. Reach to Recovery services are free and can be secured by contacting your local ACS unit.

5. Association of Brain Tumor Research
3735 North Talman Avenue
Chicago, IL 60618
(312) 286-5571

This organization works to raise funds for brain tumor research and patient education materials. The purposes are to raise funds for brain tumor research, raise the level of public awareness about the prevalence of brain tumors, and to help the victims of the disease and their families by making them aware that they are not alone and by disseminating information to them. ABTR furnishes on request a list of experimental treatment centers and brain tumor study groups. Twelve publications, in lay language, are available free of charge to patient and family members. Organizations may purchase these pamphlets:
Chemotherapy of Brain Tumors
A Primer of Brain Tumors
Radiation Therapy of Brain Tumors Part 1: A Basic Guide
Radiation Therapy of Brain Tumors Part 2: Background and Research Guide
Living With a Brain Tumor
Coping With a Brain Tumor
When Your Child is Ready to Return to School
Shunts
Tumor Specific
About Glioblastoma Multiforme and Malignant Astrocytoma
About Medulloblastoma
About Meningioma
About Oligodendroglioma

6. Cancer Care
1180 Avenue of the Americas
New York, NY 10036
(212) 221-3300

Founded approximately 44 years ago, this organization offers services to cancer patients and their families and friends at all stages of the disease to help them cope with the emotional, psychological, and financial impact of cancer. This social service agency directly provides professional counseling and offers referrals for nursing care, homemakers, home health aides, and housekeepers to patients with cancer and their supportive others. They also distribute cancer education materials. Although they primarily serve New York City and its tristate, metropolitan region, they answer letters and telephone calls from all over the United States, providing information and referrals to these inquiries whenever possible. The pamphlet "Listen to the Children" (a study of the impact on children's mental health when a parent has a catastrophic illness) is available from Cancer Care.

7. Cancer Information Service
1-800-4-CANCER
Hawaii: Oahu 524-1234 (call collect from neighbor islands)
Alaska: 1-800-638-6070
National Office: 1-800-638-6694

The Cancer Information Service is a program of the NCI. It is a network of regional offices with trained staff and volunteers that provide accurate and confidential telephone information to questions concerning cancer (rehabilitation, research, causes, prevention and detection, diagnosis, treatment, support services, etc) from patients and their supportive others, health care professionals, and the public.

8. Candelighters Childhood Cancer Foundation
Suite 1001
1901 Pennsylvania Avenue
Washington, DC 20006
(202) 659-5136

Candelighters began in April 1970 as a group of parents of young cancer patients at local hospitals and clinics in the Washington, DC, area. The group's focus is children, adolescents, and teens. There are presently 250 chapters in the United States. Candelighters have two primary goals: to obtain consistent and adequate federal support for cancer research and to help parents and other family members who share the particularly difficult experience of living with a child with cancer. A national newsletter is published quarterly, which serves as a communication link among parents and parents' groups and concerned professionals. A quarterly youth newsletter is also published to provide information to young cancer patients. The free newsletters include information about research in childhood cancer, bibliography materials, and group activities. Local groups usually have their own newsletter. Candelighters also publishes a resource list of childhood cancer education materials. All the above information is available free on request.

9. Children's Hospice International
1101 Kings Street, Suite 131
Alexandria, VA 22314
(800) 24-CHILD
(703) 684-0330

The purpose of Children's Hospice International is to "create a world of hospice support for children, providing medical and technical assistance, research and education for these special children, families and health care professionals." Membership (individual is $35) includes a quarterly newsletter titled, *CHI*, 10% discount on publications and other purchases, national conference discount, and update information mailings. Also available are two teddy bears (one with a tape player and special tapes that can be purchased) and dolls, one of which, Zaadi, is an overstuffed soft cloth doll with embroidered insides (heart, ribs, lungs, etc) that is useful in teaching children.
A partial list of publications is as follows:
Home Care for Children: A Manual for Parents
Palliative Pain and Symptom Management for Children and Adolescents
My Life, Melinda's Story

10. Concern for the Dying
250 West 57th Street
New York, NY 10107
(212) 246-6962

A nonprofit organization, founded in 1967, Concern for the Dying is an educational council that advocates an individual's right to participate in the decisions regarding her or his treatment, particularly those decisions when a person is near death. Concern for the Dying developed the Living Will, a document that specifies one's wishes concerning life-sustaining measures. This organization offers the Living Will, up-to-date information on the current laws of each state, and registration of the will in the Living Will Registry. Other services provided include assistance to terminally ill patients whose wishes are not being honored, a quarterly newsletter for annual contributors of $5 or more, a staff attorney and legal advisors committee for assistance with patients' rights issues, conferences on death and dying (professional and lay), audiovisual materials (purchase or rent), publications, an extensive library, and a multidisciplinary forum for health care professionals in educational settings to address issues related to the terminally ill.

11. Corporate Angel Network, Inc.
Westchester County Airport
Building One

White Plains, NY 10604
(914) 328-1313

CAN is a nonprofit organization that arranges free air transportation for cancer patients going to or from recognized treatments, consultations, or checkups. The program uses available seats on corporate aircraft. A person must be in stable condition, able to board unassisted, and have back-up reservations on commercial airlines, since travel is not guaranteed. This service is available regardless of financial need.

12. Encore
National Board, YWCA
726 Broadway
New York, NY 10003
(212) 614-2827

Encore is a national program offered by the YWCA and sponsored by local YWCAs. It provides floor and pool exercises as well as discussion and support groups for women recovering from breast cancer surgery. The reader is encouraged to contact the local YWCA for details of program availability and cost.

13. International Association of Laryngectomees
c/o American Cancer Society
Tower Place
3340 Peachtree Road, NE
Atlanta, GA 30026
(404) 320-3333

The International Association of Laryngectomees was founded in 1952 and affiliated with the ACS and consists of 257 domestic and 14 foreign clubs whose members are laryngectomees. For the location of the "Lost Chord," "New Voice", or "Anamile" club nearest you, write the IAL or contact your local ACS. The goal of these lost chord clubs is to assist newly laryngectomized persons to make early adjustments to loss of voice and to overcome psychosocial problems. They accomplish this by serving as hosts for newly laryngectomized persons at club meetings and by collaborating with surgeons in preoperative and postoperative speech orientations. Members of the Lost Chord Club visit new laryngectomee patients in the hospital (at the invitation of the physician). The Lost Chord Club member discusses with both the spouse and the patient early home adjustment, speech therapy, the need for early return to normal work and recreation, required changes in the activities of daily living, and benefits of joining a Lost Chord Club. Meetings enable patients and their spouses to discuss common problems of caring for a laryngectomee and to offer moral support and encouragement and social confidence after similar surgery. Manuals and newsletters are available to members. A laryngectomy kit is available and contains stoma covers, an emergency identification card, booklets (first aid, stoma care, tracheostomy care, speech, etc), and an erasable writing board with a pen.
Other resources for laryngectomy patients:
Bruce Medical Supply
411 Waverly Oaks Road
P.O. Box 9166
Waltham, MA 02254
(800) 225-8446
This company has a catalog of tracheostomy supplies.

Communitrach
Implant Technologies, Inc.
7900 West 78th Street

Minneapolis, MN 55435
(800) 328-0925
A trach tube is available, which allows the intubated patient to speak laryngeally.

Medic-Alert Foundation International
P.O. Box 1009
Turlock, CA 95381
(800) 344-3226
(209) 668-3333 (California)
Contact the Foundation for medic-alert bracelets.

Vocaid (Texas Instruments) and Spelling Ace (Franklin Computers) are electronic voice communication aids.

14. Leukemia Society of America
733 Third Avenue
New York, NY 10017
(212) 573-8484

This is a national voluntary health agency dedicated solely to seeking the control and eventual eradication of leukemia and allied diseases. The Society supports a three-pronged program: research, patient aid, and public and professional education. The patient-aid program provides up to $750 per year on an outpatient basis: drugs for the care, treatment or control of leukemia; laboratory service charges for blood processing, cross-matching, typing, and transfusing; up to $300 per individual for radiotherapy in the first stages of Hodgkin's disease; also, up to $300 for prophylactic radiation for children with acute leukemia. The patient-aid program is conducted through the Society's local chapters, which also give counsel and referrals to other community resources to all leukemia patients and their families regardless of financial circumstances. Some local chapters also offer family support programs for patients and family members or friends. There are 56 chapters in 31 states and the District of Columbia.

15. Make A Wish Foundation of America
2600 North Central Avenue
Suite 936
Phoenix, AZ 85004
1-800-722-9474
(602) 240-6600

This foundation grants wishes for individuals under 18 years of age who are suffering from life-threatening illnesses. The wish includes the immediate family and expenses. The local Make a Wish chapter assigns a wish team for each wish. Common wishes include trips to Disneyland, meeting celebrities, visiting relatives, and requests for material things such as videorecorders and entertainment centers. The Foundation is a nonprofit organization composed of volunteers. There are 68 chapters serving 44 states in the United States and 5 international affiliates.

16. Make Today Count
101½ South Union Street
Alexandria, VA 22314
(703) 548-9674

Make Today Count is a mutual support group for persons with life-threatening illnesses. The purpose is to allow these people to discuss their personal concerns so that they may deal with them in a positive way. By sharing and exchanging experiences of living with a life-threatening illness, it is hoped that patients and their families will live their lives as fully and meaningfully as possible. Make Today Count chapter activities include formal programs, group discussions, chapter newsletters, social activities, workshops and seminars, community projects, educational activities, and monthly meetings. It was founded by Orville Kelly, a cancer patient, in January 1974 in Burlington, IA. There are over 200 chapters in the United States, Canada, and Europe. A national newsletter and the book *Make Today Count* may be purchased through the above address. Information about local chapters or establishing a chapter in your area can be obtained from the same address.

17. Meals on Wheels Program

This service provides at least one hot meal a day and in some cases an additional cold meal. The program varies from state to state, but the cost for the meals is usually minimal, and they are delivered Monday through Friday. Some programs require a referral from a physician. Programs may be run by local health departments, church groups, or community volunteer organizations. Local hospitals can provide information on this program through their social service departments.

18. National Coalition for Cancer Survivorship
323 Eighth Street, SW
Albuquerque, NM 87102
(505) 764-9956

"The mission of NCCS is to communicate that there can be vibrant, productive life following the diagnosis of cancer." The NCCS is a relatively new organization founded in 1986. It is composed of independent groups and individuals interested in issues of cancer survivorship and support of cancer survivors and their significant others. It provides a national communication network between persons and organizations involved with survivorship, advocates issues, research and interests of cancer survivors, and collects and distributes information. NCCS is a proponent of National Cancer Survivors' Day.

19. National Hospice Organization
1901 North Moore Street
Suite 901
Arlington, VA 22209
(703) 243-5900

Established in 1978, NHO is a nonprofit organization, promoting quality care to the terminally ill and their significant others. NHO has worked over the past decade to establish hospice as a part of the health care delivery system in the United States. As a result of its efforts, hospice is now included as a Medicare/Medicaid benefit and as an employee benefit for 66% of American workers. The number of hospices has also increased from one in 1974 to over 1725 in 1990. Most hospices are members of NHO and receives NHO's technical assistance, education programs and events, publications, and advocacy and referral services. Membership has several categories and includes *The Hospice Journal* among numerous other publications and workshops.

20. Nurses' Clubs: Loan Closets

Many communities have local nurses' clubs that provide free-of-charge hospital equipment to cancer patients for use in their homes. Equipment varies with clubs but ranges from bedpans to crutches.

21. Ronald McDonald Houses
Kathy Charlton, Coordinator
500 North Michigan Avenue
Chicago, IL 60611
(312) 836-7100

The first Ronald McDonald House opened in 1974 in Philadelphia. Currently there are over 100 such houses in the United States (and in some foreign countries). The purpose of the house is to provide temporary lodging for families of children who are undergoing treatment at a nearby hospital for cancer, leukemia, and other serious illnesses. Rooms are usually available on a first-come basis. Families are asked to donate financially toward their stay if they are able (ranging from $5 to $15 per day); if unable, their lodging is free. They are also asked to keep their room clean and to do their own cooking, laundry, and grocery shopping. Each house is a partnership consisting of volunteers, community organizations, local hospital(s), and area McDonald's restaurants.

22. Society for the Right to Die
250 West 57th Street
New York, NY 10107
(212) 246-6973

The Society for the Right to Die is a national nonprofit organization in the United States that pursues a program on several fronts: legal services, legislation, and promotion for citizens' rights. It supports legislation enabling persons, while of sound mind, to execute a legally binding document directing that in the event of a terminal condition, medical procedures that prolong the dying process be withheld or withdrawn. Services include a newsletter, bibliographies, handbooks, and material related to the right to refuse treatment, journal articles, and several legislative handbooks. A physician in residence is on staff and available for consultation. A copy of a living will for each of 40 states will be sent free of charge on request. A declaration in general language is provided for those states that still lack living will legislation.

23. TOUCH
513 Tinsley Harrison Tower
University Station
Birmingham, AL 35294
(205) 934-3814

TOUCH is an acronym for Today Our Understanding of Cancer is Hope and is cosponsored by ACS Alabama Division, Inc. and Comprehensive Cancer Center, Birmingham, AL. It started in 1976 and grew from a small group to several hundred members in a number of different cities in Alabama. The program offers emotional and psychological support to cancer patients who are undergoing or have completed cancer treatment and their significant others. TOUCH's goal is to enable patients to cope with psychosocial difficulties caused by their disease such as side effects of treatment, employment, lack of adequate information, communication barriers with family or friends, and fear. Trained peer counselors offer group and individual counseling. TOUCH also seeks to combat unproved cancer treatment methods.

24. United Cancer Council
Parc Place Office Center
4010 West 86th Street, Suite H
Indianapolis, IN 46268-1704
(317) 844-6627

Founded in 1963, the purpose of the UCC is to serve cancer patients through service programs, public and professional education, and research. It is composed of 39 member agencies. Free patient services, provided by the member agencies, include counseling, financial assistance for treatment and medications, loan closets, transportation, and detection clinics. UCC offers public and professional educational services such as cancer prevention seminars, smoking clinics, screening programs, mastectomy group counseling, breast-self-examination clinics, and pamphlets. Research is funded by UCC in the form of grants to institutions.

Pamphlets available:
Reduce Your Risk of Getting Cancer: Tips for people over 50
Cancer Prevention: Fact & Fiction
Facts on Cancer Risk Factors
"How Do You Talk with Someone who Has Cancer?"
Protect Your Skin
Breast Self-Examination Guide
MEN

25. United Ostomy Association
36 Executive Park
Suite 120
Irvine, CA 92714
(714) 660-8624

Local chapters are composed primarily of ostomates who provide aid, moral support, and education to those who have a colostomy, ileostomy, or urostomy surgery. The chapter supplements the work of the surgeon by offering rehabilitation through follow-up by people who have learned to live with an ostomy. Trained members make visits to homes and hospitals, on request, with the prior consent of the patient's physician. Chapters have medical advisory boards consisting of non-surgeon physicians, surgeons, and enterostomal therapists trained in ostomy care and the use of equipment. At regular monthly meetings, open to anyone who is interested, members can exchange practical, personal experiences about their ostomies, see ostomy equipment displayed, and hear speakers who are knowledgeable about ostomy. All local chapters are volunteer organizations. A list of the chapters is available on request from the UOA. Annual chapter dues vary from no fee to $30. Each member of the UOA receives the *Ostomy Quarterly* magazine and is eligible to participate in the UOA insurance programs. The UOA has both publications and slide programs, which cover every aspect of ostomies. The following is a list of some of these booklets and programs:
Sex, Courtship and the Single Ostomate, $1.50
Sex and the Female Ostomate, $1.50
My Child Has An Ostomy, $0.25
The Ostomy Handbook, $4.50
Ileostomy: A Guide, $5
Urinary Ostomies: A Guidebook for Patients
Colostomies—A Guide, $4 (In English, Spanish, French, and Chinese)

26. We Can Do
1800 Augusta, Suite 150
Houston, TX 77057
(713) 780-1057

This program offers psychological and educational support for cancer patients and their significant others addressing long-term needs. Support groups and referral to local resources are available in California, Washington, DC, and Texas.

27. Wellness Centers/Groups

The basic philosophy of these organizations is to provide psychosocial support for people with life-threatening illnesses. Some of the centers are specifically for people with cancer and their significant others, some cater to children and adults, others include the bereaved, and a few include people without any serious illness who want to improve the quality of their lives. Other services may include information such as books or pamphlets, free second opinions, work-shops, mind-body exercises, coping skills, support groups, matching people with the same diagnosis, joke fests, hotlines (some staffed with cancer survivors), relaxation and guided imagery sessions, and social events. The reader is encouraged to contact a local Wellness Center or Group for details. The CIS (1-800-4-CANCER) provides location and telephone numbers of the nearest center or group.

Cancer Support Center
5300 Rockhill Road
Kansas City, MO 64111
(816) 932-8453 (Hotline 9 AM to 4:30 PM)

Cancer Wellness Center
9701 North Kenton, #18
Skokie, IL 60076
(312) 982-9689

Center for Hope
374 Middlesex Road
Darien, CT 06820
(203) 655-4693

Exceptional Cancer Patients
1302 Chapel Street
New Haven, CT 06511
(203) 865-8392

The Wellness Community
1235 Fifth Street
Santa Monica, CA 90401
(213) 393-1415

28. Y-ME
18220 Hardwood Avenue
Homewood, IL 60430
(312) 799-8228 Open 24 hours
(800) 221-2141 Weekdays 9 to 5

Founded in 1978 by Ann Marcou and Mimi Kaplan, two mastectomy patients, Y-ME has become the largest breast cancer support program in the USA. It provides hotlines staffed by volunteers who have personally experienced breast cancer, presurgery counseling, open door meetings, early detection workshops, speakers bureau, resource library, wigs and prosthesis bank, and inservice workshops for health care professionals. Volunteers are professionally supervised, and the information provided to patients is monitored by a medical advisory board. Contributing members receive a quarterly newsletter and an invitation to attend the Y-ME national conference at discounted rates.

Miscellaneous Consumer Groups

1. American Health Decision
Dept P 1200 Larimer
Campus Box 133
Denver, CO 80204

American Health Decisions are groups of concerned citizens in various states that tell their legislators how they want their tax dollars spent related to health care issues such as rationing of resources and other biomedical ethical questions.

2. National Alliance of Breast Cancer Organizations (NABCO)
1180 Avenue of the Americas
2nd Floor
New York, NY 10036
(212) 719-0154
(NABCO prefers written inquiries)

NABCO is a central resource of information on breast cancer. NABCO publishes a breast cancer resource list.

3. National Coalition for Cancer Survivorship
323 Eighth Street, SW
Albuquerque, NM 87102
(505) 764-9956

NCCS serves as a resource to network individuals and groups concerned with cancer survivorship issues by providing access to information, referrals, resources, educational opportunities, and professional and peer support.

AIDS-Related Organizations

1. AIDS Action Council
729 Eighth Street, SE
Suite 200
Washington, DC 20003
(202) 293-2886

The purpose of this organization is lobbying for AIDS education, research, and policy.

2. American Foundation for AIDS Research
1515 Broadway, Suite 3601
New York, NY 10036-8901
(212) 719-0033

The American Foundation for AIDS Research is a nonprofit fundraising organization for AIDS research. Funds are raised in forms of scientific and educational grants for individual researchers.

3. American Society of Psychiatric Oncology/AIDS
Mary Jane Massie, MD
Psychiatry Service
1275 York Avenue
New York, NY 10021

ASPOA established itself in November of 1988 as a national organization of psychiatrists working with patients with AIDS and cancer. It seeks to encourage research and education, enhance clinical care, and foster communication and disseminate information among its members. ASPOA will have semiannual meetings, a newsletter, and a directory. Associate membership is open to non-physicians.

4. Gay Men's Health Crisis
129 West 20th Street
New York, NY 10011
(212) 807-6655 (Hotline)
(212) 645-7470 (TTY)

GMHC is the world's first AIDS organization, founded by members of the gay community. Staffing includes 120 paid members and 1700 to 2000 volunteers. GMHC locally serves the New York City area. Its purposes are to maintain and improve the quality of life for persons with AIDS, ARC, and their care partners, to advocate for fair and effective public policies and practices concerning HIV infection, and through education and AIDS prevention programs, to increase awareness and understanding of HIV infection. Services include the buddy system (volunteers assigned to AIDS patients to help with daily chores), crisis intervention, meals, tickets to theaters, outings, exercise machines (at the facility), legal assistance, complaint department, AIDS profesional education program, and a speakers bureau. GMHC lobbys in New York City and Washington on AIDS issues. A newsletter on treatment issues and experimental drug therapies is published 10 times per year.

5. Health Education AIDS Liaison
PO Box 1103
Old Chelsea Station
New York, NY 10103
(212) 674-HOPE (Counseling)
(212) 243-3612 (Information packet—leave name and address)

Formed in 1982 to challenge the idea that AIDS is fatal, HEAL is a nonprofit organization providing holistic and alternative treatment approaches to people with AIDS. Their services include weekly information and support groups, monthly intensive healing workshops, forums, and a clearinghouse.

6. National AIDS Hotline
(800) 342-2437 (Open 24 hours, 7 days a week)
(800) 344-7432 (Spanish, live operator from 8 AM–2 PM)
(800) 243-7889 (TTY/TDD, Monday–Friday, 10 AM–10 PM)

The hotline is staffed by volunteers and paid workers with information from the CDC, Federal Government, etc. The hotline offers counseling, referrals to other agencies, hotlines and local AIDS testing sites, printed materials, and a wealth of additional information.
Sampling of pamphlets:
What About AIDS Testing
How You Won't Get AIDS
If Your AIDS Test is Positive
Surgeon General's Report on AIDS
Facts About AIDS
Understanding AIDS
Guidelines for Effective School Health Education to Prevent the Spread of AIDS
Information for Teachers and School Officials: AIDS and Children
Information for Parents: AIDS and Children
Pamphlets available in Spanish, Laotian, and Braille:
AIDS and the Safety of the Nation's Blood Supply
Caring for the AIDS Patient at Home

7. National AIDS Information Clearinghouse
PO Box 6003
Rockville, MD 20850
(800) 458-5231 (Publications)
(301) 762-5111 (Database)

This is a clearinghouse for free publications from the CDC and other organizations. A catalog is available on request. The database access provides additional information for speakers and other AIDS-related resources.
Partial list of publications:
Understanding AIDS (English, Spanish, Chinese, Braille, Portugese)
MMWR *(Morbidity and Mortality Weekly Report)*
Universal Precautions for Health Care Workers (Reprint)
Monthly Report CDC HIV/AIDS Surveillance
AIDS and Deafness Resource Directory
AIDS Education: A Business Guide (AIDS in the Workplace)

8. National AIDS Network
2033 M Street, NW
Suite 800
Washington, DC 20036
(202) 293-2437

NAN is a resource center and national voice for community-based volunteer organizations that provide AIDS services and education. Currently, 700 volunteer organizations and 200 health departments belong to the network. NAN offers

many services including technical assistance in areas such as volunteer management and buddy programs, a clearinghouse for current resources, directories, and publications.
Publications:
Network News (monthly newsletter)
NAN Multi-Cultural Notes (monthly newsletter)
NAN Monitor (quarterly newsletter)
NAN Directory of AIDS Education and Service Organizations
NAN Video Directory
NAN Directory of AIDS-Related Periodicals
AIDS Into the 90s: Strategies for an Integrated Response to the AIDS Epidemic
The CORO Report
Americans Who Care
Heads, Hearts, & Hands

9. National Association of People with AIDS
2025 Eye Street, NW
Suite 415
Washington, DC 20006
(202) 429-2856

NAPWA's members are people living with AIDS, ARC, and HIV helping themselves and others. Local chapters serve their own communities, offering housing, meals, peer support groups, information pamphlets, alternative therapies and holistic healing, forums on AIDS for health care professionals, and other programs. The national office service include the newsletter *NAPWA NEWS*, scholarships and traveling expenses to national meetings and conferences, technical assistance to local chapters in areas such as fundraising and grantwriting, and administering two funds that support education of and advocacy by people with AIDS.

10. National Minority AIDS Council
714 G Street, SE
Washington, DC 20003
(202) 544-1076

Composed of nearly 160 education and service or community-based minority AIDS organizations, NMAC is dedicated to "creating a greater, more coordinated response among People of Color to the devastating and disproportionate effect of AIDS on minority communities." It provides technical assistance to its member organizations and emerging organizations, promotes AIDS education among the minorities, influences policymakers on a community and national level, creates resources for AIDS programs and education, and acts as a national advocate for the minority response to the AIDS epidemic.

11. Project Inform
347 Dolores Street, Suite 301
San Francisco, CA 94110
(800) 822-7422 (national 10 AM to 2 PM PST)
(800) 334-7422 (California)
(415) 558-9051 (local)

This nonprofit volunteer organization gives current available information on drug treatment protocols for HIV, ARC, and AIDS. The information is available nationally and internationally free of charge with donations accepted. Project Inform publishes a quarterly newsletter, *P.I. Perspectives."*

12. San Francisco AIDS Foundation
PO Box 6182
San Francisco, CA 94101
(415) 863-2437
(800) FOR AIDS (Northern California Hotline)
(415) 864-6606 (TTY)

Locally, the foundation offers an emergency housing and food bank, case management, and support groups to persons with ARC and AIDS. It also has two special programs: (1) a bilingual multicultural program with support groups and events in Spanish and other languages and (2) a program of women's services. Another aspect of the foundation is disseminating publications and information, which is available free to local San Francisco nonprofit agencies but with some restrictions to nonprofit agencies and individuals outside the San Francisco area.
Brochures:
AIDS and Healthcare Workers
Women and AIDS
Alcohol, Drugs and AIDS
Your Child and AIDS
Risky Business (comic book for teenagers)
When a Friend has AIDS

13. The Women AIDS Network
c/o San Francisco AIDS Foundation
PO Box 6182
San Francisco, CA 94101
(415) 863-2437

The Women's AIDS Network is a coalition of women providers to individuals with AIDS. Their monthly meeting is in San Francisco. Membership is $20 for individual and $30 for institution. Benefits of membership include monthly mailings encompassing new information about women and AIDS, legislation, conferences, and education.

Organizations Devoted to Pain

1. American Academy of Pain Medicine
43 East Ohio, Suite 914
Chicago, IL 60611
(312) 645-0083

Founded in 1983, the AAPM is comprised of physicians and surgeons whose practices involve a large number of patients with chronic intractable pain. Its mission is "to enhance the practice of pain medicine in the United States." Primary goals include quality and comprehensive treatment of patients with intractable chronic pain through education and research, and promoting "a socioeconomic and political climate which will be conducive to the practice of pain medicine in an effective and efficient manner." One of the objectives of the AAPM is to be the official organization representing physicians who specialize in the field of pain medicine in the USA.

2. American Chronic Pain Association
257 Old Haymaker Road
Monroeville, PA 15146
(412) 856-9676

ACPA, founded in Pittsburgh in 1980, is now a national organization with 174 chapters. Its purpose is to provide support groups for persons with chronic pain. The focus is on coping and living with chronic pain, moving from the role of the patient back to being a person. The groups are open to chronic pain sufferers, should not be affiliated with a hospital or other institution or meet in a hospital, and the facilitator is a person with chronic pain. Professionals are not allowed to practice therapy at group meetings. Members are chronic pain sufferers. Membership entitles one to the ACPA Member's Manual and relaxation tapes at reduced rates.

3. American Pain Society
   1200 17th Street NW
   Suite 400
   Washington, DC 20036
   (202) 296-9200

   The APS, a national chapter of the International Association for the Study of Pain, is a professional multidisciplinary educational society promoting acute and chronic pain control. Membership includes the quarterly APS Newsletter, *Principles of Analgesic Use in the Treatment of Acute Pain and Chronic Cancer Pain,* meetings and special events information and discount rates at the annual meeting.

4. American Society of Clinical Hypnosis
   2250 East Devon, Suite 336
   Des Plaines, IL 60018
   (312) 297-3317

   The American Society of Clinical Hypnosis is comprised of 3500 doctorally prepared professionals (physicians, dentists, psychologists) who use hypnosis in their clinical practice. Of interest is the use of hypnosis in the treatment of pain and side effects of chemotherapy. The society publishes a quarterly journal, *American Journal of Clinical Hypnosis.* It also has a speakers bureau and a referral service.

5. Association for Applied Psychophysiology and Applied Biofeedback
   10200 West 44th Avenue
   Wheatridge, CO 80037
   (303) 422-8436

   The reader may contact this organization for resource people working with biofeedback in a particular specialty or region of the United States.

6. Commission on Accreditation of Rehabilitation Facilities
   101 North Wilmot Road, Suite 500
   Tucson, AZ 85711
   (602) 748-1212

   CARF provides national accreditation and standards on a variety of programs including chronic pain management. Many states recognize the value of CARF accreditation and require it for licensure. On request, CARF will send a list of accredited chronic pain management clinics.

7. The Committee on the Treatment of Intractable Pain
   PO Box 9553
   Friendship Station
   Washington, DC 20016
   (202) 965-6717

   The major purpose of the committee is to promote education and research on more effective management and alleviation of intractable pain, particularly pain that is beyond the control of available drugs and conventional techniques. One activity of the committee is to seek the transfer of heroin from Schedule I of the Controlled Substance Act, which designates it of no medical use, to Schedule II, which places it in the same restricted category as morphine.

8. InControl: Cancer Pain Care Association
   2320 Tracy Place NW
   Washington, DC 20008
   (202) 483-6108

   Educational and consulting services are provided for a fee to physicians, nurses, patients, and significant others on pain and pain management. Telephone consultation is available without charge.

9. International Association for the Study of Pain
   909 NE 43rd Street, Suite 306
   Seattle, WA 98105
   (206) 547-6409

The purposes of IASP are multifold and include promoting professional and public education, encouraging research, disseminating new information, developing a national and international data bank, formatting national associations for the study and treatment of pain, sponsoring world congresses, and encouraging the adoption of a uniform classification system of pain. Presently, there are 20 national chapters. Regular membership fees are salary based and include a subscription to the monthly journal *PAIN*, the IASP newsletter, and a members' directory.

10. National Chronic Pain Outreach Association, Inc.
    4922 Hampden Lane
    Bethesda, MD 20814
    (301) 652-4948

    Established in 1980, NCPOA is a nonprofit organization that receives its funds from the public. Its purpose is to reduce chronic pain suffering. Services provided include a clearinghouse for pain information and management, the quarterly newsletter *Lifeline,* seminars and lectures, local support groups for chronic pain sufferers and their families, and professional education. Membership has several categories and includes *Lifeline* and reduced rates for publications, pamphlets, and audio tapes.
    Publications:
    Recommended Reading List
    Pain Management Strategies
    Flare-up Coping Tips
    Choosing a Pain Clinic or Specialist
    The Mind-Body Dilemma
    10 Hints for Helping Your Patients with Chronic Pain
    Support Group Discussion Topics
    Arthritis and Bradykinins
    Neuropathy Pain
    Audio cassette tapes:
    Chronic Pain and Hypnosis
    Progressive Relaxation Exercise

11. National Pain Association
    Department of Family Health Care Nursing
    Pain Study Office, N411Y
    University of California, San Francisco
    San Francisco, CA 94134
    (415) 476-4400

    Founded in the bay area relatively recently, the NPA seeks to encourage education, research, and high standards of nursing care in treating patients with acute and chronic pain. The NPA also fosters communication and dissemination of information among members and with other nursing colleagues. Membership requires one to be an RN and pay annual dues of $10.

12. Society for Behavioral Medicine
    PO Box 8530
    University Station
    Knoxville, TN 37996
    (615) 974-5164

    The Society is a scientific multidisciplinary organization whose purpose is to communicate the relationship between behavior and health among researchers, academicians, and clinicians. One of its areas of research and clinical practice is chronic pain treatment. Membership has several categories and includes two quarterly journals, *Behavioral Medicine Abstracts* and *Annals of Behavioral Medicine,* as well as reduced rates on publications and the annual meeting.

13. Wisconsin Pain Initiative
    3675 Medical Sciences Center
    University of Wisconsin Medical School

1300 University Avenue
Madison, WI 53706

The Initiative started in 1986 as a statewide comprehensive effort to improve the management of cancer pain. The Initiative focuses on educating the patient, family, public, and professional, establishing patient care advocates to improve clinical cancer pain management, overcoming regulatory, legislative, and system barriers such as inadequate stocking of narcotics secondary to fear of theft, and determining through research and evaluation the success and future direction of the Initiative. The World Health Organization (WHO) designated Wisconsin as a demonstration state in the effort of worldwide cancer pain relief. *Handbook of Cancer Pain Management* can be purchased for $3 at the above address. A bimonthly newsletter, *Cancer Pain Update*, listing meetings and statewide activities can be obtained by contacting *Cancer Pain Update*, Jeanne Dosch (ed), 3717 Ross Street, Madison, WI 53705. A patient education booklet, *Cancer Pain Can Be Relieved*, is available through the ACS—Wisconsin Division, 615 North Sherman Avenue, Madison, WI 53704.

14. World Health Organization
Publications Center, USA
49 Sheridan Avenue
Albany, NY 12210

WHO sponsors the Cancer Pain Relief Program, which essentially proposes cancer pain relief as a worldwide priority. One can contact WHO to receive a booklet titled *Cancer Pain Relief*. The booklet discusses the prevalence of cancer pain, the need for education and training in pain management, legislative factors, pharmacologic guidelines, etc.

Oncology Nursing Organizations and Related Oncology Professional Organizations

1. American Association for Cancer Education
Samuel Brown, EdD
Secretary, AACE
Educational Research and Development
University of Alabama at Birmingham
401 CHSD University Street
Birmingham, AL 35294

The purpose of the AACE has been "to provide a forum for those concerned with education of groups who attempt to advance the cause of early cancer detection, promote individualized multimodality therapy, or develop programs of rehabilitation for cancer patients." This multidisciplinary organization brings together basic scientists, surgeons, internists, oncology nursing educators, pediatricians, pathologists, gynecologists, dentists, and radiation oncologists. They hold an annual fall meeting, and members receive the *Journal of Cancer Education* and other publications on cancer education.

2. American Association for Cancer Research
Margaret Foti, Executive Director
530 Walnut Street, Tenth Floor
Philadelphia, PA 19106
(215) 440-9300

AACR provides an organization of research workers for presentation and discussion of new and significant observations and problems in cancer.

3. American Cancer Society
Trish Greene, RN, MSN, Vice President, Cancer Nursing
Tower Place
3340 Peachtree Road, NE
Atlanta, GA 30026
(404) 320-3333

4. American Society of Clinical Oncology
435 North Michigan Avenue
Chicago, IL 60611-4067
(312) 644-0828

ASCO is a professional organization of physicians board-certified in neoplastic diseases and other health care professionals of the doctorate level whose interests involve biology, diagnosis, prevention, or treatment of human cancer. Affiliate membership is granted to oncology nurses, physician assistants, and other paramedical personnel involved with the care of oncology patients. Membership includes attendance at the annual meeting.

5. Association of Community Cancer Centers
Lee Mortenson, Executive Director
11600 Bevel Street, Suite 201
Rockville, MD 20852
(301) 984-9496

The ACCC acts as the national voice of community cancer care professionals. It serves as a forum on national issues and a source of information on clinical research organizations, new technology, and research results. Annual dues are $100 (1989). Members include institutions and individuals. Membership benefits include a copy of ACCC's quarterly publication, *Oncology Issues*, and an annual publication, *Community Cancer Programs in the United States*.

6. Association of Freestanding Radiation Oncology Centers
3960 Park Boulevard, Suite E
San Diego, CA 92103
(610) 692-1598

AFROC is a nonprofit organization composed of physicists, physicians, administrators, technicians, and clinical personnel working in freestanding, fully equipped radiation centers. It acts as a forum for addressing concerns and as an advocate for reimbursement and legislative policies affecting the centers. Full membership is $400, and benefits include a quarterly newsletter, *Source*, legislative information, reduced rates at the annual meeting, and current information on reimbursement, economic issues, practice development/marketing ideas, financial management, quality assurance, and more.

7. Association of Pediatric Oncology Nurses
11508 Allecingie Parkway, Suite C
Richmond, VA 23235
(804) 379-9150

APON has been in existence since 1973. Membership in the organization is open to all registered nurses who are either interested in or engaged in pediatrics or pediatric oncology. Annual dues are $55 (1989), which entitles the member to receive a copy of the quarterly journal, *J.A.P.O.N., A.P.O.N. Newsletter*, and other pertinent publications, attend all business meetings and programs at a reduced rate, and vote on all issues concerning the organization. The objectives of the organization are to promote excellence in the specialty of pediatric oncology nursing, provide opportunities for communication among all nurses who work with children who have cancer through quarterly newsletters and an annual seminar, encourage dissemination of information among nurses about the medical and nursing care of pediatric oncology patients that is used in various areas of the country, encourage members to update professional and lay literature with regard to the care of children with cancer, and encourage and support research in nursing care of children with cancer.

8. Food and Drug Administration
   Office for Consumer Affairs
   HFE-88
   5600 Fishers Lane
   Rockville, MD 20857
   (301) 443-3170

   The FDA serves as a source for information regarding FDA regulations, cosmetics, foods, drugs, health fraud, and medical devices.

9. International Society of Nurses in Cancer Care
   Carol Reed Ash, EdD, RN, FAAN
   Secretary/Treasurer
   Adelphi University School of Nursing
   Box 516
   Garden City, NY 11530
   (516) 663-1001

   Established in 1984, this society's goal is "to enable cancer nurses to share their knowledge and problems on a worldwide basis." Individual membership is $35 per year and entitles one to the bimonthly journal, *Cancer Nursing: An International Journal for Cancer Care,* and attendance at the biennial international meetings.

10. International Union Against Cancer
    (Union Internationale Contre Le Cancer - UICC)
    Rue de Conseil - General 3
    1205 Geneva, Switzerland
    Telephone: (41-22) 20 18 11

    UICC is composed of multidisciplinary cancer organizations. Its purpose is to encourage the fight against cancer worldwide, promoting communication internationally in cancer research, treatment, and prevention. It is also a certifying government of legitimate cancer-fighting organizations. Membership dues are based on an organization's ability to pay. Congresses are held biennially.

11. National Institute for Occupational Safety and Health
    US Department of Health and Human Services
    Room 714B
    200 Independence Avenue, SW
    Washington, DC 20201
    (202) 472-7134
    (800) 35 NIOSH (Clearinghouse)

    NIOSH is a federal research agency. Of interest is its research in the area of handling cytotoxic drugs and laminar airflow hoods. It also has developed guidelines for health care workers in preventing the transmission of hepatitis B virus and HIV. For information on printed materials, contact the clearinghouse.

12. National Tumor Registrars Association
    11600 Nebel Street, Suite 201
    Rockville, MD 20852
    (301) 984-1748

    The purpose of the NTRA is to provide support and promote tumor registry and its use. Both certified and noncertified tumor registrars may be members in this organization.

The NTRA will assist certified members in maintaining their credentials. Information gathered from tumor registry is used for statistics, research, epidemiology, quality assurance, screening, etc, but its main focus is the patient and quality care.

13. Oncology Nursing Society
    1016 Greentree Road
    Pittsburgh, PA 15220-3125
    (412) 921-7373

    ONS was founded in 1975 to promote the highest professional standards of oncology nursing; study, research, and exchange information, experiences, and ideas leading to improved oncology nursing; encourage nurses to specialize in the practice of oncology nursing; identify resources within the group; and establish guidelines of nursing care for patients with cancer. Annual dues are $53 (1989), which entitles a member to the society's referred journal, *Oncology Nursing Forum,* and a newsletter, *ONS News,* which are published six times per year. Members are also entitled to reduced rates for the annual Congress, an opportunity to serve on society committees, and research and travel awards. ONS publishes guidelines and standards for various aspects of oncology nursing and makes these publications available through its national office. In 1989 there were more than 100 chapters of ONS across the country.
    Partial list of publications:
    Cancer Related Resources in U.S.
    Graduate Programs in Cancer Nursing
    Patient Classification Systems: An Annotated Bibliography (1987)
    Membership Directory (1988-89)
    Standards
    Standards of Oncology Nursing Practice (1987)
    Cancer Patient Education (1982)
    Public Cancer Education (1982)
    Modules—Cancer Chemotherapy Guidelines
    Course Content and Clinical Practicum (1988)
    Acute Care Setting (1988)
    Outpatient Setting (1988)
    Home Care Setting (1988)
    Management of Extravasation and Anaphylaxis (1988)
    Monographs
    Oncology Nursing Reflections (1985)
    The Role of the Oncology Nurse in the Office Setting
    Oncology Nursing Forum
    Oncology Nursing Forum Index
    Oncology Nursing Forum Back Issues
    Annual Congress Supplement
    Audio/visual
    Those Were Hard Days
    History of ONS

14. Occupational Safety and Health Administration
    US Department of Labor
    200 Constitution Avenue, NW
    Washington, DC 20210
    (202) 523-8151

    OSHA is a federal enforcement agency. It has published guidelines for handling antineoplastic drugs (currently being updated) and other information related to health care worker safety.

GOVERNMENT AGENCIES/PROGRAMS*

Resources for Cancer Education

1. Center for Health Promotion and Education
   Centers for Disease Control
   Building 1 South, Room SSB249
   1600 Clifton Road, NE
   Atlanta, GA 30333
   (404) 329-3492

   The Center has a number of programs that emphasize prevention: providing technical assistance to state and local health departments on tracking risk factor conditions in the population; coordinating the Behavioral Risk Factor Surveillance System, a telephone-based survey on major risk factors such as smoking, alcohol, nutrition, hypertension, weight, and seat belt use; implementing School Health Education Evaluation project, an extensive evaluation of the impact of school health education programs on students' health-related behaviors; and maintaining a Health Education Database, a computer online summary of national health education efforts.

2. Clearinghouse for Occupational Safety and Health Information
   National Institute for Occupational Safety and Health
   Technical Information Branch
   4676 Columbia Parkway
   Cincinnati, OH 45226
   (513) 684-8326

   Provides technical information to the National Institute for Occupational Safety and Health research programs and supplies information to others on request.

3. Clearinghouse on Health Indexes
   National Center for Health Statistics
   Division of Epidemiology and Health Promotion
   3700 East-West Highway, Room 2-27
   Hyattsville, MD 20782
   (301) 436-7035

   Provides informational assistance in the development of health measures for health researchers, administrators, and planners.

4. Consumer Information Center
   General Services Administration
   Pueblo, CO 81009
   (303) 948-3334

   The Consumer Information Center, a mail order operation, distributes consumer publications on topics such as children, food and nutrition, health, exercise and weight control. The *Consumer Information Catalog* is available free from the Center and must be used to identify publications being requested.

5. Consumer Product Safety Commission
   Washington, DC 20207
   (301) 492-6800
   (800) 638-2772 (Hotline)

   An independent Federal regulatory agency with jurisdiction over consumer products used in and around the home, the Commission sets standards and conducts information programs on potentially hazardous products, among them carcinogens and other chronic hazards. Single copies of printed materials are available free of charge.

6. Food and Nutrition Information Center
   US Department of Agriculture
   National Agricultural Library Building - Room 304
   Beltsville, MD 20705
   (301) 344-3719

   Serving the informational needs of professionals interested in nutrition education, food service management, and food technology, the Center acquires and lends books, journal articles, and audiovisual materials.

7. National Audiovisual Center
   National Archives
   8700 Edgeworth Drive
   Capitol Heights, MD 20743-3701
   (301) 763-1896
   (301) 763-4385 (TDD)

   The National Audiovisual Center, a nonprofit public service, is the central source for federally sponsored audiovisuals. The Center distributes more than 8000 programs on over 600 topics, including cancer and the environment, breast cancer, cancer detection and smoking. Costs for these audiovisuals and accompanying printed materials range from $50 to $350.

8. Division of Cancer Prevention and Control
   National Cancer Institute
   National Institutes of Health
   Bethesda, MD 20892-4200
   (301) 496-6616

   The Division of Cancer Prevention and Control (DCPC) plans and conducts basic and applied research programs aimed at reducing cancer incidence, morbidity and mortality. Activities are carried out across five phases of research: hypothesis development, methods testing, controlled intervention trials, defined population studies, and demonstrations relevant to the prevention and management of cancer. DCPC plans, directs and coordinates the support of basic and applied research on cancer prevention and control at cancer centers and community hospitals. It also coordinates program activities with Federal and state agencies and establishes liaisons with professional and voluntary health agencies, labor organizations, cancer organizations, and trade associations.

9. Office of Cancer Communications
   National Cancer Institute
   National Institutes of Health
   Bethesda, MD 20892
   (301) 496-6631

   The Office of Cancer Communications provides information on all aspects of the cancer problem to physicians, scientists, educators, Congress, the Executive Branch, the media, and the public and fosters and coordinates a national cancer communications program designed to provide the public and health care professionals with information they need to take more responsible health actions. The CIS (1-800-4-CANCER) is located within this office, with a network of locations across the country.

10. Office of Prevention, Education, and Control
    National Heart, Lung, and Blood Institute
    National Institutes of Health
    9000 Rockville Pike
    Bethesda, MD 20892
    (301) 496-5437

*Adapted from Cancer Prevention Resource Directory, National Cancer Institute, NIH pub no. 86-2827. Bethesda, Md, US Government Printing Office, 1986.

The National Heart, Lung, and Blood Institute is congressionally mandated to develop and foster informational and educational activities designed to reduce preventable heart, lung, and blood disease morbidity and mortality. This office is responsible for initiating educational activities.

11. National Clearinghouse for Alcohol Information
National Institute on Alcohol Abuse and Alcoholism
PO Box 2345
Rockville, MD 20852
(301) 468-2600

The National Clearinghouse for Alcohol Information, a service of the National Institute on Alcohol Abuse and Alcoholism, gathers and disseminates current information on alcohol-related subjects. It responds to requests from the public, health care professionals, scientists, educators, and other professionals. The Clearinghouse provides literature searches, referrals, a library and reading room, and summaries of current alcohol-related information.

12. National Library of Medicine
National Institutes of Health
8600 Rockville Pike
Bethesda, MD 20892
(301) 496-6308 Public Information Office
(301) 496-6095 Reference Section

The National Library of Medicine collects, organizes, and disseminates both printed and audiovisual materials. The collection, technical and scientific in nature, is primarily for medical professionals. The Library offers an extensive computerized literature retrieval service. A list of bibliographies, catalogs, and indexes with specific ordering instructions is available from the Public Information Office.

13. National Maternal and Child Health Clearinghouse
38th and R Street, NW
Washington, DC 20057
(202) 625-8410

The National Maternal and Child Health Clearinghouse provides information and publications on maternal and child health and genetics to consumers and health professionals. Materials cover such topics as smoking and pregnancy and nutrition and pregnancy.

14. National Toxicology Program
National Institute of Environmental Health Sciences
M.D. B2-04, Box 12233
Research Triangle Park, NC 27709
(919) 541-3991

The National Toxicology Program develops and disseminates scientific information regarding potentially hazardous chemicals, including those that can cause cancer. The program also coordinates research conducted by four agencies of the Department of Health and Human Services. Information in the form of technical reports is available free of charge to scientists and the general public.

15. Office of Consumer Affairs
Food and Drug Administration
5600 Fishers Lane
Rockville, MD 20857
(301) 443-3170

The Office of Consumer Affairs, Food and Drug Administration, responds to consumer inquiries and serves as a clearinghouse for consumer publications on a variety of topics including pregnancy, food and nutrition, cosmetics, proper use of drugs, and health fraud. Over 250 publications are available free of charge.

16. National Health Information and Clearinghouse
Office of Disease Prevention and Health Promotion
PO Box 1133
Washington, DC 20013-1133
800-336-4797
(202) 429-9091 (in Washington, DC)

The National Health Information Clearinghouse, a service of the Office of Disease Prevention and Health Promotion, is a central source of information and referral for health questions from the public and health care professionals. It maintains a computer database of government agencies, support groups, professional societies, and other organizations that can answer questions on specific health care topics. In addition, the Clearinghouse offers a library containing medical and health reference books, directories, information files, and periodicals; database development on organizations that provide health information; and a number of publications including resource guides and bibliographies. Some publications prepared by this office are the Department of Health and Human Services (DHHS) *Prevention Abstracts*, which summarizes prevention-oriented findings in the scientific literature; the DHHS *Prevention Activities Calendar*, which highlights major prevention events for the month; the *Healthfinder Series*, which provides resource lists on specific health topics such as exercise for older Americans, health risk appraisals, health statistics and many other issues; and *Staying Healthy: A Bibliography of Health Promotion Materials*, which serves as a guide to current information on health-promotion and disease-prevention topics.

17. Office on Smoking and Health
US Department of Health and Human Services
Technical Information Center
Park Building - Room 1-10
5600 Fishers Lane
Rockville, MD 20857
(301) 443-1690

The Office on Smoking and Health produces and distributes a number of informational and educational materials. It also offers bibliographic and reference services to researchers and others. The materials and services are available free of charge. In addition, the Office produces pamphlets, posters, and public service announcements that contain various health messages.

18. Public Information Center
Environmental Protection Agency
820 Quincy Street, NW
Washington, DC 20011
(202) 829-3535

Materials on such topics as hazardous wastes, the school asbestos project, air and water pollution, pesticides, and drinking water are available from the Environmental Protection Agency's Public Information Center. The Center provides information on other Environmental Protection Agency programs and activities.

19. Publication Distribution Office
Occupational Safety and Health Administration
US Department of Labor
200 Constitution Ave, NW - Room s4203
Washington, DC 20210
(202) 523-9667

The Publication Distribution Office responds to inquiries from the general public, health care professionals, industry, educational institutions, and other sources about a limited number of job-related carcinogens and toxic substances. Single copies of materials are available free of charge.

20. Information Office
National Institute on Aging
Federal Building, 6th Floor
9000 Rockville Pike
Bethesda, MD 20892
(301) 496-1752

Distributes information for older Americans on many topics, including cancer and smoking.

21. Office of Minority Health Resource Center
PO Box 37337
Washington, DC 20013-7337
1-800-444-MHRC (6472)

An office of the Department of Health and Human Services, its activities include bilingually staffed toll-free number providing minority health information and referrals, a computerized database of materials, organizations, and programs, and a resource persons network of professionals active in the field.

Other Government Offices Related to Oncology

1. International Cancer Information Center
National Cancer Institute
Bethesda, MD 20205
(301) 496-7403

This agency provides information on the computerized databases, ie, CANCERLINE, that have been detailed previously.

2. Clinical Center of the National Institutes of Health
Bethesda, MD
(301) 496-4891—Patient Referral Service

Patients who are referred to the Clinical Center by their physician and who meet the criteria for the research studies being conducted at the Clinical Center receive free nursing and medical care. A limited number of patients are accepted.

Regional Cancer Centers

The National Cancer Act of 1971 authorized the development of new comprehensive research and demonstration centers known as comprehensive cancer centers and specialized cancer centers. Through community outreach activities, comprehensive cancer centers are to provide coordination and leadership within their geographic regions to ensure the availability of complete care for patients with cancer.

At present, there are 23 comprehensive cancer centers and 21 clinical cancer centers designated by the NCI. To receive this designation by the NCI, a treatment center must meet rigorous criteria set by the NCI, including the ability to perform advanced diagnostic and treatment methods, support a strong research program, and participate in an integrated nationwide system in prevention, diagnosis, and treatment.

The following is a list of the comprehensive* and clinical† cancer centers supported by NCI as of June 1989.

Alabama
University of Alabama Comprehensive Cancer Center*
1918 University Boulevard
Basic Health Sciences Building, Room 108
Birmingham, AL 35294
(205) 934-6612

Arizona
University of Arizona Cancer Center†
1501 North Campbell Avenue
Tucson, AZ 85724
(602) 626-6372

California
The Kenneth Norris Jr. Comprehensive Cancer Center* and
The Kenneth Norris Jr. Hospital and Research Institute
University of Southern California
1441 Eastlake Avenue
Los Angeles, CA 90033-0804
(213) 226-2370

Jonsson Comprehensive Cancer Center (UCLA)*
10-247 Factor Building
10833 Le Conte Avenue
Los Angeles, CA 90024-1781
(213) 825-8727

City of Hope National Medical Center†
Beckman Research Institute
1500 East Duarte Rd.
Duarte, CA 91010
(818) 359-8111, ext 2292

University of California at San Diego Cancer Center†
225 Dickinson Street
San Diego, CA 92103
(619) 543-6178

Charles R. Drew University of Medicine and Science (consortium)
12714 South Avalon Boulevard, Suite 301
Los Angeles, CA 90061
(213) 603-3120

Northern California Cancer Center (consortium)
1301 Shoreway Road
Belmont, CA 94002
(415) 591-4484

Colorado
University of Colorado Cancer Center†
4200 East 9th Avenue, Box B190
Denver, CO 80262
(203) 270-3019

Connecticut
Yale University Comprehensive Cancer Center*
333 Cedar Street
New Haven, CT 06510
(203) 785-6338

District of Columbia
Howard University Cancer Research Center*
2041 Georgia Avenue, NW
Washington, DC 20060
(202) 636-7610 or 636-5665

Vincent T. Lombardi Cancer Research Center*
Georgetown University Medical Center
3800 Reservoir Road, NW
Washington, DC 20007
(202) 687-2110

Florida
Sylvester Comprehensive Cancer Center*
University of Miami Medical School
1475 Northwest 12th Avenue
Miami, FL 33136
(305) 548-4850

Illinois—Illinois Cancer Council* (includes institutions listed and several other organizations)
Illinois Cancer Council
36 South Wabash Avenue
Chicago, IL 60603
(312) 226-2371

University of Chicago Cancer Research Center
5841 South Maryland Avenue
Chicago, IL 60637
(312) 702-9200

Kentucky
Lucille Parker Markey Cancer Center†
University of Kentucky Medical Center
800 Rose Street
Lexington, KY 40536-0093
(606) 257-4447

Maryland
The Johns Hopkins Oncology Center*
600 North Wolfe Street
Baltimore, MD 21205
(301) 955-8638

Massachusetts
Dana-Farber Cancer Institute*
44 Binney Street
Boston, MA 02115
(617) 732-3214

Michigan
Meyer L. Prentis Comprehensive Cancer Center of Metropolitan Detroit*
110 East Warren Avenue
Detroit, MI 48201
(313) 745-5429

University of Michigan Cancer Center†
101 Simpson Drive
Ann Arbor, MI 48109-0752
(313) 936-2516

Minnesota
Mayo Comprehensive Cancer Center*
200 First Street Southwest
Rochester, MN 55905
(507) 284-3413

New Hampshire
Norris Cotton Cancer Center†
Dartmouth-Hitchcock Medical Center
2 Maynard Street
Hanover, NH 03756
(603) 646-5505

New York
Memorial Sloan-Kettering Cancer Center*
1275 York Avenue
New York, NY 10021
1-800-525-2225

Columbia University Cancer Center*
College of Physicians and Surgeons
630 West 168th Street
New York, NY 10032
(212) 305-6730

Roswell Park Memorial Institute*
Elm and Carlton Streets
Buffalo, NY 14263
(716) 845-4400

Mt. Sinai School of Medicine†
One Gustave L. Levy Place
New York, NY 10029
(212) 241-8617

Albert Einstein College of Medicine†
1300 Morris Park Avenue
Bronx, NY 10461
(212) 920-4826

New York University Cancer Center†
462 First Avenue
New York, NY 10016-9103
(212) 340-6485

University of Rochester Cancer Center†
601 Elmwood Avenue, Box 704
Rochester, NY 14642
(716) 275-4911

North Carolina
Duke University Comprehensive Cancer Center*
PO Box 3843
Durham, NC 27710
(919) 286-5515

Lineberger Cancer Research Center†
University of North Carolina School of Medicine
Chapel Hill, NC 27599
(919) 966-4431

Bowman Gray School of Medicine†
Wake Forest University
300 South Hawthorne Road
Winston-Salem, NC 27103
(919) 748-4354

Ohio
Ohio State University Comprehensive Cancer Center*
410 West 12th Avenue
Columbus, OH 43210
(614) 293-8619

Case Western Reserve University†
University Hospitals of Cleveland
Ireland Cancer Center
2074 Abington Road
Cleveland, OH 44106
(216) 844-8453

Pennsylvania
Fox Chase Cancer Center*
7701 Burholme Avenue
Philadelphia, PA 19111
(215) 728-2570

University of Pennsylvania Cancer Center*
3400 Spruce Street
Philadelphia, PA 19104
(215) 662-6364

Pittsburgh Cancer Institute†
200 Meyran Avenue
Pittsburgh, PA 15213-2592
1-800-537-4063

Rhode Island
Roger Williams General Hospital†
825 Chalkstone Avenue

Providence, RI 02908
(401) 456-2070
Tennessee
St. Jude Children's Research Hospital†
332 North Lauderdale Street
Memphis, TN 38101
(901) 522-0694
Texas
The University of Texas M.D. Anderson Cancer Center*
1515 Holcombe Boulevard
Houston, TX 77030
(713) 792-6161 (Physicians)
(713) 792-3245 (Patients)
Utah
Utah Regional Cancer Center†
University of Utah Medical Center
50 North Medical Drive, Room 2C10
Salt Lake City, UT 84132
(801) 581-4048
Vermont
Vermont Regional Cancer Center†
University of Vermont
1 South Prospect Street
Burlington, VT 05401
(802) 656-4580
Virginia
Massey Cancer Center†
Medical College of Virginia
Virginia Commonwealth University
1200 East Broad Street
Richmond, VA 23298
(804) 786-9641

University of Virginia Medical Center†
Box 334
Primary Care Center, Room 4520
Lee Street
Charlottesville, VA 22908
(804) 924-2562
Washington
Fred Hutchinson Cancer Research Center*
1124 Columbia Street
Seattle, WA 98104
(206) 467-4675
Wisconsin
Wisconsin Clinical Cancer Center*
University of Wisconsin
600 Highland Avenue
Madison, WI 53792
(608) 263-6872

COOPERATIVE CLINICAL TRIAL GROUPS IN THE UNITED STATES

Below are the United States Clinical Trials Cooperative Groups and telephone numbers from which information can be obtained on clinical trials being conducted, eligibility criteria, treatment plan on the clinical trial and how to refer a patient to one of these trials. Currently in the United States fewer than 10% of eligible adult patients are entered on clinical trials. The result of this low percentage of patients is a delay in answering important thera-

peutic and scientific questions and in disseminating therapeutic advances to the general oncology community. There are multiple clinical trials conducted within each of the Cooperative Groups.

1. **BTCG**
Brain Tumor Cooperative Group
For patient entry information:
Lauren Rich, Data Manager, or
Marie Topor, Project Manager
Information Mgmt Services, Inc.
1400 Spring Street, Suite 500
Silver Springs, MD 20910
(301) 495-0440
2. **CALGB**
Cancer and Leukemia Group B
Emil Frei III MD, Chairman
Dana-Farber Cancer Institute
For patient entry information:
Daniel Paterson,
Clinical Research Manager
CALGB Headquarters
303 Boylston Street
Brookline, MA 02146
(617) 732-3676
3. **CCSG**
Children's Cancer Study Group
Denman Hammond, MD, Chairman
University of Southern California
For patient entry information:
John M. Weiner, Dr. PH
Administrative Director
University of Southern California
199 North Lake Avenue, 3rd Floor
Pasadena, CA 91101-1859
(213) 681-3032
4. **ECOG**
Eastern Cooperative Oncology Group
Paul P. Carbone, MD, Chairman
Wisconsin Clinical Cancer Center
University of Wisconsin
For patient entry information:
Barbara Miller, Coordinator
Medical Science Center, Room 4765
420 North Charter Street
Madison, WI 53706
(608) 263-6650
5. **GOG**
Gynecologic Oncology Group
For patient entry information:
George Lewis Jr., MD, Chairman
GOG Headquarters
1234 Market Street, 19th Floor
Philadelphia, PA 19107
(215) 854-0770
6. Intergroup Rhabdomyosarcoma Study
For patient entry information:
Harold M. Maurer, MD, Chairman
Professor and Chairman
Department of Pediatrics
Virginia Commonwealth University
Medical College of Virginia
MCV Box 646
Richmond, VA 23298
(804) 786-9602

7. LCSG
Lung Cancer Study Group
E. Carmack Holmes, MD, Chairman
UCLA School of Medicine
For patient entry information:
Sherrill Long
Administrative Coordinator
IMS, Inc.
6110 Executive Boulevard, Ste 310
Rockville, MD 20852
(301) 984-3445

8. NSABP
National Surgical Adjuvant Project for Breast and Bowel
Cancers
Bernard Fisher, MD
Project Chairman
University of Pittsburgh
For patient entry information:
Mary Ketner, RN, Assistant Director for Clinical Affairs
University of Pittsburgh
914 Scaife Hall, 3550 Terrace Street
Pittsburgh, PA 15261
(412) 648-9720

9. NWTSG
National Wilms' Tumor Study Group
Guilio D'Angio, MD, Chairman
Children's Cancer Research Center
Children's Hospital of Philadelphia
For patient entry information:
Juanita Guagenti, Administrator
Children's Cancer Research Center
Children's Hospital of Philadelphia
3400 Civic Center Boulevard
Ninth Floor
Philadelphia, PA 19104
(215) 387-5518

10. NCCTG
North Central Cancer Treatment Group
Charles G. Moertel, MD, Chairman
Mayo Clinic
For patient entry information:
Mrs. Rose Smith, Supervisor
Mayo Clinic
200 First Street, SW
Rochester, MN 55905
(507) 284-8384

11. POG
Pediatric Oncology Group
Teresa J. Vietti, MD, Chairman
The Edward Mallinckrodt
Department of Pediatrics
Washington University School of Medicine
For patient entry information:
Patricia Gensel, Administrator
4949 West Pine Street, Suite 2A
St. Louis, MO 63108
(314) 367-3446

12. RTOG
Radiation Therapy Oncology Group
James Cox, MD, Chairman
M.D. Anderson Cancer Center
For patient entry information, contact:
Sharon Hartson, Coordinator
RTOG Headquarters
American College of Radiology
1101 Market Street, 14th Floor
Philadelphia, PA 19107
(215) 574-3205

13. SWOG
Southwest Oncology Group
Charles A. Coltman, MD, Chairman
Cancer Therapy & Research Center
San Antonio, TX
For patient entry information:
Ms. Marj Godfrey, Coordinator
5430 Fredericksburg Road
San Antonio, TX 78229-3533
(512) 366-9300